# THEOLOGICAL ISSUES IN BIOETHICS

# THEOLOGICAL ISSUES IN
# BIOETHICS

An Introduction with Readings

*Edited by*

**Neil Messer**

DARTON·LONGMAN+TODD

*To Janet*

First published in 2002 by
Darton, Longman and Todd Ltd
1 Spencer Court
140–142 Wandsworth High Street
London SW18 4JJ

ISBN 0–232–52441–6

A catalogue record for this book is available from the British Library.

Designed by Sandie Boccacci
Set in 9.75/12.75pt Palatino
by Intype London Ltd
Printed and bound in Great Britain by
The Cromwell Press, Trowbridge, Wiltshire

# Contents

**PREFACE**                                                           ix
**INTRODUCTION**                                                       1

**1   THEOLOGICAL VISIONS**                                            9

Introduction                                                          9

Christian Vision                                                     13
GILBERT MEILAENDER

Facing Bioethical Dilemmas Theologically                             19
JOHN BRECK

Introduction to *Evangelium Vitae*                                   26
JOHN PAUL II

Science, Technology, Power and Liberation Theology                   31
LEONARDO BOFF

**2   RESPECT FOR LIFE**                                              37

Introduction                                                         37

The Quality of Life, the Sanctity of Life                            39
RICHARD McCORMICK

The Sacredness and Sanctity of Human Life                            45
JOHN BRECK

Alien Dignity: The Legacy of Helmut Thielicke for Bioethics          50
KAREN LEBACQZ

Case Study: Baby Doe and Others                                      63

**3   PERSONS, BODIES AND WHY THEY MATTER**                           65

Introduction                                                         65

The Moral Status of the Embryo                                       68
MAUREEN JUNKER-KENNY

Who Is My Neighbor? The Good Samaritan as a Source for
Theological Anthropology                                        76
IAN A. McFARLAND

'Embodiment' and Moral Critique: A Christian Social Perspective    85
LISA SOWLE CAHILL

Case Study: A Dilemma about Abortion                            102

4   **HEALTH, DISEASE AND WHOLENESS**                          **103**

Introduction                                                   103

The Strength for Human Life                                    107
KARL BARTH

A Blind Person's Conversations with the Bible                  117
JOHN M. HULL

Case Study: Cochlear Implants for Deaf Children                123

5   **DEATH**                                                  **125**

Introduction                                                   125

Religious Concepts of Brain Death and Associated Problems      128
STANLEY HAUERWAS

The Vision of Death                                            139
VIGEN GUROIAN

Case Study: The Right to Die?                                  152

6   **PROFESSIONAL–PATIENT RELATIONSHIPS**                     **153**

Introduction                                                   153

The Medical Covenant: An Ethics of Obligation or Virtue?       156
WILLIAM F. MAY

Empowerment in the Clinical Setting                            172
KAREN LEBACQZ

Case Study: The Alder Hey Affair                               188

**7 ECONOMICS AND BIOETHICS** 191

Introduction 191

A Human Lottery? 195
PAUL RAMSEY

Power, Ethics and the Poor in Human Genetic Research 202
MÁRCIO FABRI DOS ANJOS

Case Study: Anti-AIDS Drugs in Developing Countries 212

**8 HUMANS AND OTHER ANIMALS** 215

Introduction 215

From 'Animal Rights: A Critique' 217
OLIVER R. BARCLAY

Animal Rights: A Reply to Barclay 223
ANDREW LINZEY

Imaging God Through Peace with Animals: An Election for Blessing 228
SCOTT BADER-SAYE

Case Study: Cc the Cloned Kitten 238

**9 HUMANS AND NATURE** 239

Introduction 239

Flawed Beauty and Wise Use: Conservation and the
Christian Tradition 242
MARGARET ATKINS

Women, Economy and Ecology 254
ARUNA GNANADASON

Case Study: Direct Action Against GM Crops 261

**10 CHRISTIANS AND PUBLIC DEBATE ON BIOETHICS** 263

Introduction 263

Case Study: Vote for the Common Good 270

**Glossary** 271
**Acknowledgements** 277
**Index** 280

# Preface

This book grew out of a course entitled 'Issues in Bioethics' that I taught in the Queen's Foundation, Birmingham in 1998 and 1999, but my interest in thinking theologically about bioethical issues goes back much further. In the late 1980s, as a Christian, an active church member and a research student in molecular biology, I felt that I should have opinions about the controversies, even then attracting considerable public attention, over human genetics, the new reproductive technologies and related topics. However, I found myself singularly ill-equipped to think theologically about such things, and when a call to ordination in the United Reformed Church led me from molecular biology into theological training, I was eager to re-visit some of these problems. A theological interest in bioethics has remained with me through my subsequent years as a local church minister and a theological teacher.

In editing this book, I have incurred many debts, and I hope I will be forgiven for any that I fail to acknowledge. Many teachers, colleagues and students have influenced me over the years: Michael Banner did more than anyone else to encourage me to think theologically about Christian ethics; Kenneth Wilson first suggested compiling this reader; Bill Mahood insistently encouraged me to work at it; its shape and content owe much to discussions with colleagues and students at Queen's; Sheila Russell provided a superb resource in the Queen's Foundation Library; and since 2001, the Department of Theology, Religious Studies and Islamic Studies in Lampeter has proved a very congenial environment for this kind of work.

I am very grateful to Katie Worrall, Kathy Dyke, Helen Porter and their colleagues at DLT for bringing their enthusiasm, expertise and patience to bear on this project, and to Petter Larsson for helping at short notice with the index. At various stages, I received valuable advice, encouragement and information from two anonymous readers and from Caroline Berry, Nigel Biggar, Alastair Campbell, the Catholic Media Office, David Clough, Peter Conley, Celia Deane-Drummond, Robin Gill, John Hull, Dave Leal, Oliver O'Donovan, Ben Quash, Esther Reed, Adrian Thatcher and Grant Vallance. What I have failed to learn from them and from others is, of course, entirely my own responsibility.

Finally, I thank my wife Janet and our children Fiona and Rebecca for their love and good humour while I have been preoccupied with this book. Fiona and Rebecca have been very tolerant when I have annexed the computer, and Janet's encouragement has helped me see the project through. One practical expression of her support was to produce well over half the typescript, which means that she has read more about bioethics than she ever intended to. In the hope that she is not thoroughly tired of it, this book is dedicated to her.

*Neil Messer*
UNIVERSITY OF WALES, LAMPETER
JULY 2002

# INTRODUCTION

## What is Bioethics?

The term 'bioethics' is a relatively recent invention: it was first coined in the early 1970s by the cancer researcher Van Rensselaer Potter, who defined it 'the science of survival'. A more typical definition is offered by Childress (1986): 'the application of ethics to the biological sciences, medicine, health care, and related areas as well as the public policies directed towards them'. This definition is itself open to debate – for example, some would question the notion that there is something 'pure' called 'ethics' which is then 'applied' to the biological sciences, medicine, etc. Nonetheless, it is a helpful starting point in understanding what we are talking about.

The activity of bioethics, like the term itself, has a fairly short history. Jonsen (1993) identifies a number of events which can be said to mark the birth, or at any rate the emergence, of bioethics in North America. First, a number of technological advances in medicine in the second half of the twentieth century raised acute ethical dilemmas. For example, the development of kidney dialysis brought questions about the allocation of scarce resources to public attention, and the development of transplant surgery using organs from dead donors raised questions about how death should be defined and identified. Second, the ethics of research on human subjects began to attract attention, partly because of the trials of Nazi doctors at Nuremberg after the Second World War and partly because of worries about the conduct of research even in democratic societies. Third, with the publication of books like Paul Ramsey's *The Patient as Person* (1970) bioethics began to emerge as a new academic discipline, albeit one which drew on much older traditions of ethical reflection.

'Bioethics' is sometimes described as a peculiarly American activity (cf. Jonsen 1993, S3–4), but the same issues are vigorously debated in other parts of the world. In Britain, these debates more frequently come under the

heading of 'medical ethics', which raises questions of terminology to which
I shall return later. Be that as it may, new (and not so new) developments in
medicine, biology and biotechnology continue to raise issues for public policy,
professional practice, academic discussion and popular debate.

Many dilemmas in medicine and biotechnology are questions of *public
policy* as well as ethics. In agricultural biotechnology, the question of GM
crops exercises policy-makers, pressure-groups and the general public, as the
case study in chapter 9 illustrates. In medicine, recent developments such
as cloning and stem-cell technology have prompted debate and legislation
(Donaldson 2000, *Hansard* 2000, 2001) while older issues like euthanasia
continue to attract attention (see the case study in chapter 5). Policy discussion goes on internationally as well as within nations: international
regulation of medical ethics goes back to the post-Second World War period
(Crawley and Hoet 1999) and has continued with more recent agreements
such as the Council of Europe's Bioethics Convention (Council of Europe
1996).

Many bioethical issues are matters of *professional practice* as well as law.
Health care professionals are those who must deal with many of these issues
on a day-to-day basis and incarnate general principles, ideals and visions in
the complex and untidy realities of their work. Increasingly, questions of
professional practice are debated not only in the journals and by professional
associations, but by ethics committees and boards in which these matters are
scrutinised by members of the public as well as professional colleagues.

*Academic discussion* of bioethical questions also flourishes, as a glance at
the contents pages of journals like the *Journal of Medical Ethics* and *Bioethics*
shows. It is often pointed out that bioethics is necessarily an interdisciplinary
exercise: doctors, nurses, scientists, philosophers, lawyers, theologians and
others besides have an interest in these academic discussions. And of course,
these debates are not just the province of professional scholars, but are echoed
week by week in the general news media and the public arena.

So far, I have said almost nothing about the relationship of theology to
bioethics. As Robert Veatch (1993) points out, it is striking that particularly
in the United States, many of the pioneers of bioethics were theologically
trained, especially in the Protestant tradition. Paul Ramsey is perhaps the
most notable example. Veatch suggests that important aspects of the bioethics
agenda, such as the emphasis on the patient's rights and the affirmation of
the role of 'lay' people in medical decision-making, 'read directly ... from
Protestant theological themes' (ibid., S7). Stanley Hauerwas, however, questions how far the religious convictions of these theological thinkers have
influenced their work in bioethics: 'it is interesting to note how seldom they
raise issues of the meaning or relation of salvation and health, as they seem
to prefer dealing with questions of death and dying, truth telling, etc.'
(Hauerwas 1986, 70). Hauerwas is well known for calling attention to the

danger that 'medical ethics' or 'bioethics' will become an autonomous activity, detached from the traditions and narratives without which it cannot ultimately be sustained or rendered intelligible (cf. Hauerwas 1993, 1996). He claims that medicine needs a community very like the church, not just to give it the intellectual resources to think through ethical dilemmas, but to sustain it in its primary calling of being present and giving care to those who are sick and in pain (Hauerwas 1986). In chapter 10 I shall return to the question of how theology should engage with public debates in bioethics. For the present I shall simply note that this book is one of those that is intended to take up Hauerwas' concern, and make a range of Christian theological voices heard in discussions of bioethical issues.[1]

## What This Book is About

At the beginning of this introduction, I quoted Childress' definition of bio-ethics as 'the application of ethics to the biological sciences, medicine, health care and related areas as well as the public policies directed towards them'. Often, public (and church) discussion of these questions focuses on specific dilemmas and conundrums: is it legitimate to clone human beings, or experiment on embryos? Should euthanasia be permitted, and if so, on what conditions? What procedures do we need for informed consent in medicine? When, if ever, is it permissible to experiment on animals? But behind these specific questions lie more basic issues, which often recur in a number of different contexts: why is life important (if it is)? What individuals are entitled to our respect and care, and why? What qualities should characterise the relations between health professionals and their patients? What duties do we have concerning the natural world, and why?

From a Christian perspective, these are profoundly theological questions. That is to say, they demand reflection in the light of the distinctive resources of the Christian faith: the Scriptures, the churches' traditions and the corporate life and worship of Christian communities today. Furthermore, Christians and churches seeking to think about bioethics may well find that their distinctive resources suggest different questions, or at least that familiar questions should be posed in different ways. For example, as one of the readings in chapter 3 argues, the right question may not be 'What individuals are entitled to our respect and care (and what individuals are not so entitled)?' but 'What kind of person am I called to be, and what kind of care and respect am I called to display to others?'

It is this conviction – that Christian resources can offer distinctive answers to basic questions about bioethics, and suggest some distinctive questions of their own – that has led me to compile a collection of previously published readings from a variety of authors and sources under the title *Theological Issues in Bioethics*. This book does not seek to address specific bioethical problems such as abortion, euthanasia, human cloning and GM crops in any detail, but to lay bare some of the fundamental theological and ethical issues underlying these specific problems. The specific problems come and go, but as I have already suggested, the same basic issues often recur under the guise of many different bioethical problems. Therefore, I have as far as possible chosen readings that reflect on the fundamental theological and ethical issues. The introductions and case studies in each chapter suggest connections between these basic issues and some current problems; the reader is invited to make other connections from his or her own experience, media reports and the medical and ethical literature. By taking this approach, I have sought to demonstrate some ways in which the specific ethical debates might be re-connected with the traditions of reflection needed to sustain ethical practice in these areas, and so to go some way towards addressing Hauerwas' concern that medical ethics or bioethics is becoming detached from those necessary sources of sustenance.

I have hinted already that there is a question as to the scope of 'bioethics'. Sometimes it is taken to mean much the same as 'medical ethics'. Sometimes it is interpreted more narrowly, as being particularly concerned with new technological developments in medicine, such as reproductive technologies, genetic engineering and cloning. However, Childress' definition, quoted earlier, suggests that bioethics has a *broader* scope than medical ethics, and in this I agree with Childress for two reasons. First, many of the same ethical and theological issues appear in medical and other contexts. To give two examples: the question 'Who is a person?' is asked with reference both to human patients and to non-human animals; hi-tech medicine and hi-tech agriculture both attract discussions about 'playing God' or 'interfering with nature'. It would seem odd, therefore, to restrict discussion of these issues to their outworking in the context of human medicine. Second, the Christian tradition has often been criticised (rightly or wrongly) for tending to exclude the non-human from the scope of its ethical concern. Bringing issues relating to medicine, animal welfare and ecology together in one book might serve as a reminder that Christian theology will not allow us to ignore any of these areas of concern.

Therefore, this book is intended to address ethical and theological issues raised by the biological and medical sciences, as these sciences affect human medicine and health care, the human treatment of non-human animals, and our treatment of the whole created world in which we live (the 'environment', as it is often rather unsatisfactorily called). It is intended to offer a reasonably short and accessible introduction to bioethics and to the range of distinctively Christian approaches one might take to bioethical questions. This gives it a somewhat different purpose from other books in the field, notably the comprehensive and highly respected collection edited by Stephen Lammers and Allen Verhey (1998). To keep the present book short enough to be an accessible entry point to bioethics for a wide range of readers, I have restricted the range of topics covered. It is perfectly possible to think of other topics which would meet my criterion of basic ethical and theological issues raised by the biological and medical sciences, but I hope that the chapters I have included will offer some pointers as to how these approaches might be extended to other issues.

The need for brevity has also limited the number of readings that could be included, and I have had to make some hard choices. Within the constraints of space, I have sought to make the collection as theologically and humanly diverse as possible. I have also tried to select readings that make significant contributions to the debates, or that are good examples of the traditions and perspectives they represent. The reader must judge how far I have succeeded.

The book consists of ten chapters, nine of which include readings from two or more authors. Chapter 1, 'Theological Visions', includes four readings which articulate different theological traditions. The purpose of this chapter is not to address any particular issue, but to introduce the reader to some of the major theological approaches that can be found in later chapters. Chapter 2, 'Respect for Life', raises the question of what it is that makes human life valuable, and what kind of ethical response this entails. The next chapter, 'Persons, Bodies and Why They Matter', examines the related concept of the 'person', often used as a key ethical category in bioethical discussions. Two readings offering different perspectives on this concept are followed by one which emphasises the importance of our embodiment for bioethics. Chapter 4, 'Health, Disease and Wholeness', asks what we mean by concepts that we very often take for granted, but which are central to the self-understanding and practice of the health care professions. Chapter 5, 'Death', deals with a reality with which health care unavoidably confronts us, namely our own mortality. The readings in this chapter offer complementary aspects of a Christian vision of death which eschews too-easy acceptance, on the one hand, and despair and denial, on the other. Chapter 6 is concerned with the relationships which are at the heart of the practice of health care, between professionals and their patients. The two readings discuss these relationships from contrasting perspectives, one examining the character and practice of the professional, the other taking the perspective of the patient.

Chapters 2–6 focus mostly on issues underlying the practice of human medicine. Chapter 7 begins to broaden the focus by recognising that economic factors and pressures are highly important for many aspects of bioethics. One reading in this chapter deals with the allocation of scarce resources within a health care system, while the other raises questions of economics, power and the position of the world's poor in relation to genetic research. Though this reading specifically discusses *human* genetic research, it is not hard to imagine how the same concerns extend to other areas such as agriculture. Chapter 8 discusses human attitudes to, and treatment of, non-human animals: the first reading in this chapter consists of a debate about the concept of animal rights, while the second reading takes the theological discussion beyond the question of rights and explores the relevance of another fundamental theological theme, the image of God. Chapter 9 asks how Christians should understand the relation between humans and the rest of the created world, and how our understanding should influence our ethical stance towards ecological questions. The final chapter, 'Christians and Public Debate on Bioethics', is a shorter chapter without readings from other sources. It is intended to conclude the book by asking how distinctively Christian reflections should interact with public debate on bioethics and outlining a range of possible answers.

With the exception of chapter 1, each chapter concludes with a case study and some questions for discussion. The purpose of the case studies is to help the reader make connections between the basic issues discussed in the chapters and specific bioethical problems to which these basic issues are relevant.

In editing this collection, I have had several groups of readers in mind. First, the book is intended for general readers who wish to explore bioethical issues in a systematic way for the first time, or to deepen their exploration or take it in new directions. Second, it is intended for Christian health professionals who wish to bring Christian thinking to bear on issues which they encounter almost daily in their professional lives, and for professionals who are not Christians, but wish to understand what a Christian perspective on such issues might entail. Third, it is intended for students of theology, ethics or bioethics, and for their teachers. As it is intended for a range of different readers, so it could be used in a variety of ways. Readers wishing to gain an overview of Christian perspectives on bioethics could read the book from beginning to end. For such readers, the readings in each chapter would be the main resource, though the case studies might help to focus and assimilate what has been learned from the readings. Those interested in particular topics could select relevant chapters to read, and perhaps to work through case studies. For students and their teachers, the book could again be read as a general introduction or used as a quarry of sources, but could also form the basis of a course in bioethics or a bioethics section of a general course in Christian ethics.

The pace of change in biotechnology and medicine shows no immediate signs of slackening, and each new development brings its own ethical questions in its wake. It is my conviction that the Christian tradition contains great resources for addressing these questions, and that if bioethical discussions become detached from these resources, they cannot but be impoverished. If this book enables its readers to draw more fully on these resources in addressing some of the most perplexing questions of our time, it will have done its work.

## References and Further Reading

Tom L. Beauchamp and James F. Childress, *Principles of Biomedical Ethics*. 5th ed., Oxford and New York: Oxford University Press, 2001.

James Childress, 'Bioethics', in John Macquarrie and James F. Childress (eds.), *A New Dictionary of Christian Ethics*, 61. London: SCM, 1986.

Council of Europe, *Convention on Human Rights and Biomedicine* (1996). Reproduced in *Bulletin of Medical Ethics* 125, 13–19 (February 1997).

Francis Crawley and Joseph Hoet, 'Ethics and Law: the Declaration of Helsinki Under Discussion', *Bulletin of Medical Ethics* 150, 9–12 (August 1999).

Liam Donaldson (Chair), *Stem Cell Research: Medical Progress with Responsibility* (report from the Chief Medical Officer's Expert Group). London: Department of Health, 2000.

Robin Gill (ed.), *Euthanasia and the Churches*. London: Cassell, 1998.

*Hansard (House of Commons Daily Debates)* 19 December 2000, column 266.

*Hansard (House of Lords Daily Debates)* 22 January 2001, column 124.

Stanley Hauerwas, 'Salvation and Health: Why Medicine Needs the Church', in *Suffering Presence: Theological Reflections on Medicine, the Mentally Handicapped, and the Church*, 63–83. Edinburgh: T & T Clark, 1986.

——, 'Why I Am Neither a Communitarian nor a Medical Ethicist', in Albert R. Jonsen (ed.), 'The Birth of Bioethics', Special Supplement, *Hastings Center Report* 23, no. 6, S9–10 (1993).

——, 'How Christian Ethics Became Medical Ethics: The Case of Paul Ramsey', in Allen Verhey (ed.), *Religion and Medical Ethics: Looking Back, Looking Forward*, 61–80. Grand Rapids: Eerdmans, 1996.

Albert R. Jonsen (ed.), 'The Birth of Bioethics', Special Supplement, *Hastings Center Report* 23, no. 6 (1993).

Stephen E. Lammers and Allen Verhey (eds.), *On Moral Medicine: Theological Perspectives in Medical Ethics*. 2nd ed., Grand Rapids: Eerdmans, 1998.

Paul Ramsey, *The Patient as Person: Explorations in Medical Ethics*. New Haven: Yale University Press, 1970.

Robert M. Veatch, 'From Forgoing Life Support to Aid-in-Dying', in Albert R. Jonsen (ed.), 'The Birth of Bioethics', Special Supplement, *Hastings Center Report* 23, no. 6, S7–8 (1993).

Allen Verhey and Stephen E. Lammers (eds.), *Theological Voices in Medical Ethics*. Grand Rapids: Eerdmans, 1993.

## Notes

1. It is only right to pay tribute to the pioneering work of Allen Verhey and Stephen Lammers in this respect: see (e.g.) Verhey and Lammers 1993, Lammers and Verhey 1998.

# 1

# THEOLOGICAL VISIONS

## Introduction

In their book *Principles of Biomedical Ethics*, widely considered a standard text in the field, Tom Beauchamp and James Childress set out what has become known as the 'four-principles' approach to bioethics (Beauchamp and Childress 2001). They deliberately avoid basing their approach on any one philosophical theory of ethics. Instead, they articulate four principles which must be considered and balanced in any decision-making in biomedical ethics: *respect for autonomy* (that is, a person's entitlement to make decisions for him or herself), *non-maleficence* (not doing harm), *beneficence* (doing good) and *justice*. Beauchamp and Childress argue that these principles are rooted in a 'common morality' which holds good for all persons in all cultures, and that it offers better prospects for consensus on difficult bioethical questions than any philosophical theory (ibid., 2–4, 404–405).

Different Christian thinkers vary in their assessments of Beauchamp and Childress' project. Courtney Campbell suggests that it may be justified theologically: 'there may be *theological* reasons for not doing medical ethics theologically' (Campbell 1993, 127; italics original), whereas others such as Stanley Hauerwas are much more sceptical about it (cf. Hauerwas 1996, 63–68). Beauchamp and Childress themselves acknowledge that there is 'community-specific' as well as common morality, and that a principle-based account does not exclude other types of theory (Beauchamp and Childress 2001, 3–4, Beauchamp 2001). Presumably, therefore, even if the four-principles approach can be shown to be universally applicable, there is more that can be said about bioethical issues from a distinctively Christian theological perspective.[1] Before examining particular areas of bioethics in this light, however, it is worth considering the general question of *how* a Christian theological vision might shape our thought about more particular issues in bioethics. In this chapter, therefore, I have selected four readings that offer contrasting examples of theological visions and whose authors relate them explicitly to the area of bioethics.

The principal sources for Christian ethical reflection are often taken to be *Scripture* (the books of the Hebrew Bible/Old Testament and of the New Testament), *tradition*, which has been defined as 'the church's time-honored practices of worship, service and critical reflection' (Hays 1997, 210), human *reason* and one's own or others' *experience*. Much discussion of Christian ethical method has to do with the ways in which these sources should be used, the relative weight that should be given to each and the ways in which the sources should be related to each other (for one recent discussion of this typology, see Hays 1997, 209–211, 295–298). The four readings in this chapter come from different Christian traditions, and illustrate a variety of possible answers to the question of how Scripture, tradition, reason and experience should inform distinctively Christian ethical reflection on medicine and bio-technology.

The reading by Gilbert Meilaender represents a Protestant tradition that gives a high priority to Scripture, while drawing in various ways on all the other three sources. Meilaender uses Scripture in a variety of ways, most importantly to shape a 'Christian vision', which guides and directs the formu-lation of more specific rules and principles. Rules and principles, though, are also of great importance in Meilaender's scheme. Some key principles can be found in Scripture; at other times, Meilaender draws from the Bible what Richard Hays calls 'paradigms': stories that offer the reader models and examples either to follow or to avoid (Hays 1997, 209). He also draws on Christian *tradition* in shaping his Christian vision, uses *experience* in the form of case studies and examples to raise issues and challenge preconceived notions, and engages critically with other positions on their own terms.

John Breck is an Eastern Orthodox theologian, who describes 'Orthodox Christian ethics' as a relatively new enterprise that has grown up in response to the perplexing issues that Christians and others face in the contemporary world. However, Orthodox Christian ethics draws on the much older tradition of 'moral theology', whose primary focus is to help and guide the spiritual growth of Christians. Addressing ethical questions is to be seen as an aspect of 'ascetic' life, the life of spiritual discipline in the power of the Holy Spirit by which the believer journeys towards the ultimate goal of *theosis* ('deification' or union with God). Thus, in words quoted by Breck, 'the answers to the medical ethical problems that each Orthodox Christian may encounter in his lifetime will best be answered in the course of his own spiritual labors' (p. 24, note 2). The Church's reflection on these questions is to help Christians find these answers and to enable pastors to give guidance and help to those in their care who are wrestling with such questions. Orthodox Christian thinking is done in the light of 'Holy Tradition', which includes the Scriptures (recognised as the authoritative word of God), the teaching of the early church's leaders (considered the most faithful interpreters of Scripture), Church law and the Church's worship.

The reading by Pope John Paul II is taken from the introduction to *Evangelium Vitae*, a document setting out official Roman Catholic teaching on a variety of bioethical subjects. In the extract reproduced here, various influences can be discerned which play a key part in the teaching developed through the rest of the encyclical and illustrate some important features of Catholic moral theology. First, appeals to *Scripture* are prominent: commentators have remarked that John Paul II's 'moral encyclicals' (*Evangelium Vitae* and the earlier *Veritatis Splendor* [1993]) make more extensive and creative use of the Bible than previous papal documents (see the articles by Donfried and Wannenwetsch in Hütter and Dieter 1998). Second, references to previous Church documents show how an encyclical like this self-consciously stands in the Church's theological and moral *tradition*. An important aspect of this is the understanding that the Church has a divinely given authority, focused in the papacy, to teach on matters of faith and morality. This authority is often referred to as the Church's 'Magisterium', and it is evident in this extract in the Pope's statement that 'the Cardinals . . . asked me to reaffirm *with the authority of the Successor of Peter* the value of human life . . .' (p. 29, italics mine). Third, human *reason* has an important place in Catholic moral theology, largely because the so-called 'Natural Law' tradition has played a major part in Catholic moral theology. Natural Law theory holds that God's law is reflected to some extent in the created order, and can be discerned by 'every person sincerely open to truth and goodness' (p. 27). This extract claims that 'the sacred value of human life' can be so discerned, appealing to Romans 2:14–15 to support the claim that God's law is written in human hearts (ibid.; see Fairweather and McDonald 1984, 141–169 for a helpful summary and discussion of Natural Law theory). Jean Bethke Elshtain has also shown how John Paul II's moral encyclicals are strongly influenced by his own philosophical understanding of the human person (in Hütter and Dieter 1998, 14–37).

Leonardo Boff is a Latin American liberation theologian, a leading representative of an approach to theology that has achieved widespread influence since the 1960s. It takes the experience of the poor, oppressed and marginalised as the starting point for theological reflection, and interprets the Bible and Christian tradition deliberately from the perspective of the poor. It is radically critical of much traditional Christian thought and practice, and stresses 'orthopraxy' (right action) more than 'orthodoxy' (right belief). For some further comments on liberation theology, see chapter 10.

Liberation theology has been very influential outside its original home of Latin America, and theologies arising from the experience of Black people, Asian people, women and people with disabilities, among others, are sometimes described as theologies of liberation. All these theologies have differences of emphasis and approach, since liberation theologies are essentially *contextual* – that is to say, they are rooted in the concrete experience of people in a particular group or community, and are intended to give rise to renewed discipleship and action in that particular context (cf. Bevans 1992).

In the reading selected for this chapter, Boff reflects from the standpoint of Latin American liberation theology on the implications of science and technology, particularly in the context of ecology. The reading by Aruna Gnanadason in chapter 9 gives another illustration of how a related approach might inform Christian reflection and practice about ecology. For some indications of how such an approach might guide medical ethics, see the readings by Karen Lebacqz in chapters 2 and 6 and John Hull in chapter 4 (see also Campbell 1995).

### References and Further Reading

Tom L. Beauchamp, 'Principlism and its Alleged Competitors', in John Harris (ed.), *Bioethics*, 479–493. Oxford: Oxford University Press, 2001.

Tom L. Beauchamp and James F. Childress, *Principles of Biomedical Ethics*. 5th ed., Oxford and New York: Oxford University Press, 2001.

Steven B. Bevans, *Models of Contextual Theology*. Maryknoll, NY: Orbis, 1992.

Alastair V. Campbell, *Health as Liberation: Medicine, Theology and the Quest for Justice*. Pilgrim Press/United Church Press, 1995.

Courtney S. Campbell, 'On James Childress: Answering That of God in Every Person', in Allen Verhey and Stephen E. Lammers (eds.), *Theological Voices in Medical Ethics*, 127–156. Grand Rapids: Eerdmans, 1993.

Ian C. M. Fairweather and James I. H. McDonald, *The Quest for Christian Ethics: An Inquiry into Ethics and Christian Ethics*. Edinburgh: Handsel Press, 1984.

Gustavo Gutiérrez, 'The Task and Content of Liberation Theology', in Andrew Bradstock and Christopher Rowland (eds.), *Radical Christian Writings: A Reader*, 335–342. Oxford: Blackwell, 2002.

Stanley Hauerwas, 'How Christian Ethics Became Medical Ethics: The Case of Paul Ramsey', in Allen Verhey (ed.), *Religion and Medical Ethics: Looking Back, Looking Forward*, 61–80. Grand Rapids: Eerdmans, 1996.

Richard B. Hays, *The Moral Vision of the New Testament*. Edinburgh: T & T Clark, 1997.

Reinhard Hütter and Theodor Dieter (eds.), *Ecumenical Ventures in Ethics: Protestants Engage John Paul II's Moral Encyclicals*. Grand Rapids, MI/Cambridge: Eerdmans, 1998.

Thomas L. Schubeck, S.J., *Liberation Ethics: Sources, Models and Norms*. Minneapolis: Fortress Press, 1993.

### Notes

1. The notion of the 'distinctiveness' of Christian ethics is easily misunderstood: 'distinctive', for example, does not necessarily mean 'idiosyncratic' or 'sectarian'. In chapter 10, I explain briefly what I mean by a 'distinctively' Christian ethic, making use of Vincent MacNamara's helpful distinction between 'distinctiveness' and 'specificity'; see below, p. 263.

# Christian Vision

GILBERT MEILAENDER

Although a great deal of the best work in bioethics has involved the application of certain ethical principles – such as respect for autonomy, beneficence, and justice – to particular issues of concern, there is no way to apply principles in a vacuum. How we understand such principles, and how we understand the situations we encounter, will depend on background beliefs that we bring to moral reflection – beliefs about the meaning of human life, the significance of suffering and dying, and the ultimate context in which to understand our being and doing. Our views on such matters are shaped by reasoned argument and reflection less often than we like to imagine. Our background beliefs are commonly held at a kind of prearticulate level. We take them in with the air we breathe, drink them in from the surrounding culture. It is therefore sometimes useful to call to mind simply and straightforwardly certain basic assumptions in a Christian view of the world – to remind ourselves of how contrary to the assumptions of our culture that vision may be . . .

## Individuals in Community

Bioethics talk is often talk about rights. Such talk is absolutely essential in many contexts. To ignore it is to ignore the just claims of others upon our attention and our care. But for Christians the relation of individual and community is too complex to be dealt with by such language alone, and I therefore begin with a different language.

In baptism we are handed over to God and become members of the Body of Christ. That is language about a community; yet, perhaps paradoxically, the first thing to note about baptism is that it is a deeply individualizing act. Our parents hand us over, often quite literally as when sponsors carry us as infants to the font. Deeply bound as we are and always will be to our parents, we do not belong to them. In baptism God sets his hand upon us, calls us by name, and thereby establishes our uniquely individual identity and destiny.

From *Bioethics: A Primer for Christians*, pp. 1–10. Grand Rapids, MI: Eerdmans, 1996/ Carlisle: Paternoster, 1997.

We belong, to the whole extent of our being, only to God, whom we must learn to love even more than we love father or mother. What makes us true individuals therefore is that God calls us by name. Our individuality is not a personal achievement or power, and – most striking of all – it is established only in *community* with God. We are most ourselves not when we seek to direct and control our destiny but when we recognize and admit that our life is grounded in and sustained by God.

If the first thing to say about baptism is that it establishes our individual identity, we must immediately add that it brings us into the community of the church – with all those whom God has called by name. It is utterly impossible to exist in relation to God apart from such a bond with all others who have been baptized into Christ's Body. We are called to bear their burdens as they are called to carry ours. Sometimes we are reluctant to shoulder theirs. At least as often, perhaps, we are reluctant to have them shoulder ours, so eager are we to be masterful and independent. That others within the Body should burden us and that we should burden them is right and proper if the life of the Body is one. Nor should such mutual burdensomeness be ultimately destructive, since Jesus has been broken by these burdens once for all.

If baptism is the sacrament of initiation into Christian life, it should inform our understanding of 'individualism.' We should not suppose that any individual's dignity can be satisfactorily described by the language of autonomy alone – as if we were most fully human when we acted on our own, chose the course of our 'life plan,' or were capable and powerful enough to burden no-one.

There will still remain – and should remain – a place within the political realm for the language of independent individualism. Christians should recognize that, in a world deeply disturbed by sin, great evil can be done in the name of community . . . Because sin distorts every human relationship, because, in particular, it leads the powerful to abuse and diminish the weak and voiceless in the name of high ideals or the common good, every individual's dignity must be protected. Because every person is made for God, no-one is – to the whole extent of his or her being – simply a member of any human community.

## Freedom and Finitude

A fuller understanding of our person requires an appreciation – and affirmation – of the created duality of our nature. That is, we are created from the dust of the ground – finite beings who are limited by biological necessities and historical location. We are also free spirits, moved by the life-giving Spirit of God, created ultimately for communion with God – and therefore soaring beyond any limited understanding of our person in terms of presently 'given' conditions of life.

This duality should not become a dualism, as if the person were *really* only the spirit or only the body. On the contrary, the person simply is the place where freedom and finitude are united. Body and spirit cannot be separated in our understanding of human beings; yet, because of the two-sidedness of our nature, we can look at the person from each of these angles.

Drop me from the top of a fifty-story building and the law of gravity takes over, just as it does if we drop a stone. We are finite beings, located in space and time, subject to natural necessity. But we are also free, able sometimes to transcend the limits of nature and history. As I fall from that fifty-story building, there are truths about my experience that cannot be captured by an explanation in terms of mass and velocity. Something different happens in my fall than in the rock's fall, for this falling object is also a subject characterized by self-awareness. I can know myself as a falling object, which means that I can to some degree 'distance' myself from that falling object. I cannot simply be equated with it . . . Likewise, I am the person constituted by the story of my life. I cannot simply be someone else with a different history. Yet I can also, at least to some degree, step into another's story, see the world as it looks to her – and thus be free from the limits of my history. That freedom from nature and history is, finally, our freedom for God. Made for communion with God, we transcend nature and history – not in order that we may become self-creators, but in order that, acknowledging our Creator, we may recognize the true limit to human freedom.

Understanding our nature in this way, we learn something about how we should evaluate medical 'progress.' It cannot be acceptable simply to oppose the forward thrust of scientific medicine. That zealous desire to know, to probe the secrets of nature, to combat disease – all that is an expression of our created freedom from the limits of the 'given,' the freedom by which we step forth as God's representatives in the world. But a moral vision shaped by this Christian understanding of the person will also be prepared to say no to some exercises of human freedom. The never-ending project of human self-creation runs up against the limit that is God. It will always be hard to state in advance the precise boundaries that ought to limit our freedom, but we must be prepared to look for them. We must be prepared to acknowledge that there may be suffering we are free to end but ought not, that there are children who might be produced through artificial means but ought not, that there is valuable knowledge that might be gained through use of unconsenting research subjects but ought not.

In short, an ethic shaped by Christian vision will, in its general form, be what moralists term 'deontological.' Such an ethic does not evaluate actions only in terms of progress, only in terms of beneficial goals that might be achieved. It encourages us to exercise our freedom in search of such goals –

but always within certain limits. It reminds us that others can be *wronged* even when they are not *harmed*. The only freedom worth having, a freedom that does not finally trivialize our choices, is a freedom that acknowledges its limits and does not seek to be godlike. That freedom, a truly *human* freedom, will acknowledge the duality of our nature and the limits to which it gives rise.

## Person and Body

Suppose a child is born who, throughout his life, will be profoundly retarded. Or suppose an elderly woman has now become severely demented. How shall we describe such human beings? We might say, as many will today, that, although they may be living human beings, they are not persons. But we might also say – and I think we should say – that they are severely disabled persons, the weakest among us.

In the last several decades it has become common to define personhood in terms of certain capacities. To be a person one must be conscious, self-aware, productive . . . Not all living human beings will qualify as persons on such a view – and, we must note, it is persons who are now regarded as bearers of rights, persons who can have interests that ought to be protected.

One might argue that such a view follows from the duality of our created nature. If the body dies, we no longer think that the living person is present. Why not reach the same conclusion if the spirit seems to have died – or never to have been present? . . .

The logic of this suggestion is not, however, as neat as it seems. For one thing, the duality of our nature is such that we have no access to the free spirit apart from its incarnation in the body. The living body is therefore the locus of personal presence. More important, our personal histories – precisely as histories of embodied spirits – do not require the presence of 'personal' capacities throughout. Our personal histories begin in dependence – first within our mother's womb and then as newborns. Often our life also ends in the dependence of old age and the loss of capacities we once had. Person-hood is not something we 'have' at some point in this history. Rather, as embodied spirits or inspirited bodies, we are persons throughout the whole of that life. One whom we might baptize, one for whom we might still pray, one for whom the Spirit of Christ may still intercede 'with sighs too deep for words' (Rom. 8:26) – such a one cannot be for us less than a person. Dependence is part of the story of a person's life.

## Suffering

At the heart of Christian belief lies a suffering, crucified God. Yet in recent years some have argued that Christian emphasis upon a suffering Jesus is too dangerous, that it gives rise to an ideology that encourages those who suffer oppression simply to accept that suffering. There are more things wrong with this argument than I can take up here, but it is not surprising that such arguments should arise in a culture devoted to self-realization. In such a setting, the cross must always be countercultural.

Suffering is not a good thing, not something one ought to seek for oneself or for others. But it is an evil out of which the God revealed in the crucified and risen Jesus can bring good. We must therefore always be of two minds about it. We should try to care for those who suffer, but we should not imagine that suffering can be eliminated from human life or that it can have no point or purpose in our lives. Nor should we suppose that suffering must be eliminated by any means available to us, for a good end does not justify any and all means.

Unless we are thus of two minds, understanding suffering as an evil that can nonetheless have meaning and purpose, medicine is likely to go awry. It seeks *h*ealth – but not *H*ealth. The doctor is a caregiver, but not, we must remind ourselves, a savior. Ultimately, all of medicine is no more than the attempt to provide care for suffering human beings. That care, however, cannot by itself offer the Health and Wholeness we ultimately need and desire. If we respect the moral limits that ought to bind us, we will not always be able to give people what they desire. We may not be able to give the infertile couple a child, the elderly man an old age free of dependence, the young woman freedom from the child she has conceived, parents the healthy and 'normal' child they had wanted, the terminally ill patient a painless death. But we can and should assure them that the story of Jesus is true – that the negative and destructive powers of the universe are not the ultimate powers we worship.

Part of the pain of human life is that we sometimes cannot and at other times ought not do for others what they fervently desire. Believing in the incarnation, that in Jesus God has stood with us as one of us, Christians must try to learn to stand with and beside those who suffer physically or emotionally. But that same understanding of incarnation also teaches us that to make elimination of suffering our highest priority would be to conclude mistakenly that it can have no point or purpose in our lives. We should not act as if we believe that the negative, destructive powers of the universe are finally victorious. Those who worship a crucified and risen Lord cannot give themselves over to such a vision of life.

## Disease and Healing

In chapters 14–16 of 2 Chronicles we read of Asa, one of the kings of Judah. His reign, not surprisingly, was a mix of good and bad, but, in the eyes of the Chronicler, it ended badly. Rather than trusting Israel's God to bless his political aims, Asa used the temple treasure to forge an alliance with Syria in his time of need. For that he was denounced by the prophet Hanani.

A few years later Asa became severely ill; 'yet,' writes the Chronicler, 'even in his disease he did not seek the Lord, but sought help from physicians' (2 Chr. 16:12). Shortly thereafter Asa died. The Chronicler's point – in both the political and medical examples – is clear, but it is also difficult to understand. Its clarity lies in the starkness with which we are required to ask ourselves whether the measures we take to secure ourselves – politically, medically or in other ways – bespeak a lack of trust and confidence in God. Its difficulty, however, lies in the suggestion that God's defending and healing work is always *im*mediate, never mediated through the work of human agents.

The warning alerts us not to ask of medicine more than it can offer. Through doctors, God often treats our diseases and sometimes treats even our more general feeling that, although we have no identifiable disease, we are not well, not whole. But doctors are not saviors, and the best doctors know that, even if they only think of themselves as cooperating with the powers of nature. They may heal our diseases but increase thereby our sense of invulnerability – a healing that would be disastrous for our spiritual Health. They may be unable to heal our diseases, but, accepting suffering and dependence as a part of our personal history, we may be drawn closer to God. Thus there is no perfect correspondence between *h*ealth and *H*ealth.

We need not, I think, fear that seeking medical help necessarily demonstrates lack of trust or faith on our part. Rather, it indicates only that we trust God to care for us mediately – through the love and concern of others. But at the same time we should not suppose that medical caregivers can finally provide the wholeness that we need. They stand beside us, but they have not voluntarily shared our fate. They are lordly and awesome in their technical prowess, but they are not the Lord whom death could not hold.

# Facing Bioethical Dilemmas Theologically

JOHN BRECK

## Facing Moral Dilemmas

... It has often been pointed out that 'Christian ethics' is a Western category. 'Eastern' Orthodoxy, on the other hand, traditionally focuses on 'moral theology,' which is basically traditional ascetic theology: exposition of the interior struggle toward sanctification through the grace and transfiguring power of the indwelling Holy Spirit. The new discipline of Orthodox Christian ethics has come into being to help us as pastors and lay people to deal effectively and faithfully, in the light of authentic 'living Tradition,' with moral dilemmas raised in modern technological societies. Its aim is above all to develop criteria that will enable us to make good, right, just and appropriate moral choices: choices that conform to the will and purpose of God for ourselves and for the world in which we live.

Today's world is one that poses radically new and extraordinarily difficult ethical dilemmas for all of us. This is particularly true in those areas where modern technology has created problems and possibilities that were never envisioned or addressed by either Scripture or patristic tradition. A few examples will suffice to illustrate the problem.

1. Prodigious developments in the area of *biomedical technology* have raised new questions concerning such matters as procreation and the meaning of 'parenting,' terminal life-support and euthanasia, together with the burning issue of physician-assisted suicide.

Introduction ... of the RU-486 pill is opening the way to do-it-yourself abortions, and other combinations of chemicals will soon permit a woman to abort an embryo or fetus in the privacy of her own bathroom. Extra-uterine conception has become routine, and its consequences in the realm of sexuality are dramatic. If the pill separated sex from procreation, *in vitro* fertilization (IVF) has separated procreation from sex. As a result, the covenantal, unitive value of conjugal relations, as a means of participating in God's own creative activity, has been largely obscured. Marriage is no longer perceived as an eternal bond of mutual faithfulness, responsibility

From *The Sacred Gift of Life*, pp. 11–18. Crestwood, NY: St Vladimir's Seminary Press, 1998.

and devotion. Prenuptial contracts, live-in experimentation, and quickie divorce are becoming increasingly the norm. We should hardly be surprised, then, at the exponential growth in ersatz homosexual 'marriages,' teen-pregnancies with single-parenting, and prime-time sexual exploitation.

Then again, respirators, dialysis machines and other routine instruments of modern medicine pose awesome questions regarding the allocation of limited resources and the selection of those who will receive and those who will be denied treatment. Medical advances such as antibiotics, ventilators and vital organ transplants have made it possible to sustain biological existence almost indefinitely, even when the patient is in a deep coma or 'persistent vegetative state' (PVS), conditions that in former generations would have allowed the terminally ill to pass quietly into the hands of God. (Only the oldest of us remember when pneumonia was welcomed as 'the dying man's friend.') Each of these areas involves us in ethical dilemmas: 'hard choices' made necessary by advances in biomedicine. Consequently, it is incumbent upon us as members of the Body of Christ to *reflect together* with medical professionals and theologians, to determine proper uses and limitations of modern medical technology.

2. A second area of grave ethical concern is that of *genetic engineering*, and particularly the 'human genome initiative.' The ability to identify and restructure genetic material has created the possibility to manipulate life, both human and otherwise, at its most fundamental level. One frightening consequence of these developments is the inevitable reaction of insurance companies, which will refuse to pay for the support of a child that could have been determined *in utero* to be 'genetically defective' and therefore subject to legal abortion.

Another potential danger concerns genetic manipulation in the interests of 'eugenics,' which seeks genetic improvement of the human species. Negative or therapeutic eugenics promises to prevent or cure diseases that up to now were either severely debilitating or lethal. Positive or 'innovational' eugenics, which would enhance positive traits and capacities, proved disastrous in the hands of the Nazis and bodes little better for our own day. Some are asking: If we can create new life forms in agriculture and lower animals, why shouldn't we improve the human stock by increasing intelligence, physical strength, and the like? The dilemma, of course, lies in deciding precisely which characteristics will be deemed appropriate to what the eminent Protestant ethicist Paul Ramsey so aptly described as 'fabricated man.' In the modern world, where competition is a dominant force in motivating human behavior and one's survival often depends on 'one-upmanship' while protecting oneself from physical threat and emotional stress, the criteria for determining which 'qualities' should be enhanced in the human species are not likely to be determined by reference to the Ten Commandments or the Sermon on the Mount.

3. The Church is faced with equally grave problems created by the *popular media* and the computer-based explosion of *information*. The so-called 'information superhighway' offers a remarkable potential for good, making possible interactive education, jobs done at home rather than at a distant workplace, and access to global interconnected resources. But that same superhighway can lead directly to the undermining of social and spiritual values: for example, TV mind-control, which means conformity to the lowest common denominator; or the power of the media concentrated in too few hands, leading to increasingly 'managed' news; or the airing of grievances over the Internet, in violation of the most elementary rights of privacy; or the growing interface between universities, the military and business, resulting in a 'military-industrial-academic complex' which is highly detrimental to academic and personal freedom.

A consequence of no little significance of this information explosion is that it focuses all of our attention and resources on *technology as such*, as we see so dramatically today in our secondary schools and universities. Together with 'computer centeredness' goes a corresponding decrease in appreciation for philosophy, art and literature. To write a program today is vastly more important, and lucrative, than to write a poem. This is a tragic state of affairs that has seriously diminished our capacity for creativity and has led to a severe spiritual crisis, both individual and collective. Consequently, it needs to be treated as a 'bioethical' issue of the first importance.

4. *Modern psychology* has also led to developments which must be judged both good and evil. On the one hand, it has provided us with new and important insight into specific behaviors traditionally attributed to 'the will acting in freedom.' For example, we now recognize that alcoholism is a disease rather than the product of a 'weak will'; that chronic anger is often an expression of suppressed rage resulting from childhood abuse; and that certain forms of criminality, and many cases of suicide, result from imbalances in the brain's neurotransmitters. In addition, insights provided by the study of psychology have led to the production of drug therapies that have significantly improved the quality of life for people who suffer from what in former generations were wholly debilitating mental diseases.

The negative consequences of our fascination with modern psychology are basically spiritual. By stressing the neuro-chemical correlates of various antisocial behaviors – from alcoholism, through child abuse, to suicide – psychological explanations of our behavior can very well lead to sheer relativism and to the rejection of personal responsibility. The primary question provoked by much modern psychology is the one raised many years ago by Dr. Karl Menninger: 'Whatever became of sin?' If Orthodox Christians are to overcome their traditional suspicion of the science of psychology, it cannot be at the expense of minimizing our awareness of the power of sin and the importance of responsibility in our personal and social affairs.

## Biomedical Ethics as a Theological Discipline

These are just some of the issues that have led theologians and philosophers, as well as members of the medical and legal professions, to create the field of 'bioethics.' The term itself is unfortunate, since it is so easily distinguished and divorced in the popular mind from considerations developed in the traditional discipline of moral theology: considerations grounded on the premise that human life is indeed a sacred gift, whose meaning and end can only be described by the vocabulary of asceticism, sanctification, illumination, perfection and deification.[1]

[Before we turn to specific bioethical issues,] it is necessary to indicate why, from an Orthodox point of view, medical ethics needs to be understood and developed as a *theological* discipline.

Generally speaking, 'ethics' studies human behavior. It is normally regarded as a *descriptive* science that attempts to discern and analyze the underlying principles and values that govern human conduct. 'Moral theology,' on the other hand, is usually considered to be *prescriptive*: it proposes the 'oughts' that shape the moral life in response to God's commandments and purposes as they are revealed in Scripture and other sources of Holy Tradition. To speak of specifically 'Christian' ethics, however, complicates the matter, since it suggests that the purpose of the field is not only to analyze our behavior but to propose a cure for our moral illness, our sin. In common usage, then, Christian ethics and Christian moral theology are virtual equivalents, since the act of making ethical judgments involves by its very nature a striving towards sanctity or holiness.

This is true as well with regard to the relatively new discipline of medical or 'biomedical' ethics. The expression could refer simply to the way physicians and other health care specialists treat patients. As such it would either be purely descriptive (analyzing the values, motives and intentions of the medical team); or, if it ventures into the realm of prescription (how the team should behave and why), its moral directives would be governed by the ethicist's own philosophical outlook. 'Christian medical ethics,' on the other hand, if it is in any sense 'orthodox,' presupposes a value system grounded in certain truths, or rather in 'the Truth' that has revealed itself and continues to reveal itself within the Church, meaning the all-embracing reality of God's presence and purpose within creation.

Orthodox ethics, and particularly medical ethics or bioethics that deals specifically with issues of life and death, is based on at least the following presuppositions:

1.   God is absolutely sovereign over every aspect of human existence, from conception to the grave and beyond. This conviction is well expressed in a popular morning prayer, attributed variously to St. Philaret of Moscow (d. 1867) or to spiritual fathers of the Optino Monastery: 'Teach me to treat

all that comes to me throughout the day with peace of soul and with firm conviction that thy will governs all . . . In unforeseen events, let me not forget that all are sent by thee.' The divine imperative to 'Choose life!' is fulfilled by loving the Lord, obeying his voice and cleaving to him (Deut. 30:19); that is, by offering ourselves in total surrender to his sovereign authority and purpose. That authority is precisely what requires Orthodox Christians to reject 'abortion on demand,' active euthanasia, and any procedure that means taking life (and death) into our own hands.

2. The Holy Trinity – characterized by 'community and otherness,' by essential unity and personal distinctiveness – should serve as the model or icon of every human relationship. Bound together by our shared humanity in the communion of the ecclesial Body, yet serving one another with differing spiritual gifts, we are called to 'responsibility': to *respond* to one another with a self-giving love that reflects the boundless love of the three Persons of the Godhead, shared among themselves and 'poured into our hearts by the Holy Spirit' (Rom. 5:5).

3. Growth in the moral life is only possible insofar as we experience the 'eschatological tension' of eternal life present in our midst. 'The hour is coming and now is,' when the sole meaning and value of human existence is to 'worship the Father in Spirit and truth' (John 4:23–4). Christian ethics is essentially 'teleological' – in the profoundly biblical sense – with its focus on realizing in the here and now the beauty, truth and perfection of life in the Kingdom of God.

What do these three principles or presuppositions imply with regard to medical ethics? Given the climate in which we live today, the following points stand out.

Health and wholeness have ultimate meaning only within the perspective of God's eternal purpose, the divine economy to be fulfilled at 'the second and glorious coming' of Jesus Christ. Medical care, therefore, should serve not only the proximate goal of restoring or improving bodily health; it should strive to provide optimal conditions for the patient's spiritual growth at every stage in the life cycle. This means curing disease; but it also means, particularly in terminal cases, easing pain and distress by any appropriate means in order to allow the patient, through prayer, confession and communion, to surrender him/herself into the hands of God. 'Medical heroics' result all too often from the prideful attempt on the part of caregivers to avoid 'failure,' defined as 'losing' the patient to death. Such hubris is responsible for a great deal of unnecessary suffering on the part of patients and their families, and it represents idolatry of the worst sort insofar as the medical team assumes the role of God.

Then again, matters of 'informed consent' and 'patient's rights' need to be evaluated in the light of the Gospel's teaching on freedom and responsibility. Some Christian ethicists today are suggesting that our unity in the Body of

Christ implies a mutual commitment that in certain cases transcends the need for informed consent and transforms the self-centered notion of personal 'rights' into the self-giving gesture of care offered to others in love. While this raises the specter of the 'slippery slope' towards paternalism in a stark and perhaps dangerous way, thus potentially jeopardizing patient autonomy and the very principle of informed consent, the theological vision behind the suggestion is profoundly 'evangelical.' It recognizes that from the point of view of health care, ultimate meaning and value in life lie not in the mere preservation of biological existence, but in the total surrender of self to the loving sovereignty of God. And it grounds personal relationships – between doctor and patient as between the medical team and the patient's family – in the ultimate relationship of love, trust and mutual devotion shared by the three Persons of the Holy Trinity.

Modern medical technology has performed wonders for which many of us will be forever grateful. But like any human invention, that technology and its application must be subject to constant reevaluation and judgment in the light of Holy Tradition. To paraphrase a well-worn maxim, 'ethics is too important to be left to the ethicists.' At its core, Christian ethics is a function of the worshiping, serving Church. This means that the work of doing ethics is a communal, ecclesial work for which each of us is responsible. Just as each Christian is called to be a theologian by offering self and the world to God in prayer, each is called to be an ethicist, a 'moral theologian' in the proper sense. Informing ourselves of the issues, discussing them in family, parish and on the job, and taking a stand, both public and personal, that reflects our understanding of the Gospel and of God's imperative in our life, we can faithfully and usefully serve the many dedicated health care professionals who live to serve us, while providing them with the guidance and discernment they seek. Thereby 'medical ethics' can be restored to its proper place as a *theological discipline* that serves the glory of Christ and the spiritual health of the members of his Body.[2]

## Notes

1. For a highly perceptive analysis of 'bioethics in the ruins,' resulting from the 'content-less moral vision' of so many of its current practitioners, see the introduction of H. Tristram Engelhardt's *The Foundations of Bioethics*, 2nd ed. (New York: Oxford University Press, 1996), pp. 3–31. This is a valuable contribution by a leading medical ethicist whose entry into the Orthodox Church led to a thoroughgoing revision of the first edition of this work. It is one of those rare books whose endnotes are as informative as the text.
2. Edward B. Andersen, M.D., raises in a perceptive and provocative way the very question, 'Is There an "Orthodox Medical Ethic"?', *Epiphany Journal* 12/3 (spring 1992), 13–17. He answers the question with a qualified negative, pointing out quite rightly that the Church has never proposed 'an overarching system of medical ethics.' In a few deft strokes he then offers opinions on a variety of bioethical issues including

abortion, reproductive technologies, contraception, organ transplants, sexuality, and euthanasia. In so doing, he is obeying an intuition common to those Orthodox who are interested in ethical issues and feel called to express their views to others: to interpret, insofar as possible, the theological (ascetic, mystical, liturgical) tradition of the Church, in an effort to guide the moral conscience of the faithful. As he well recognizes, such guidance . . . needs to be constantly submitted to the 'mind of the Church,' beginning with the judgment of our bishops and qualified theologians. If there is indeed an 'Orthodox medical ethic,' its content can only be provided by Holy Scripture, together with the sacramental and liturgical experience of the believing community: provided, that is, by God himself. Consequently, although it may reach some of the same conclusions as found in a system of religious or secular 'ethics,' the ethics of Orthodox Christianity is grounded in a very different presupposition. In Dr. Andersen's words, 'the answers to the medical ethical problems that each Orthodox Christian may encounter in his lifetime will best be answered in the course of his own spiritual labors.'

# Introduction to *Evangelium Vitae*

POPE JOHN PAUL II

1.   The Gospel of Life is at the heart of Jesus' message. Lovingly received day after day by the Church, it is to be preached with dauntless fidelity as 'good news' to the people of every age and culture.

At the dawn of salvation, it is the Birth of a Child which is proclaimed as joyful news: 'I bring you good news of a great joy which will come to all the people; for to you is born this day in the city of David a Saviour, who is Christ the Lord' (Luke 2:10–11). The source of this 'great joy' is the Birth of the Saviour; but Christmas also reveals the full meaning of every human birth, and the joy which accompanies the Birth of the Messiah is thus seen to be the foundation and fulfilment of joy at every child born into the world (cf. John 16:21).

When he presents the heart of his redemptive mission, Jesus says: 'I came that they may have life, and have it abundantly' (John 10:10). In truth, he is referring to that 'new' and 'eternal' life which consists in communion with the Father, to which every person is freely called in the Son by the power of the Sanctifying Spirit. It is precisely in this 'life' that all aspects and stages of human life achieve their full significance.

## The Incomparable Worth of the Human Person

2.   Man is called to a fullness of life which far exceeds the dimensions of his earthly existence, because it consists in sharing the very life of God. The loftiness of this supernatural vocation reveals the *greatness* and the *inestimable value* of human life even in its temporal phase. Life in time, in fact, is the fundamental condition, the initial stage and an integral part of the entire unified process of human existence. It is a process which, unexpectedly and undeservedly, is enlightened by the promise and renewed by the gift of divine life, which will reach its full realization in eternity (cf. 1 John 3:1–2). At the same time, it is precisely this supernatural calling which highlights the *relative character* of each individual's earthly life. After all, life on earth is not an 'ultimate' but a 'penultimate' reality; even so, it remains a *sacred reality* entrusted to us, to be preserved with a sense of responsibility and brought

From John Paul II, *Evangelium Vitae*, pp. 3–9. London: Catholic Truth Society, 1995.

to perfection in love and in the gift of ourselves to God and to our brothers and sisters.

The Church knows that this *Gospel of life*, which she has received from her Lord,[1] has a profound and persuasive echo in the heart of every person – believer and non-believer alike – because it marvellously fulfils all the heart's expectations while infinitely surpassing them. Even in the midst of difficulties and uncertainties, every person sincerely open to truth and goodness can, by the light of reason and the hidden action of grace, come to recognize in the natural law written in the heart (cf. Rom. 2:14–15) the sacred value of human life from its very beginning until its end, and can affirm the right of every human being to have this primary good respected to the highest degree. Upon the recognition of this right, every human community and the political community itself are founded.

In a special way, believers in Christ must defend and promote this right, aware as they are of the wonderful truth recalled by the Second Vatican Council: 'By his incarnation the Son of God has united himself in some fashion with every human being'.[2] This saving event reveals to humanity not only the boundless love of God who 'so loved the world that he gave his only Son' (John 3:16), but also the *incomparable value of every human person*.

The Church, faithfully contemplating the mystery of the Redemption, acknowledges this value with ever new wonder.[3] She feels called to proclaim to the people of all times this 'Gospel', the source of invincible hope and true joy for every period of history. *The Gospel of God's love for man, the Gospel of the dignity of the person and the Gospel of life are a single and indivisible Gospel.*

For this reason, man – living man – represents the primary and fundamental way for the Church.[4]

## New Threats to Human Life

3.   Every individual, precisely by reason of the mystery of the Word of God who was made flesh (cf. John 1:14), is entrusted to the maternal care of the Church. Therefore every threat to human dignity and life must necessarily be felt in the Church's very heart; it cannot but affect her at the core of her faith in the Redemptive Incarnation of the Son of God, and engage her in her mission of proclaiming the *Gospel of life* in all the world and to every creature (cf. Mark 16:15).

Today this proclamation is especially pressing because of the extraordinary increase and gravity of threats to the life of individuals and peoples, especially where life is weak and defenceless. In addition to the ancient scourges of poverty, hunger, endemic diseases, violence and war, new threats are emerging on an alarmingly vast scale.

The Second Vatican Council, in a passage which retains all its relevance today, forcefully condemned a number of crimes and attacks against human life. Thirty years later, taking up the words of the Council and with the same forcefulness I repeat the condemnation in the name of the whole Church, certain that I am interpreting the genuine sentiment of every upright conscience: 'Whatever is opposed to life itself, such as any type of murder, genocide, abortion, euthanasia, or wilful self-destruction, whatever violates the integrity of the human person, such as mutilation, torments inflicted on body or mind, attempts to coerce the will itself; whatever insults human dignity, such as subhuman living conditions, arbitrary imprisonment, deportation, slavery, prostitution, the selling of women and children; as well as disgraceful working conditions, where people are treated as mere instruments of gain rather than as free and responsible persons; all these things and others like them are infamies indeed. They poison human society, and they do more harm to those who practise them than to those who suffer from the injury. Moreover, they are a supreme dishonour to the Creator'.[5]

4.  Unfortunately, this disturbing state of affairs, far from decreasing, is expanding: with the new prospects opened up by scientific and technological progress there arise new forms of attacks on the dignity of the human being. At the same time a new cultural climate is developing and taking hold, which gives crimes against life a *new and – if possible – even more sinister character*, giving rise to further grave concern: broad sectors of public opinion justify certain crimes against life in the name of the rights of individual freedom, and on this basis they claim not only exemption from punishment but even authorization by the State, so that these things can be done with total freedom and indeed with the free assistance of health-care systems.

All this is causing a profound change in the way in which life and relationships between people are considered. The fact that legislation in many countries, perhaps even departing from basic principles of their Constitutions, has determined not to punish these practices against life, and even to make them altogether legal, is both a disturbing symptom and a significant cause of grave moral decline. Choices once unanimously considered criminal and rejected by the common moral sense are gradually becoming socially acceptable. Even certain sectors of the medical profession, which by its calling is directed to the defence and care of human life, are increasingly willing to carry out these acts against the person. In this way the very nature of the medical profession is distorted and contradicted, and the dignity of those who practise it is degraded. In such a cultural and legislative situation, the serious demographic, social and family problems which weigh upon many of the world's peoples and which require responsible and effective attention from national and international bodies, are left open to false and deceptive solutions, opposed to the truth and the good of persons and nations.

The end result of this is tragic: not only is the fact of the destruction of so many human lives still to be born or in their final stage extremely grave and disturbing, but no less grave and disturbing is the fact that conscience itself, darkened as it were by such widespread conditioning, is finding it increasingly difficult to distinguish between good and evil in what concerns the basic value of human life.

## In Communion With All the Bishops of the World

5.  The *Extraordinary Consistory* of Cardinals held in Rome on 4–7 April 1991 was devoted to the problem of the threats to human life in our day. After a thorough and detailed discussion of the problem and of the challenges it poses to the Christian community, the Cardinals unanimously asked me to reaffirm with the authority of the Successor of Peter the value of human life and its inviolability, in the light of present circumstances and attacks threatening today.

In response to this request, at Pentecost in 1991 I wrote a *personal letter* to each of my Brother Bishops asking them, in the spirit of episcopal collegiality, to offer me their cooperation in drawing up a specific document.[6] I am deeply grateful to all the Bishops who replied and provided me with valuable facts, suggestions and proposals. In so doing they bore witness to their unanimous desire to share in the doctrinal and pastoral mission of the Church with regard to the *Gospel of life*.

In that same letter, written shortly after the celebration of the centenary of the Encyclical *Rerum Novarum*, I drew everyone's attention to this striking analogy: 'Just as a century ago it was the working classes which were oppressed in their fundamental rights, and the Church very courageously came to their defence by proclaiming the sacrosanct rights of the worker as a person, so now, when another category of persons is being oppressed in the fundamental right to life, the Church feels in duty bound to speak out with the same courage on behalf of those who have no voice. Hers is always the evangelical cry in defence of the world's poor, those who are threatened and despised and whose human rights are violated'.[7]

Today there exists a great multitude of weak and defenceless human beings, unborn children in particular, whose fundamental right to life is being trampled upon. If, at the end of the last century, the Church could not be silent about the injustices of those times, still less can she be silent today, when the social injustices of the past, unfortunately not yet overcome, are being compounded in many regions of the world by still more grievous forms of injustice and oppression, even if these are being presented as elements of progress in view of a new world order.

The present Encyclical, the fruit of the cooperation of the Episcopate of every country of the world, is therefore meant to be a *precise and vigorous reaffirmation of the value of human life and its inviolability,* and at the same time a pressing appeal addressed to each and every person, in the name of God:

*respect, protect, love and serve life, every human life!* Only in this direction will you find justice, development, true freedom, peace and happiness!

May these words reach all the sons and daughters of the Church! May they reach all people of good will who are concerned for the good of every man and woman and for the destiny of the whole of society!

6.   In profound communion with all my brothers and sisters in the faith, and inspired by genuine friendship towards all, I wish to *meditate upon once more and proclaim the Gospel of life*, the splendour of truth which enlightens consciences, the clear light which corrects the darkened gaze, and the unfailing source of faithfulness and steadfastness in facing the ever new challenges which we meet along our path.

As I recall the powerful experience of the Year of the Family, as if to complete the Letter which I wrote 'to every particular family in every part of the world',[8] I look with renewed confidence to every household and I pray that at every level a general commitment to support the family will reappear and be strengthened, so that today too – even amid so many difficulties and serious threats – the family will always remain, in accordance with God's plan, the 'sanctuary of life'.[9]

To all the members of the Church, *the people of life and for life*, I make this most urgent appeal, that together we may offer this world of ours new signs of hope, and work to ensure that justice and solidarity will increase and that a new culture of human life will be affirmed, for the building of an authentic civilization of truth and love.

## Notes

1. The expression 'Gospel of life' is not found as such in Sacred Scripture. But it does correspond to an essential dimension of the biblical message.
2. Pastoral Constitution on the Church in the Modern World *Gaudiam et Spes*, 22.
3. Cf. John Paul II, Encyclical Letter *Redemptor Hominis* (4 March 1979), 10: *AAS* 71 (1979), 275.
4. Cf. *ibid.*, 14: *loc. cit.*, 285.
5. Pastoral Constitution on the Church in the Modern World *Gaudiam et Spes*, 27.
6. Cf. Letter to all my Brothers in the Episcopate regarding the 'Gospel of Life' (19 May 1991): *Insegnamenti* XIV, 1 (1991), 1293–1296.
7. *Ibid., loc. cit.*, p. 1294.
8. Letter to Families *Gratissimam sane* (2 February 1994), 4: *AAS* 86 (1994), 871.
9. John Paul II, Encyclical Letter *Centesimus Annus* (1 May 1991), 39: *AAS* 83 (1991), 842.

# Science, Technology, Power and Liberation Theology

LEONARDO BOFF

Liberation theology represents the mind of the parts of the church that have adopted the people's struggle so that they can make sure that society changes sufficiently to satisfy fundamental needs and allow the exercise of basic human rights. It arose, and continually arises, from the confrontation of human misery with the gospel, and of collective injustice with a thirst for justice; and it starts from a definite practice of liberation focused on the poor themselves as subjects of change.

## The Dependent Capitalist System and Unsatisfied Needs

The specific and cruel experience of organized popular groups from the 1960s onward, which has been shared by many Christians . . ., is that the thrust of the present socio-economic system has hindered (as it continues to hinder) the satisfaction of basic needs and respect for the person, and the social rights of the vast majority of the population.

Development may follow one of three models: that of an alliance between the bourgeoisie of a certain country with its people (populism); that of a pact between national groups and multinational trusts (alliance for progress); or, more recently, that of a modern, transnational, and populist neo-liberal state (modernization). In each case it takes place at the cost of an increasing impoverishment of the masses. If they are part of the system, they are exploited by it; if not, they are excluded from it.

In Latin America today the most crucial problem is not that of the poor within the dominant system, but that of the 30 to 40 percent of the population, the mass of the urban proletariat, who are excluded from it. They count for nothing economically, for their production and consumption are marginal in GNP terms. They do count politically, for they can vote and decide the outcome of elections, as happened recently in Argentina, Peru, Brazil, and Mexico. They vote for the candidates who speak to their profound awareness, and who can articulate fundamental deficiencies with the myth of a great

From Leonardo Boff, *Ecology and Liberation: A New Paradigm*, pp. 123–130. Maryknoll, NY: Orbis, 1995.

father (with the characteristics of a protective mother), or of a hero, the savior of his country, who can give them bread, a roof over their heads, health care, and leisure. This is how the new populism is born; it manipulates these desires cleverly, but its ability to put them into effect is weak.

The non-satisfaction of basic needs is seen as oppression. It not only seems unlikely but has been shown to be impossible for the present socio-economic system applied in the Third World to satisfy the fundamental demands for life – and ongoing life – of most of the population.

Experience shows that within the dependent liberal-capitalist system . . ., there is no salvation for the poor, no respect for basic rights, and no satisfaction of basic needs. Therefore we have to abandon this system. The alternative may not be clear, but there is irrefutable evidence that we can expect no solution within the logic of capitalism for wage-earners or for those excluded from the system.

The pope's recent statement in *Centesimus annus* that the alternative to capitalism in the Third World should be sought not in socialism but in an improved form of capitalism (no. 42) has dashed the hopes of the oppressed. With the papal blessing, capitalists can now calmly condemn the poor of the world to another hundred years (*centesimus annus!*) of blood, sweat, and tears. The papal magisterium has never been so far from the truth and from compassion with the wretched of the earth.

The iron logic that constitutes the secret power of capitalism is that of the greatest profit in the shortest possible time. Any business that does not observe this law runs the risk of failing in competition with those that do. This logic can soften only if the stability of the market is guaranteed, or under exceptional circumstances, such as temporary collaboration to bring down the rate of inflation. Today, with continental economies and a global market, this law remains in force; it is absolutely necessary to observe it. Those who are not successful in the marketplace go under. What is not in the marketplace does not exist.

Faced with this bleak prospect for the poor, we seek liberation. Liberation is real only if political conditions for exercising justice are created. Social justice presupposes power and a different quality in its exercise. We therefore seek power for the people in order to obtain social justice and to satisfy people's basic needs efficiently and effectively. Otherwise, what freedom can we achieve for society as a whole?

## Popular Power to Satisfy Needs and Ensure Freedom

Liberation theology locates science and technology within the triangle formed by the satisfaction of basic needs, justice for society, and power . . .

Consequently, science and technology are seen not as neutral elements standing alone (instrumental rationalization), but as dependent on the way in which society, politics, economics, and culture are organized. From the viewpoint of the poor of the Third World, science and technology today are the new caravelles, the main weapons for upholding political dependence and ensuring economic dominance over nations and their populations that do not control the production, distribution, and sale of goods. This statement does not amount to a rejection of science and technology. We need them to satisfy present-day basic human needs on a global scale. But we want to see them politically integrated in a society that sets itself better goals than unlimited growth (with the ecological violence this entails) and the greatest profit in the shortest time (leading to the marginalization and exclusion of the masses).

Liberation theology is in communion with the political aspirations of many social groups that seek a society concentrated on the dignity of the human person and on a form of participation that, through labor, satisfies the basic needs of food, shelter, health, education, and leisure, and opens up areas of freedom for creativity and the collective building up of society. Because of this, liberation theology is opposed to the technological messianism (the gospel of technocracy) of the ruling system. This claims to resolve the problems of underdevelopment, and its failed solution, which produced libertarian thinking in politics and in the churches. It seeks to do this by making intensive use of science and technology to produce food and everything else necessary for human sustenance, and by distributing them to those who are without them. Biotechnology has set itself such a goal.

This is the providentialist and assistentialist solution on a world scale. It is an agenda for guaranteeing survival (by providing food), but not for promoting life (by creating conditions for people to produce their food). Liberation theology is opposed to this kind of erroneous good will.

## Technological Messianism Versus Participatory Politics

The problem cannot be reduced to guaranteeing survival, as though human beings were simply hungry animals (beings full of needs). Instead, it supposes an adequate vision of what human life is (human beings are made for freedom, for solidarity, for unlimited relationships, and with a capacity for communication, even with God). The logic of human life does not merely obey the instinct to reproduce, but seeks the advancement and expansion of systems of life. This logic is built on freedom, participation, communication, and creativity.

It is not enough, therefore, to distribute bread, which can be done by technological messianism. If we want to respect human nature, we have to create the appropriate conditions for producing food. That is, we have to provide work by means of participatory politics . . . [Human beings] do not want to be simply creatures helped by the decisions of others, in a history made by others. They want to share in decision making and in a history which they themselves have helped to shape. That is, they want to construct their own individualities and their collective subjectivity. Only thus will they feel human and build up their own historical, ecological and social humanity.

Finally, liberation theology seeks to throw light on society's agenda. In doing so it reflects on the power expressed through science and technology, which is deeply problematical. In effect, it is exercised with a capitalist agenda that produces a bad quality of life, both in the so-called First World and in the world in which two-thirds of the population live in poverty. The current process of globalization is being pursued within the capitalist ambit, yet not by means of religion, ethics, or ideology, but through the global market (in general, the needs of the market are not those of human beings).

Left to its own devices, the market eventually puts a price on everything and sets aside everything that is not profitable. Therefore, even if the great trusts, with their masses of technicians and technostructures, were to succeed in satisfying basic human needs, the question of the nature of human beings, their freedom, creativity, sharing, and the meaning of their lives, which goes well beyond material needs, would remain unanswered.

## Requisites of a New Global Political Economy

Liberation theology insists on this orientation: Technological globalization should be directed toward a worldwide political agenda (a new political economy), including a minimum of humanization, citizenship, equity, human, and ecological welfare, and respect for cultural differences and openness to cultural reciprocity and complementarity. I shall examine each of these elements briefly.

*A minimum of humanization.* All human beings should have the basic right to existence. This means that they should be able to eat at least one meal a day, have a roof over their heads, and be helped with basic health care. Present regimes do not focus on whole persons, but only on their work effort (muscles, brains, the athlete's feet, and so on). It is revolutionary nowadays to say that we have to nourish love and friendship for human persons as such, beyond their ethnic, religious, or cultural attributes. The novelty of human rights movements in the Third World consists in reclaiming them primarily for the victims, and in taking as their motto: 'Serve life, beginning with the most threatened.'

*Citizenship.* Social systems should not tend to exclude people. All people should feel themselves to be potentially citizens of the world, used to thinking globally while acting locally in their own countries (with their own cultural roots). Citizenship implies anti-authoritarianism and the intrinsic acceptance of plurality.

*Equity.* This implies the certainty of being able to enjoy social benefits and of being able to overcome an established relationship between the contribution which certain citizens can make and what they receive in exchange. Equity seeks a greater realization of the political ideal of equality, which becomes a utopian goal in the positive sense of the term (a reference that makes relative all embodiments and continually invokes new ones). Solidarity among groups and nations alleviates the harshness of social inequalities.

*Human and ecological welfare.* The best projects, practices, and organizations are those that do not aim exclusively at the quality of goods and services, but at the quality of life, in order to make that life truly human. Society as a whole should make a life of this kind its goal. The alliance that is in the course of establishment between men and women and nature, in terms of brother-sisterhood and veneration, also forms part of human well-being. Another component is spirituality, in the sense of the capacity to communicate with the deepest subjectivity of other persons, and all other entities, including the otherness of all created beings and the absolute Otherness of God. Another, final, component is the pluralist expression of the values and visions of life, of history, and the ultimate goals and confines of the universe.

*Respect for cultural differences.* Human beings live in history. They have worked out their responses to the meaningful questions about their passage here on earth in different ways. Just as we have an external ecology (environmental and social ecology), so we have an internal ecology (profound ecology). We interpret, evaluate, and dream our existence on the basis of our cumulative experience. All this diversity reveals the richness of the venture and adventure that being human is. We have been able to communicate this, to the enrichment of all. In spite of the tendency of science and technology to homogenize everything, new singularities are constantly emerging from specific cultural appropriations of such processes. Each culture has a different way of combining work and leisure, and of articulating great dreams with harsh reality. Science and technology are stages in this mode of inhabiting the earth and experiencing our integration in a greater ecological whole.

*Cultural reciprocity and complementarity.* It is not sufficient to recognize otherness. This act of respect is truly fulfilled when we accept the values of others, develop reciprocity (the exchange of experience and understanding), and reciprocally complement others. No one culture expresses the entire human creative potential. This means that one culture can complement another. All cultures together demonstrate the versatility of human beings and our various ways of fulfilling our humanity. In this way, every culture proffers an inestimable richness of language, philosophy, religion, and arts, as well as techniques and technologies – a whole way of living in the world. This is true whether we speak of a simple culture, such as that of the Amazonian tribes, or the 'modern' scientific-technological forms of culture.

In conclusion, liberation theology sees science, technology, and power as part of the program of redemption, construction, consolidation, and expansion of human life and freedom, starting with those who have the least life and freedom. Life and freedom are the greatest and most desirable goods in existence, without which we always feel enslaved to need, but with which we can feel that we are sons and daughters of happiness.

# 2

# RESPECT FOR LIFE

## Introduction

In discussing many bioethical issues, such as abortion, care of the newborn, care of the dying, and euthanasia, it is common for Christians and others to appeal to the 'sanctity of [human] life' – the notion that human life is in some sense 'sacred' or has an absolute value. It may be argued, for example, that the sanctity of the foetus' life forbids abortion, or that the sanctity of the dying person's life rules out active euthanasia.

But can we say that human life in and of itself possesses 'sanctity' or 'absolute value'? In recent years, a number of philosophers have argued that it is not the mere fact that a human individual is alive that demands our respect, but rather the capacity, potential or quality of an individual's life. Thus, a severely disabled newborn infant may be judged to have such a poor quality of life that she should be allowed to die or even be killed (Kuhse and Singer 1985); a terminally ill patient may request euthanasia because her life is 'not worth living', or it may even sometimes be right for others to make that decision on her behalf if she is incapable of making it for herself (Glover 1977, 182–202). So is the sanctity or the quality of life the better moral criterion to bring to bear on difficult decisions at the margins of life?

In the first reading in this chapter, the Catholic theologian Richard McCormick takes up the question of quality *versus* sanctity of life, and argues that this is a false dichotomy. His conclusion is that it is possible to make 'a quality-of-life judgment in a way that both expresses and reinforces our concern for the sanctity of life' (p. 43). However, in order to reach this conclusion, he develops a somewhat different understanding from the traditional notion of the sanctity of life. His account is partly based on a Christian opposition to what he calls 'vitalism' – that is, the notion that life itself is an absolute value or the highest human good.

John Breck, too, argues that 'quality *versus* sanctity' is a false debate, but he collapses the distinction in a very different way from McCormick. From an Orthodox Christian perspective, he distinguishes between the 'sacredness' and 'sanctity' of life. Every human life is 'sacred' because we are created by God who loves us and calls us to participate in the divine life. 'Sanctity' is the result of our growth in holiness towards that ultimate goal. This is not a merely human achievement, but the result of God's work in us, and it is this work of God that can give our lives true quality even in the midst of pain and suffering.

The Protestant feminist theologian Karen Lebacqz takes a somewhat different line through the discussion. She wishes to defend the 'dignity' of human life as a basis for respecting and protecting the lives of individuals regardless of their ability or potential. But, following Helmut Thielicke, she denies that this dignity is an intrinsic property of human life: rather, it is an 'alien dignity' conferred upon us all by a loving God. She argues that such alien dignity, contrary to our usual intuitions, provides a *more* secure foundation for the protection of human life and well-being than would a notion of intrinsic dignity or value. Intrinsic dignity would inevitably depend on some property or capacity, and any individual lacking that property or capacity (for example, on some accounts, a severely disabled infant or a patient with severe dementia) would lose the right to some or all of the respect normally accorded to human life. Alien dignity, by contrast, does not depend on any ability or potential we possess, but on God's free and undeserved love for us all. It is God's gift which we cannot earn; neither can we lose it or deny it to others.

The question of the sanctity of life is closely related to the question 'who is a person?', which often appears in the same medical-ethical debates. The question of personhood and its significance for bioethics is the subject of chapter 3. The sanctity-of-life and personhood debates are also related to the question of the status of non-human animals. Some philosophers hold that the concept of the sanctity of human life is 'speciesist': it represents a prejudice in favour of humans simply because they belong to the species *Homo sapiens* (Singer 1993, 55–68). The status of non-human animals, and the relations between humans and other animals, will be taken up in chapter 8.

### References and Further Reading

Jonathan Glover, *Causing Death and Saving Lives*. Harmondsworth: Penguin, 1977.
John Paul II, *Evangelium Vitae*. London: Catholic Truth Society, 1995.
Helga Kuhse and Peter Singer, *Should the Baby Live?* Oxford: Oxford University Press, 1985.
Paul Ramsey, *Ethics at the Edges of Life*. New Haven: Yale University Press, 1978.
Peter Singer, *Practical Ethics*. 2nd ed., Cambridge: Cambridge University Press, 1993.

# The Quality of Life,
# the Sanctity of Life

RICHARD McCORMICK

[In the first part of the chapter from which this reading is taken, McCormick has surveyed the work of several other writers on the issue of the quality and sanctity of life. The chapter concludes with his personal reflections, which are reproduced in this reading.]

Before spelling out the direction I believe this discussion ought to be taking in the future, let me note several introductory points that cling to it.

*Life as a condition for other values and achievements.* It is clear that, before any human experiences, responses, or achievements are possible, there must be life. In this sense, life is a condition for all other values and experiences. Some theologians have stated therefore that life is a value to be preserved precisely because it makes other achievements possible. When, because of the condition of the patient, no experience or interrelation is possible, then (so the formulation goes) that life has achieved its potential. As Kautzky words it: 'Since human life is the condition for the realization of human freedom, it should be prolonged with all appropriate and reasonable means insofar as prolongation according to a competent estimate can serve this goal.'[1]

William May has leveled the following objection against this reasoning: 'In other words ... life itself, in the sense of physical or biological life, is what an older tradition would have called a *bonum utile*, not a *bonum honestum*.'[2]

Two possible responses can be made. First, one could insist that to say life is a good to be preserved insofar as it contains some potentiality for human experience is not to make life a *bonum utile*, or merely a useful good, and therefore a kind of negotiable thing. Rather, it is to talk about our duties – and especially the why of those duties – towards the preservation of a *bonum honestum* – that is, a good in itself, the dying human person, and to admit that these duties may differ depending on the conditions of that *bonum honestum*.

Second, and perhaps even more to the point, it could be counterstated that the usage of 'useful good' and 'good in itself' plays upon the ambiguity

From *How Brave a New World? Dilemmas in Bioethics*, pp. 395–401. London: SCM, 1981.

of the term 'life.' 'Life' can mean two general things: (1) a state of human functioning (or capacity thereof), of well-being; or (2) the existence of vital and metabolic processes with no human functioning or capacity. We do not, in Christian perspectives, preserve these functions *for their own sake*; we are not vitalists. In this second sense of 'life,' then, one could argue that it is indeed a useful good only, though it is not clear to me how such terminology illuminates the matter. Where one draws the line between the two senses of the 'life' is crucial, of course. But once it is drawn, I have no problem with referring to life beyond that line as a useful good, though I see no gain in doing so.

Very close to this is the insistence of some discussants (such as Weber) that use of quality-of-life criteria means that 'life is not good or worthwhile or meaningful anymore.'[3] Similarly, this move is seen as implying that 'life is not good in itself.'[4] Or again, it is argued that for the infant 'just to be alive may be a great success.' Such statements are subject to the distinction made above. Concretely, if 'life' means *only* metabolism and vital processes, then what is meant by saying that this is a 'good in itself'? If that means a good to be preserved independently of any capacity for conscious experience, I believe it is a straightforward form of vitalism – an approach that preserves life (mere vital processes) no matter what the condition of the patient. One can and, I believe, should say that the *person* is always an incalculable value, but that at some point continuance in physical life offers the person no benefit. Indeed, to keep 'life' going can easily be an assault on the person and his or her dignity. Therefore, phrases such as 'the good of life in itself' are misleading in these discussions.

*Sanctity of life v. quality of life.* Some who compare 'sanctity of life' and 'quality of life' approaches see the former as more satisfactory.[5] It focuses our attention on obligations to preserve life and avoids degrees of discrimination in quality-of-life criteria. Actually, the two approaches ought not to be set against one another in this way. Quality-of-life assessments ought to be made within an over-all reverence for life, as an extension of one's respect for the sanctity of life. However, there are times when preserving the life of one with no capacity for those aspects of life that we regard as *human* is a violation of the sanctity of life itself. Thus to separate the two approaches and call one *sanctity* of life, the other *quality* of life, is a false conceptual split that very easily suggests that the term 'sanctity of life' is being used in an exhortatory way.

*Quality-of-life criteria and equality of value.* It is argued that quality-of-life language implies 'that not all lives are equally good or equally deserving of protection.'[6] Thus it is essentially discriminatory. As Weber puts it: 'Can one really use a condition-of-life criterion and still insist that every life is of equal value regardless of condition?'[7]

While speaking in terms of 'every life' being of 'equal value' reveals a legitimate concern (that medical treatment be not denied or withheld in a way violative of the rights of individuals), that is not the issue. Every *person* is of 'equal value.' But not every *life* (once again, the distinction noted above) is of equal value if we are careful to unpack the terms 'life,' 'equal,' and 'value.' If 'life' means the continuation of vital processes in a persistent vegetative state; if 'value' means 'a good to the individual concerned'; if 'equal' means 'identical' or 'the same,' especially of treatment, then I believe it is simply false to say that 'every life is of equal value.'

What the 'equal value' language is attempting to say is legitimate: We must avoid *unjust* discrimination in the provision of health care and life supports. But not all discrimination (inequality of treatment) is unjust. *Unjust* discrimination is avoided if decision-making centers on the benefit to the patient, even if benefit is described largely in terms of quality-of-life criteria.

*The means approach and sanctity of life.* It is occasionally argued that emphasis on means better protects the equal value of all lives because it stresses *'objective* indications' and 'puts the whole question in the context of the goodness of life.'[8] Thus Weber states: 'Focus on the means is a constant reminder that we should not decide who should live or die on the basis of the worth of someone's life.'[9]

Here it must be pointed out that the terms 'ordinary' and 'extraordinary' are so relative that they are equally capable of abuse as quality-of-life language. The famous Johns Hopkins case (in which a baby with Down's syndrome, needing minor surgery, was allowed to die on the grounds that the surgery would be extraordinary) is a well-known instance. What is important in these matters is that the line be drawn in the proper place. Language itself does not draw such lines. Both the 'means approach' and the 'quality-of-life approach' can be abused. But they need not be. Indeed, if treatment decisions are often quality-of-life decisions, as Weber admits, then the greater danger may be to disguise this fact with the language of ordinary/ extraordinary, for it means we are not attending to the line-drawing process and its criteria. And not attending to it could easily lead to allowing that line to slip around in a way that is ultimately unfair to the incompetent patient. In sum, then, I would seriously question whether 'means language' better protects human life.

This discussion is far from ended. Indeed, in a sense it is just beginning, for one thing is increasingly clear: Technological and medical advances bring, for some individuals, mixed blessings at best. In the contemporary literature one sees a move away from the language of ordinary/extraordinary means as being increasingly confusing, ambiguous, and circular. I myself, with Veatch, favor the terms 'reasonable/unreasonable treatment.' These terms are themselves of course empty, but they do achieve two things. First, and negatively, they move us away from a terminology (ordinary/ extraordinary) that suggests too easily and to too many that 'usualness' is the key and crucial factor in these decisions, whereas that notion very often disguises the real character of the decision.

Second, and more positively, the terms 'reasonable/unreasonable' point in the direction of what will be in the future the crucial referrent in these decisions – the judgment of the reasonable person. In the Quinlan case, the New Jersey Supreme Court argued: (1) that Karen Quinlan had a right to self-determination (the court said 'privacy') where treatment is concerned; (2) that she is in a noncompetent and vegetative state, leaving her incapable of exercising her right to withdraw treatment; (3) that it may be exercised on her behalf by her family and guardian. Then most interestingly it stated: 'If their (family) conclusion is in the affirmative their decision should be accepted by a society *the overwhelming majority of whose members would, we think, in similar circumstances, exercise such a choice in the same way for themselves or for those closest to them*' (emphasis added).[10] This is an appeal to what most of us, in similar circumstances, would do – as reasonable people with healthy outlooks on the meaning of life and death.

That is a formal criterion, of course, and in itself leaves untouched the criteria that reasonable people would use in making decisions. The judgment of reasonable people is not *constitutive* of the rightness of the decision. It is merely *confirmatory* that the criterion is close to the mark. In deciding what those criteria are, we must distinguish carefully with Veatch between competent and noncompetent patients. For competent patients, refusal of treatment may be considered reasonable 'wherever they can offer reasons valid to themselves – that is, out of concern about physical or mental burdens or other objectives . . .'[11] In other words, the appropriate mix of values during dying, how one shall live while dying, belongs to the patient. And here patients may and do differ within the range of morally acceptable options.

Of the three values copresent (preservation of life, human freedom, lack of pain), some will choose to maximize freedom, others to minimize pain even with the diminution of freedom.[12] Still others will manage their dying with a controlling view of the financial and/or psychological condition of their dear ones. That is the meaning of 'reasons valid to themselves.' These cannot and need not be specified further. Treatment that conforms to such wishes and perspectives may be considered reasonable (morally appropriate), always allowing for legal appeal by physician or hospital if a patient is judged to be frivolously jeopardizing life.

For the incompetent patient, obviously this decision must be made by proxy (family or guardian). When the incompetent (unconscious) patient is an adult, there may exist warrants in past statements and clearly known perspectives that aid the proxies in determining what is reasonable treatment. When these are not present, I believe that the judgment of reasonable people may be used as an aid to a morally acceptable decision – that is, if the situation is such that most or very many of us would not want life-preserving treatment *in that condition*, it would be morally prudent (reasonable) to conclude that life-preserving treatment is not morally required for this particular patient. But once again, it is not the consensus that *constitutes* the reasonableness. Rather, reasonable people can be presumed to be drawing the line on the kind of life being preserved at the right place – in the best over-all interests of the patient.

The matter becomes even more difficult when the patient is an infant, for the simple reason that it is all but impossible for *healthy adults* to extrapolate backward on what kind of life will be acceptable to the infant. Yet, if we are to avoid vitalism in practice, these judgments must sometimes be made. I agree with Judson G. Randolph (surgeon in chief, Children's Hospital National Medical Center, Washington, D.C.) when he states: 'I think it is well within the guidelines of right and wrong to make certain qualitative judgments about human life . . .'[13] Randolph continues: 'If a severely handicapped child were suddenly given one moment of omniscience and total awareness of his or her outlook for the future, would that child necessarily opt for life? No-one has yet been able to demonstrate that the answer would always be "yes".' In my judgment, the perspectives of the Christian tradition on life and its meaning would suggest that in some instances the answer would be 'no.' In some cases the reason would be the continuing burden to the patient of treatment. But in others, the reason is that in this tradition mere life (vital processes, metabolism) has not been viewed as a value *in itself* . . .

Our main task is to discover as a community of reasonable persons where the line is drawn and why. When we do so, we will have discovered the differences between reasonable and unreasonable treatment, especially for those who cannot make the decision themselves but depend for their well-being on us. In other words, we will have made a quality-of-life judgment in a way that both expresses and reinforces our concern for the sanctity of life.

## Notes

1. R Kautzky, 'Der Arzt,' *Arzt und Christ*, 15 (1969), 138.
2. William May, 'Ethics and Human Identity: The Challenge of the New Biology,' *Horizons*, 3 (1976), 35.
3. Leonard J. Weber, *Who Shall Live?* (New York: Paulist Press, 1976), 83.
4. Ibid., 81.
5. Leonard J. Weber (see below), and Eugene F. Diamond, ' "Quality" vs. "Sanctity" of Life in the Nursery,' *America*, 135 (1976), 396–98.
6. Weber, *Who Shall Live?* 78.
7. Ibid., 82.
8. Ibid., 84.
9. Ibid., 85.
10. *In the Matter of Karen Quinlan, an Alleged Incompetent*, A-116 (Mar. 31, 1976), 24. [Editor's note: Karen Ann Quinlan, a young New Jersey woman, entered an irrevers-

ible coma following an accident. She was originally on a respirator, but the New Jersey Supreme Court ruled that it was permissible for a guardian to withdraw life support and allow her to die. However, after the respirator was disconnected, she continued to live for nearly ten years, sustained by artificial feeding. See Tom L. Beauchamp and James F. Childress, *Principles of Biomedical Ethics*, 125–126. 5th ed., Oxford and New York: Oxford University Press, 2001.]

11. Robert M. Veatch, *Death, Dying, and the Biological Revolution* (New Haven, Conn.: Yale University Press, 1976), 100.
12. See the helpful article of Albert Ziegler, 'Sterbehilfe – Grundfragen und "Thesen",' *Orientierung*, 39 (1975), 39–41, 55–58.
13. As cited by J. G. Randolph in 'Ethical Considerations in Surgery of the Newborn,' *Contemporary Surgery*, 7 (1975), 17–19.

# The Sacredness and Sanctity of Human Life

JOHN BRECK

'The glory of God is a living person and the life of the person is the vision of God.' (St. Irenaeus)

'Abba Lot went to see Abba Joseph and said to him, "Abba, as far as I can I say my little office, I fast a little, I pray and meditate, I live in peace and as far as I can, I purify my thoughts. What else can I do?" Then the old man stood up and stretched his hands towards heaven. His fingers became like ten lamps of fire and he said to him, "If you will, you can become all flame!" ' (Joseph of Panephysis)

'Ascend, brothers, ascend eagerly, and be resolved in your hearts to ascend and hear Him who says: Come and let us go up to the mountain of the Lord and to the house of our God, who makes our feet like hinds' feet and sets us on high places, that we may be victorious with His song.' (St. John Climacus)

Orthodox Christianity affirms that life is a *gift*, freely bestowed by the God of love. Human life, therefore, is to be received and welcomed with an attitude of joy and thanksgiving. It is to be cherished, preserved and protected as the most sublime expression of God's creative activity. God has brought us 'from non-being into being' for more than mere biological existence. He has chosen us for Life, of which the ultimate end is participation in the eternal glory of the Risen Christ, 'in the inheritance of the saints in light' (Col. 1:12; Eph. 1:18).

In the language of the Eastern Church Fathers, this transcendent destiny or *telos* of human existence is expressed as *theosis* or 'deification.' To the patristic mind, God in his innermost being remains forever transcendent, beyond all we can know or experience. An unbridgeable gulf separates the creature from the Creator, human nature from divine nature. The Orthodox teaching on *theosis* nevertheless affirms that our primal vocation or calling is to *participate* in divine life itself, to 'ascend to the house of our God,' where we shall enjoy eternal communion with the three Persons of the Holy Trinity.

From *The Sacred Gift of Life*, pp. 5–11. Crestwood, NY: St Vladimir's Seminary Press, 1998.

How does Orthodox teaching resolve this tension between the absolute trans-cendence of God and his accessibility in the life of faith? We can answer the question, briefly and schematically, in the following way.

From the inner mystery of his absolute 'otherness,' the total inaccessibility of his divine nature or being, God reaches out to the created world and to his human creatures, to save, restore and heal all that is sinful and corrupt. By means of what St. Irenaeus calls his 'two hands' – the Son and the Spirit – God the Father assumes and embraces human life, filling it with his attributes or 'energies' of love, power, justice, goodness and beauty. Thereby he opens the way for our ascension into the realm of his holiness, where those who live and die in Christ join with the saints of all ages, to offer their worship of praise and thanksgiving before the divine glory and majesty. Human life, therefore, finds its ultimate fulfilment beyond death, in the boundless communion of 'righteousness, peace and joy in the Holy Spirit' that consti-tutes the Kingdom of God (Rom. 14:17).

Yet the apostle Paul, like the evangelist John and other New Testament authors, speaks of the Kingdom as a reality that is presently accessible to us: the Kingdom is 'among' us, 'in our midst' or even 'within' the depths of our being . . . (Luke 17:21). Although its fullness can be known only after our physical death, our present life within the Church offers us a very real foretaste of the ineffable joy to come. 'Righteousness, peace and joy' are qualities St. Paul believes should characterize the ecclesial community on earth as well as life within the eternal 'communion of saints.' In the Gospel of John, Jesus speaks to those who are tempted by apostasy . . . He addresses them in the present tense, in the midst of their immediate, present-day experience: 'Truly, truly I say to you, he who hears my word and believes him who sent me *has* eternal life and does not come into judgement, but has passed from death to life' (John 5:24). From this perspective the Kingdom of God is not merely the object of our future hope. It is a present reality, inaugurated by baptism and nourished by communion in the Body and Blood of the glorified Lord. It is a 'sacramental' reality that radically transforms our understanding of the origin and the ultimate destiny of human existence. Life now is experienced as an ongoing pilgrimage marked by inner struggle. It becomes at its heart an *askesis* or spiritual warfare between, on the one hand, sickness, sin and death, and on the other, wholeness, sanctity and eternal blessedness. It is this struggle, and its ultimate victory, that constitute the 'life in Christ.'

Created by God as the most sublime expression of his divine love, we are called to enjoy everlasting communion with him in the fellowship of those who reflect through all eternity his radiant sanctity. Yet like those saints who have gone on before us – the myriad of martyrs, 'confessors' and other holy people who have 'fought the good fight' and emerged victorious – we can only attain to divine sanctity through the exercise of faithful *stewardship*, offering 'ourselves and each other and all our life to Christ our God.' Admonishing members of the church in Corinth who were tempted to give in to the lure of fornication, the apostle Paul asks rhetorically, 'Do you not know that your body is a temple of the Holy Spirit within you, which you have from God?' Then he makes the startling assertion: '*You are not your own*; you were bought with a price. Therefore glorify God in your body!' (1 Cor. 6:19–20). Christian stewardship demands that we 'render unto God that which is God's.' As the parable of the talents makes clear, stewardship of this kind involves not mere caretaking, but the bearing of fruit: rendering to God what is his, with interest, for the glory of God and the salvation of his world.

Created in the divine image and called to assume the divine 'likeness' by becoming 'perfect' as our heavenly Father is perfect, Christian believers assume, as an inescapable aspect of their life and calling, an arduous, ascetic struggle against demonic powers of sin, death and corruption. Bearing the cross of Christ daily, they embark on an inward pilgrimage that leads, through continual repentance, from death to life and from 'glory to glory,' to attain at the end everlasting communion with God. This is their God-given vocation, just as it is their unique source of ultimate meaning and personal value.

It is this sublime vocation that confers upon human existence its *sacredness* or *sanctity*. It alone endows human life with eternal value, from conception, through physical death, to resurrected existence in the Kingdom of God. Accordingly, any reflection on the moral issues that shape and influence human life must presuppose an anthropological perspective, faithful to the Church's Tradition, which acknowledges and honors that sanctity.

To speak of the sanctity or sacredness of human life is also to speak of 'personhood.' One is truly a person only insofar as one reflects the 'being-in-communion' of the three Persons of the Holy Trinity. This is a much-misunderstood concept in present-day America, where the 'person' has been thoroughly confused with the 'individual.' Individual characteristics distinguish us from one another, whereas authentic personhood *unites* us in a bond of communion with each other and with God. We can truly claim to be persons only insofar as we embody and communicate to others the beauty, truth and love that unite the three Persons – Father, Son and Spirit – in an eternal tri-unity. The Trinitarian God is thus the model, as well as the source and ultimate end, of all that is authentically *personal* in human experience.

It is as personal beings that we bear the ineradicable *image* of God; in fact, that image determines our personhood. Yet we are fulfilled as persons, and thus actualize within ourselves authentic sanctity, through the arduous work of ongoing repentance and ascetic struggle that leads to personal growth in the divine *likeness*. The 'sacredness' of life, in other words, is intrinsic to our very nature; yet it is 'actualized,' made concrete and effective in daily existence, through our ceaseless effort to affirm and preserve an authentic 'sanctity' or holiness of life. Acquisition of sanctity, therefore, requires our active participation, a 'synergy' or cooperation with divine grace that involves 'putting off the old Adam' and 'putting on the new.' St. Paul expresses the dynamic quality of this ongoing inner conversion in these terms: 'Put off your old nature which belongs to your former manner of life and is corrupt through deceitful lusts, and be renewed in the spirit of your minds, and put on the new nature, created after the likeness of God (*ton kata theon*) in true righteousness and holiness' (Eph. 4:22–24, RSV).

'Sacredness' and 'sanctity' are often used synonymously to speak of the divine origin and purpose of human existence. In light of what we have just stressed, however, it might be preferable to speak of our life as 'sacred' by virtue of its created *nature* that embodies and gives expression to the divine 'image.' The life of every person is 'sacred,' insofar as it is created by God with the purpose of participating in his own holiness, and possesses the capacity to reflect the presence and glory of God from its depths. (However much that capacity may be diminished by sin and wilful rejection of God, Orthodox anthropology affirms that the divine image can be obscured but never eradicated; there is no 'total depravity,' however morally depraved an individual may in fact be.) 'Sanctity,' on the other hand, would refer to the *personal* or 'hypostatic' qualities that one attains through ascetic struggle against temptation and sin, as well as through the acquisition of virtue. Sacredness would thus be considered a function of 'nature' and sanctity, as a function of 'person.'

Christian existence is nevertheless paradoxical: although our personal struggle, our 'spiritual warfare,' is indispensable and unavoidable in the life of faith, its fruits depend entirely on the grace of God. Orthodoxy insists that a 'synergy' between God and his human creatures is essential to the work of sanctification, of attaining 'sanctity.' Still, sanctity remains a gift, wholly unmerited and wholly unattainable by our own efforts. While the quest for sanctity requires a profound sense of responsibility on our part, the fruit of that quest is produced by God alone. As 'it is no longer I who live, but Christ who lives in me' (Gal. 2:20), so it is not I who achieve holiness, but rather the 'Spirit of holiness' (Rom. 1:4) who dwells in me and who alone works out my salvation.

Endowed with 'sacredness' from its conception, human life thus finds its ultimate sense, its deeply 'spiritual' meaning, in the quest for 'sanctity' or holiness. This distinction between sacredness and sanctity is useful, and it conforms to Orthodox anthropology. Modern ethical discourse nevertheless tends to confuse the terms. This is especially evident in the impassioned discussions between those who represent either a 'sanctity of life' or a 'quality of life' perspective in assessing moral issues.

There has been a tendency in recent years to oppose these two perspectives, setting 'sanctity' and 'quality' over against each other in an unresolvable tension. Proponents of the 'sanctity of life' principle, according to a popular caricature, will want to preserve biological existence at all cost, irrespective of the degree of suffering endured by the person concerned. 'Quality of life' proponents, according to the same caricature, strive above all to avoid debilitating pain and suffering. Therefore they favor procedures such as 'abortion on demand' and 'physician-assisted suicide,' to assure control over the 'quality' of life experienced by a pregnant woman or a terminally ill patient. In reality, the former position represents a philosophical view known as 'vitalism.' This is a form of bio-idolatry that by its very nature violates the 'sanctity' of life, since God-given life is ultimately fulfilled beyond the limits of biological existence. And insofar as the radical 'quality of life' position places the avoidance of mental and physical pain above every other value, it deprives human life of its innate God-given value, purpose and destiny.

. . . Rather than set the 'sanctity of life' and the 'quality of life' in opposition to each other, we need to see the two as complementary. Christian experience knows that pain and suffering are potentially redemptive. While certain levels of physical and emotional anguish can appear to be 'dehumanizing,' even those who suffer intractable pain are in the hands of God and can experience his loving care and mercy. It is precisely these gifts of divine love and mercy that assure the true *quality* of human life in any condition or circumstance. Similarly, it is the free gift of God's own holiness that suffuses human life with authentic *sanctity*. If both the sanctity and the quality of human life are seen to derive from divine grace, then the opposition reflected in the current debate is simply false. The true 'quality' of personal existence is defined by its attainment of 'sanctity'; and authentic 'sanctity' derives only from a particular 'quality' of life, conferred by knowledge of and participation in the loving mercy of an infinitely compassionate God.

This complementarity between the quality of life and the sanctity of life is possible because human life by its very nature is 'sacred.' Its origin, purpose and ultimate end are given and determined by God alone. Once again, 'sacredness' and 'sanctity' need to be distinguished, the former referring to the essential goodness and infinite value of human life created in the divine image, and the latter to the arduous yet blessed struggle of the human person to attain and reflect the divine likeness.

# Alien Dignity: The Legacy of Helmut Thielicke for Bioethics

KAREN LEBACQZ

> This experience of rejection made me think that there was no God, because in moments of rejection like that one I feel I am no good. And if I am no good, how can there be any God? Am I not made in the image and likeness of God?[1]

With these haunting words, Ada Maria Isasi-Diaz points not only to the painful realities of racism and sexism in our midst but also to the centrality of the image of God for theological ethics and to the intimate link between that image and the valuation of human beings. 'If I am no good, how can there be any God? Am I not made in the image and likeness of God?' What does it mean to be made in the image and likeness of God and how does it relate to our valuation as persons?

No modern ethicist has elaborated the link between the image of God and the valuing of persons with more care than the great German theologian Helmut Thielicke ... In 'The Doctor as Judge of Who Shall Live and Who Shall Die,'[2] Thielicke suggested that there are two ways to view people: in terms of their utility, or in terms of their 'infinite worth.' Thielicke opted for their infinite worth, and based that option on his understanding of the 'alien dignity' of persons.

In this essay, I will explore briefly the theological roots and meaning of 'alien dignity' in Thielicke's thought, and then develop the legacy of this term for the task of health care ethics today by illustrating its implications in several arenas of medicine and health care. Although there are problems with the concept of alien dignity, I will argue that it provides a rich legacy for protecting and equalizing human beings, for requiring personal responsibility, for attending to structural problems in health care, and for seeing humans as fundamentally relational.

From Allen Verhey (ed.), *Religion and Medical Ethics: Looking Back, Looking Forward*, pp. 44–60. Grand Rapids, MI: Eerdmans, 1996.

## Alien Dignity and the Image of God

The 'incommensurable, incalculable worth of human life,'[3] argued Thielicke, does not reside in any immanent quality of human beings, but in the fact that we are created and redeemed by God. Our worth is imparted by the love bestowed on us by God. Human worth is thus an 'alien dignity,' given in the relationship between humans and God. It is the image of God in us that gives us our alien dignity.

The image of God in humans was not, for Thielicke, a given attribute or property, such as rationality or even freedom.[4] Rather, 'the divine likeness rests on the fact that God remembers [us] . . . '[5] The image of God is not our own immanent or ontic dignity, not some quality such as rationality that 'imitates' the character of the divine, but rather a statement of our relationship to God. To speak of the *imago Dei* is to speak of God's love for us. God creates us in love, calls us in love, and redeems us in love; and it is this love that creates the image of God in us and gives us our worth. The image of God is not substantive, but relational.

Human worth is therefore 'alien' in the sense that it comes to us from God. It is 'that alien dignity which is grounded in and by [the one] who does the giving.'[6] As a *proprium*, a true ontic possession or attribute in the strict sense, it belongs only to Christ.[7] The divine likeness of human beings is fulfilled only in Christ. Only in Christ is there the immediacy of relation to God that constitutes the *imago Dei*, and that was destroyed in the 'Fall.' The immediacy thus lost is restored in Christ, and so we participate in the divine likeness through Christ. God 'remembers' us and draws us back into proper relationship, and herein lies the image of God.

The image of God is therefore ineffable and difficult to describe concretely, since it does not consist in specific characteristics or attributes that can easily be named.[8] For Thielicke, the divine image in humans was like a mirror reflecting the glory of God. Like a mirror, the image goes dark when the source of light is withdrawn: 'it possesses only borrowed light.'[9]

The *imago Dei* is thus, substantively, a representation of agape – of God's love for humans. It is therefore also agape that recognizes and realizes the *imago Dei*, seeing the other person in her standing before God rather than in her 'utility' value for me. It is agape that allows us to love our enemies, not identifying them with their opposition to us, but seeing in them the children of God.[10]

For Thielicke, then, to speak of the alien dignity of human beings is to speak of their infinite worth. It is to speak of their relationship to God, and of the love with which they are held by God. It is to speak of what God has 'spent' on human beings, the love poured out that creates an unimpeachable worth possessed by 'even the most pitiful life.'[11] To speak of alien dignity is to speak of the individual destiny received from God, of the invisible totality of the person, of the person's standing in the eyes of God.

## Problems with Alien Dignity

'Alien dignity' may not be a comfortable term today, especially for feminists and others from oppressed groups. Two problems are immediately evident. First, to speak of dignity as 'alien' is to imply that it is not truly 'ours.' If the source is outside humans, then it seems something that is 'not us.' If it is only reflective of a light that originates elsewhere, then it seems that it could too easily be removed. To see dignity as 'alien' thus seems to remove it too much from the *humanum* and to make it precarious.

In our post-Enlightenment world, and particularly since the human potential movement, the Western world has tended to stress the dignity and potential that are inherent to humans. We want a dignity that is *precisely* ours, that is so much a part of us that there can never be any recognition of us without an acknowledgement of that dignity. To suggest that one's dignity is 'alien' and comes from outside us may perhaps make us think that it is therefore vulnerable to attack or erosion. We are probably more comfortable today with a notion of *intrinsic* dignity, as this notion would imply something so inbuilt that it can never be taken away.

Second, Thielicke's notion that alien dignity is like the reflection of a mirror in which all light comes from outside may appear to posit human beings as empty vessels. All value, all light, all dignity appear to come from God and from God alone. Thielicke's God seems distant and omnipotent. The gulf between the divine and the human seems virtually unbridgeable. Thielicke's alien dignity, the mirror reflecting God's light, seems to pose an all-powerful God and an all-empty human being: 'the *imago Dei* depends on the reflecting of alien light, a process which is always under the control of the glory of God which casts the reflection.'[12] Any sense of divine-human partnership seems fragile at best. We appear to have a process in which humans are at most pawns in a game controlled by God.

Such a transcendent, omnipotent God has been abandoned in many contemporary theologies. Liberation and feminist theologians tend instead to speak of a vulnerable God who suffers with us or of a partnership between humans and God. How else are we to explain the suffering of children who are abused by their parents or of oppressed peoples everywhere? An omnipotent God who fails to intervene in human suffering seems a cruel hoax.[13]

We might wonder, then, whether Thielicke's notion of alien dignity is theologically and ethically adequate. Does it create too fragile a dignity, not sufficiently rooted in human nature itself? Does it pose a God too remote and removed for an age of liberation that needs a God who suffers with us?

Within the scope of this essay, I cannot fully address these questions. Nonetheless, I believe that such doubts may arise from a misreading of the implications of Thielicke's work, and that Thielicke's core notion of alien dignity offers protections and insights badly needed today. I will illustrate this claim by pointing to five implications of alien dignity and their application in bioethics.

## Implications of Alien Dignity for Ethics
### 1. *Alien Dignity* **Protects People**

That human dignity is 'alien' does mean that it comes from outside me; it does not arise from within me. But for Thielicke, it is also integral to me. Since it is given to me in my very creation by God, since it is bestowed from the beginning with God's love, it is always present with me. It is therefore intimately mine, as truly mine as any of my characteristics and far more enduring. My youth will surely pass, my beauty will fade, but my alien dignity does *not* dim, in Thielicke's view.

Precisely because human dignity is 'alien,' it does not have to be *earned*, and it cannot be *lost*. It does not depend on my skin color, my sex, my sexual orientation, my intelligence, or any other particular characteristic or achievement. It does not depend on 'works.'[14] Precisely because it is 'alien' to me, it cannot be given away by me or taken away by others. It is both alien and inalienable. It is indelible, a mark put on us by God's love that permeates our being to the core. Since the alien dignity of humans depends only on God's love, and since God's love is constant and enduring, so is the dignity of each person.

To speak of alien dignity is therefore precisely a way of securing the basic inalienable worth of every person. Alien dignity *protects* people. They are inviolable. 'Even the most pitiful life' retains its dignity, and its incommensurable, incalculable worth. Because of this worth, humans may not be subjected to the dictatorial rule of technical capacities.[15]

The concept of alien dignity thus provides a strong base for responding to difficult bioethical questions such as when to cease treatment. In 'House Calls to Cardinal Jackson,' David Schiedermayer struggles to explain why he continues to treat a 79–year-old woman who has been 'mindless, lights-are-on-but-nobody's-home' for over ten years.[16] In trying to explain why he does not withdraw her feeding tube, Schiedermayer speaks of the daughter's love for the old woman and also of the fire that still burns in her green eyes. Then he asks:

> What is it that gives a person dignity? What is that inner grace that projects out toward the doctor, so that he, despite his intellect and

education and training and skills, is taken aback? . . . You can't take
dignity away from the dignified.[17]

Schiedermayer speaks here of the dignity of a woman who no longer functions as she once did. There is something about Cardinal Jackson that makes
her inviolable to him, in spite of her advanced age and her mental incompetence. This something, which Schiedermayer calls her dignity, is what
Thielicke would have called her alien dignity. For Thielicke, it is the worth
that does not fade with age nor dim with incompetence because it comes
from God.[18] Schiedermayer finds it hard to name the source of the dignity.
He mentions not the love of God but the love of Cardinal Jackson's daughter,
the hardship of Cardinal Jackson's life, the sense that we cannot abandon
her after her history of discrimination and mistreatment.

While Schiedermayer does not name the same source of dignity that Thielicke would name, his understanding of the inviolability conferred by that
dignity comes very close to Thielicke's. For Thielicke, alien dignity of humans
means that others can never be treated simply for their instrumental value.
They cannot be a means to an end for me. Their technical or utilitarian
capacities do not define their worth. Hence, they do not lose their worth
when they cease to function or when their capacities diminish.

In *The Ethics of Sex*,[19] for example, Thielicke argues against prostitution
because it entails the instrumentalization of a human being. Such instrumentalization – turning the other into an instrument for my pleasure or
satisfaction – is contrary to the alien dignity that prevents another from
simply being a means to my ends.

Elsewhere, Thielicke argues that one can never fully possess another
human being. To try to do so would be to destroy him at the center of his
being.[20] One cannot split off parts of a person or objectify the person, but
must deal with the whole person, with the 'indivisible totality of a human
being.'[21] Only this is recognition of the alien dignity of the other.

Nor are others subject to the fickle nature of our emotions. To see another
as the bearer of an alien dignity means that our regard for that other will
remain even when her or his importance for us diminishes.[22]

Thus, in none of these ways can we take away the dignity of the other.
Alien dignity protects the other from our vagaries, from objectification or
instrumentalization, from our lust for possession or for power, from our
imposition of our goals and purposes. If Cardinal Jackson's daughter tired
of caring for her mother and ceased to love her, the old woman would not
lose her dignity, in Thielicke's view.

In the medical arena, the inviolable worth of the other means that no one
could simply be used, for example, as an organ bank. It means that research
on human beings must respect those persons as whole beings, even if they
are convicted criminals or the 'most pitiful' of mental patients.[23] The notion

of alien dignity provides fundamental protections against using persons as means to the ends of others, against objectifying people, against the intrusions of power to oppress the powerless.

## 2. *Alien Dignity* Equalizes People

If the first implication of alien dignity is the protection of persons, the second is the equalization of persons. Since human worth is not earned or achieved, but given by God, no one is 'worth' more than others. All were bought for a price, and therefore all carry an incalculable value. The worth of human life for Thielicke was 'incommensurable' – it is not possible to measure one person's worth against another. Genuine agape, which recognizes the alien dignity in the other, 'does not degrade the other person.' Rather, it honors the other, and puts the other 'on the same level' as the one doing the loving.[24] Alien dignity has an equalizing effect.

This is reinforced by understanding that alien dignity would never allow the other to be dealt with simply in utilitarian terms. The 'use value' or 'social contribution value' of the person is not the person's true value. Only the alien dignity, the love poured out by God, represents the true value of the person. This value is unique, individual, incommensurable.

Operating out of this understanding of alien dignity would therefore prevent some approaches to the allocation of health care resources. In his study of medical directors of kidney dialysis and transplant facilities, John Kilner found that 'more than half of the directors would assess the different social value of various candidates' for dialysis or transplant, and 'less than a third would institute a more egalitarian random selection.'[25] Thielicke's understanding of alien dignity would suggest that such attempts to measure the social worth of candidates for dialysis violates the incommensurable dignity of each.

In 'The Doctor as Judge of Who Shall Live and Who Shall Die,' Thielicke tackled directly the problem of insufficient resources to help those who might live with medical intervention. He recognized explicitly that at times, difficult choices must be made and some must be chosen to live while others die. Under these circumstances, humans will make the best choices they can. Considerations of social worth may in fact enter those choices. But there can never be, for Thielicke, an easy conscience about this choice. 'One must simply run the risk of making the decision – and be prepared in doing so to err, and thereby to incur guilt.'[26] When we must choose some to live at the price of death for others, we should experience that choice as wounding. These are the wounds that 'must not be allowed to heal.'[27] They touch on a deep 'metaphysical' guilt that is built into the very structure of human existence[28] and that, ironically, makes us sound and healthy. Not to experience such guilt would be a sign that we forget the alien dignity and hence equality of all; to experience it is a sign that we recognize the alien dignity and equal worth of each. To do so is to be in partnership; thus, experiencing metaphysical guilt means that we remain fundamentally in relationship and hence healthy.

To say that alien dignity equalizes people is not to say that it makes everyone the same. The great diversity of human life is not denied by Thielicke. Indeed, he held to some traditional notions, for example of the differences between men and women and of the roles appropriate to them. But even in the midst of recognizing these differences, Thielicke held that women were right to demand respect because their alien dignity makes them 'equal before God.'[29] Women's different *roles* did not affect women's basic *worth* or *equality* with men, which is secured by their alien dignity. Similarly, people's different roles or status in life do not affect their basic value, which is secured by their alien dignity. Precisely because we are made in the image and likeness of God, we cannot be rejected as being 'no good.' Whatever our race, color, sex, class or social status, we are all equal in the eyes of God.

From the notion of alien dignity, then, might come an appreciation not only of the protectability of humans, but of their equality within diversity. As the Human Genome Project continues to locate and define the many genes that make up human beings, it will be increasingly important to find a grounding for understanding equality in the midst of diversity. Our history of genetic discrimination indicates all too graphically how easy it is for human communities to establish genetic norms and discriminate against those who do not fit the norm.[30] As the Human Genome Project progresses, there is the danger that we will make judgments of social worth based on individual genomes. Troy Duster charges that we are opening a 'backdoor' to eugenics, legitimizing social discrimination under the name of genetic science as we seek to correct 'defective' genes.[31] Some will be judged not to have 'normal' genes, others to have 'superior' genes. Such judgments are exactly what the concept of 'alien dignity' prevents. To accept diversity and yet affirm equality may be the most important challenge that lies before us in the realm of genetics. Thielicke's notion of alien dignity captures the underlying premise of equal worth amidst differing manifestations of human life.

### 3. Alien Dignity Requires Personal Response

For Thielicke, the alien dignity of the other required an 'I-Thou' relationship. Agape must be immediate, improvisational, non-routinized.[32] For Thielicke, there is no escaping personal responsibility by assuming that institutions or others will take over. The institutionalization of agape was therefore problematic: 'Does not the Samaritan's ministry of mercy become inconceivable, is it not altered in its very substance, the moment it is institutionalized? . . .'[33] Thielicke cautioned against the 'welfare state,' because 'no one is ever summoned personally' or need take personal responsibility in it.[34] In the welfare state, care would be 'rationalized,' and this very rationalization would kill the agape element in it.[35] Thus, the agape that responds to the alien dignity of the other, and in so responding realizes that dignity, must always be a personal response.

In the arena of health care, such a view may be an important corrective to the assumption that 'others' or 'the system' will provide. In the United States, for example, 95 percent of elderly people live not in nursing homes but in the community, dependent on care by family, friends, or hired workers. More than 80 percent are cared for by families, and in 75 percent of these cases, the caregiver is a woman. Most of these women are over the age of 50 and not always in the best of health themselves.[36]

On the one hand, Thielicke would probably applaud these women. They have chosen positively, lovingly, and willingly to care for elderly spouses or parents. They exhibit agape. They assume personal responsibility.

On the other hand, the fact that 75 percent of the care is being done by women should make us ask, Where are the men? In Thielicke's view, no one should escape from personal response to and responsibility for the needs of others. A society that allows some to escape responsibility while others carry the burden would not meet with Thielicke's approval. Since Thielicke did not believe that a ministry of mercy could be institutionalized without losing something of its basic character, the institutionalization of caring as 'women's work' or a 'female function' might also violate his understanding of the need for personal responsibility. Thus, alien dignity could provide correctives to some societal arrangements.

### 4. *Alien Dignity Requires* Structural Response

Thielicke's resistance to the institutionalization of care might be particularly problematic today for liberation theologians who stress the structural nature of injustice. It might seem at first glance that Thielicke's understanding of alien dignity would militate against nationalized health care . . .

Yet before we draw this conclusion, some nuancing is in order. It is true that Thielicke argued against the welfare state. The rationalization or routinizing of care, he asserted, ran counter to what is characteristic of Christian love of the neighbor.[37] He was particularly troubled by the argument that the welfare recipient could 'claim' welfare as a right, and that claiming such a right would be seen to honor the dignity of the person in ways that offering charity or agape does not.[38] But one must understand why Thielicke was troubled in order to understand the structural implications of his reflections on the welfare state. In spite of his reservations, his understanding of the implications of alien dignity pushes in the direction of a structural response to social and personal ills.

Thielicke's resistance to 'rights' and preference for agape or charity was based on the understanding that love never degrades the other, but must treat the other as a true partner. 'Rights' or claims separate people and force them into antagonistic relationships. Not antagonism, but a partnership 'in the ultimate dimension' was, for Thielicke, the goal of all Christian action.[39] Precisely because of the alien dignity of the other, that other is meant to be seen as a person in the sight of God, never merely as an object. But if the other is a subject, contended Thielicke, then the other can never be left as the mere passive recipient of our actions. To do so is to degrade the other.

By the same token, poverty can never be accepted as the other person's fate.[40] The other must not simply be helped or sustained in poverty, but must 'be restored to economic independence.'[41] I have argued elsewhere that such restoration is implied by the Jubilee image of justice.[42] Such restoration requires structural undergirding. Rehabilitation was, for Thielicke, a proper undertaking of the state.[43]

In fact, for Thielicke the other must not simply be restored and helped to move out of poverty, but must be prevented from moving into poverty in the first place. 'What is more urgently needed is preventive action.'[44] Prevention, however, requires structural response: 'a social order in which the right to gainful employment is assured and in which possibilities are created for the attainment of economic independence by way of education, financial credits, and the like.'[45] Only such a structural, preventive response would constitute in Thielicke's view a genuine partnership or expression of agape.

Thus it is true that Thielicke argued for a limited role for the state and would not have condoned either the Marxist analysis or the more extensive welfare state supported in some liberation treatises today. At root, he understood agape to be a deeply personal response, and he shied away from any institutional response that would relieve personal responsibility. He feared the 'impersonal machine' that would take away direct person-to-person care.[46] Nonetheless, his understanding of alien dignity also required preventive and structured response, in order to support the dignity of the other and the true partnership between people and between people and the state. Most significantly, it required not simply 'charity' but moving people to a place of restored autonomy and self-support. Thielicke recognized the structural components of poverty and other human ills, and his understanding of alien dignity required attention to these components. To argue that the social order must guarantee 'a right to gainful employment' is to take a large step toward structural justice.

By extension from this reasoning, I believe that we could also see in Thielicke's work the structural demands for a system of universal health care. If, as President Clinton said . . . , health care is crucial to the security necessary in order for people to make free choices and take risks for the future, then health care would be one of the structural demands of agape. Universal access to basic health care would recognize the alien dignity of all.

### 5. *Alien Dignity is* Relational

It is clear by now that Thielicke's concept of alien dignity is relational through and through. To have dignity is to be in relation.

First, it is to be in relation to God, who gives the dignity by investing love in people. Thus, one cannot speak of alien dignity without speaking of God's relationship to humankind. The very concept depends on relationality. Indeed, it connotes relationality, since for Thielicke alien dignity is not an 'ontic' possession but precisely a statement of our relationship to God.

Second, to have alien dignity is to be in relation to people. It is others who realize our dignity by acting out agape, out of a perspective of who we are before God. The term thus implies not only our 'vertical' relation to God but also our 'horizontal' relation to others.

Alien dignity is therefore very *personal*, but it is not *private* or atomistic. Dignity derives *between* beings – between humans and God, between humans and other humans. Thielicke called alien dignity 'teleological, not onto-logical.'[47] By this he meant that it does not refer to human characteristics or status, but to the purposes for which we are created by God. The term implies connections between beings and a fundamental covenant of life with life. To speak of alien dignity is therefore always to point us to relationship, interdependence, and covenant.

In this relationality, love is central. It is God's love that establishes the alien dignity of humans. It is human love that recognizes and realizes it. Once we know that God, like every mother, loves precisely the vulnerable and weak ones, then we know how irrevocable is the dignity of the poor and outcast. 'If I am no good, how can there be any God? Am I not made in the image and likeness of God?' Our fate is sealed not by our actions or by the judgments of others about us, but by the love of God for us. Alien dignity is a Christological concept for Thielicke.

This notion of relationality also has important implications for contem-porary bioethics. Criticisms of the current stress on 'autonomy' are now legion.[48] Increasingly, bioethicists are searching for an approach to ethics that neither isolates the individual nor manufactures a false autonomy, but places the individual in a social context, recognizing the role of family, of fiduciary relationships, of diminished autonomy. Feminists have been particularly keen on stressing caring and relationship as central to the tasks of ethics.

Thielicke's notion of alien dignity fits well with these concerns. Cardinal Jackson's dignity was not dependent on her mental capacity, but rather on her relationships. Significantly, as Schiedermayer struggled with what gave

Jackson her dignity, he pointed both to past relationships and to present ones, both to relationships of harm and to relationships of love. Cardinal Jackson's unassailable dignity came for him in part because of the love that her daughter still held for her. But it also came because a history of discrimination and mistreatment required a form of reparations – of refusing to abandon now one who had been abandoned in the past. In his own way, Schiedermayer attempts to establish a covenant that would assure Cardinal Jackson and her family that her dignity remained evident and appreciated. Cardinal Jackson does not have to have autonomy in order to be in relationship, to be the recipient of duties such as reparations on the part of others, to be loved and recognized. Her dignity – what Thielicke would call her alien dignity – is relational and implies covenant.

In response to Isasi-Diaz, Schiedermayer might say that the fact that she has experienced racist rejection in the past is precisely what gives her an inviolable dignity, just as it has contributed to that dignity for Cardinal Jackson. A relationship need not be one of love in order to remind us of the inviolable dignity of the other. Alien dignity requires a relational understanding of human life.


## Conclusions

[When Helmut Thielicke wrote 'The Doctor as Judge of Who Shall Live and Who Shall Die'], health care ethics was in its infancy. The Human Genome Project, Kevorkian's 'suicide machine' – these were unknowns. Abortion was not legal in the United States, in vitro fertilization clinics were not dotting the landscape as they do now. Much has changed in the intervening years.

Yet much has also remained the same. The genome project, assisted suicide, legalized abortion, in vitro fertilization – these modern developments raise ancient questions: should there be limits to human intervention in nature; when if at all is it permissible to take human life; should human bodies be bought and sold? At the root of these questions lies the ever present dilemma of the valuing of human life. What does it mean to be human, and what gives human life its worth?

It is to these foundational questions that Thielicke addressed his understanding of alien dignity. 'If I am no good, how can there be any God? Am I not made in the image and likeness of God?' queries Isasi-Diaz. For Thielicke, being made in the image and likeness of God meant that each person gained an alien dignity that stamped a fundamental worth on that person – a worth so central and ineradicable that nothing done by oneself or others could ever remove it. If there is a God, and God is good, then so are we, for we are made in the image of God.

To be sure, Thielicke's precise formulation of alien dignity raises some problems. Although he speaks of partnership 'in the ultimate dimension,' it is not clear whether his understanding of alien dignity implies a true partnership between humans and God. His God seems distant and wholly 'other,' his human beings perhaps a bit too empty. Human dignity seems removed, perhaps a bit too alien.

Yet in spite of these problems, there is an enduring legacy here to which we would do well to attend. The notion of alien dignity provides considerable protection to human beings. It keeps us from being used as objects of others' desires or schemes and from being swept up in the instrumentalization of human life. This may be important for our consideration as we move toward increasing technological imperatives. Alien dignity also has a powerful equalizing vector, which may be important as we struggle to understand how to do ethics in the midst of diversity. Alien dignity requires both the immediacy of love and personal responsibility on the one hand, and on the other hand structures that undergird true partnership. It neither lets us off the hook nor reduces ethical action to mere sentimentality.[49] Finally, alien dignity requires a relational view of human beings. Such a focus on relationality is consonant with many feminist approaches to bioethics, and provides an important corrective to the contemporary stress in bioethics on autonomy.

## Notes

1. Ada Maria Isasi-Diaz, 'Las Palmas Reales de Ada,' in Katie G. Cannon et al. (The Mudflower Collective), *God's Fierce Whimsy* (New York: Pilgrim Press, 1985), 106.
2. Helmut Thielicke, 'The Doctor as Judge of Who Shall Live and Who Shall Die,' in Kenneth Vaux, ed., *Who Shall Live? Medicine, Technology, Ethics* (Philadelphia: Fortress Press, 1970).
3. Thielicke, 'Doctor as Judge,' 170.
4. Helmut Thielicke, *Theological Ethics, Volume 1: Foundations*, ed. William H. Lazareth (Philadelphia: Fortress Press, 1966), 151.
5. Thielicke, *Theological Ethics*, vol. 1, 165.
6. Thielicke, *Theological Ethics*, vol. 1, 170.
7. Thielicke, *Theological Ethics*, vol. 1, 171.
8. Thielicke, *Theological Ethics*, vol. 1, 159.
9. Thielicke, *Theological Ethics*, vol. 1, 177.
10. Helmut Thielicke, *The Ethics of Sex*, trans. John W. Doberstein (New York: Harper & Row, 1964), 32.
11. Thielicke, 'Doctor as Judge,' 172.
12. Thielicke, *Theological Ethics*, vol. 1, 180.
13. See, e.g., Wendy Farley, *Tragic Vision and Divine Compassion: A Contemporary Theodicy* (Louisville, KY.: Westminster/John Knox Press, 1990); Joanne Carlson Brown and Carole R. Bohn, eds., *Christianity, Patriarchy, and Abuse: A Feminist Critique* (New York: Pilgrim Press, 1989).
14. It also does not depend on faith, but only on the image of God. Thus, even the nonbeliever would have dignity.
15. Thielicke, 'Doctor as Judge,' 186.
16. David Schiedermayer, 'The Case: House Calls To Cardinal Jackson,' *Second Opinion* 17, no. 4 (April 1992): 35–40.

17. Scheidermayer, 'The Case,' 39.
18. Indeed, for Thielicke, her dignity would remain even if there was no fire in her eyes and no love proffered by her daughter.
19. Thielicke, *Ethics of Sex*, 33.
20. Thielicke, *Ethics of Sex*, 61.
21. Thielicke, *Ethics of Sex*, 63.
22. Thielicke, *Ethics of Sex*, 27.
23. See The National Commission for the Protection of Human Subjects, *Research Involving Those Institutionalized as Mentally Infirm*, DHEW #OS-78–0006, and *Research Involving Prisoners*, DHEW #OS-76–131.
24. Helmut Thielicke, *Theological Ethics, Volume 2: Politics*, ed. William H. Lazareth (Philadelphia: Fortress Press, 1969), 305.
25. John F. Kilner, 'Selecting Patients when Resources are Limited: A Study of U.S. Medical Directors of Kidney Dialysis and Transplantation Facilities,' *American Journal of Public Health* 78, no. 2 (1988): 146.
26. Thielicke, 'Doctor as Judge,' 166.
27. Thielicke, 'Doctor as Judge,' 173.
28. Thielicke, 'Doctor as Judge,' 164.
29. Thielicke, *Ethics of Sex*, 12.
30. Troy Duster, *Backdoor to Eugenics* (New York: Routledge, 1990). See also John Horgan, 'Eugenics Revisited,' *Scientific American* 268, no. 6 (June 1993): 122–31.
31. Duster, *Backdoor to Eugenics*, 122–31.
32. Thielicke, *Theological Ethics*, vol. 2, 291.
33. Thielicke, *Theological Ethics*, vol. 2, 291.
34. Thielicke, *Theological Ethics*, vol. 2, 292.
35. Thielicke, *Theological Ethics*, vol. 2, 294.
36. See Tish Sommers and Laurie Shields, *Women Take Care: The Consequences of Caregiving in Today's Society* (Gainesville, Fla.: Triad Publishing, 1987), 21.
37. Thielicke, *Theological Ethics*, vol. 2, 300.
38. Thielicke, *Theological Ethics*, vol. 2, 304.
39. Thielicke, *Theological Ethics*, vol. 2, 305.
40. Thielicke, *Theological Ethics*, vol. 2, 306.
41. Thielicke, *Theological Ethics*, vol. 2, 306.
42. See Karen Lebacqz, *Justice in an Unjust World* (Minneapolis: Augsburg Publishing House, 1987), ch. 7.
43. Thielicke, *Theological Ethics*, vol. 2, 307.
44. Thielicke, *Theological Ethics*, vol. 2, 306.
45. Thielicke, *Theological Ethics*, vol. 2, 306.
46. Thielicke, *Theological Ethics*, vol. 2, 313.
47. Thielicke, *Theological Ethics*, vol. 1, 154.
48. See, e.g., Marshall B. Kapp, 'Medical Empowerment of the Elderly,' *Hastings Center Report* (July–August 1989): 5–7, George J. Agich, 'Reassessing Autonomy in Long Term Care,' *Hastings Center Report* (November–December 1990): 12–17.
49. Some feminist texts that take 'caring' or love as central to ethics do run the risk of dealing only with immediate relationships and failing to provide structural supports. See, for example, Nel Noddings, *Caring: A Feminist Approach to Ethics and Moral Education* (Berkeley: University of California Press, 1984).

# CASE STUDY:
# Baby Doe and Others

'Baby Doe' was born in Indiana, USA, with Down's syndrome and a digestive tract that was not properly formed, so that he could not feed by mouth. This digestive complication could have been corrected by surgery, but his parents refused consent. Afterwards they explained that they had decided surgery would not be in his or his family's best interests. Their decision was upheld by their county court and state Supreme Court, and Baby Doe died before the case could go to the US Supreme Court.

Subsequently the US Congress passed legislation defining the 'withholding of medically indicated treatment' from children as child abuse. However, it allowed that life-sustaining treatment was optional if the infant was irreversibly comatose, if treatment would not correct a life-threatening condition or if it would be futile and inhumane.

British cases have established that there is no duty to provide active treatment which would be futile or which would merely prolong a patient's terrible suffering, though in a similar case to Baby Doe's, the court ruled that surgery should be performed because the baby's life would not be 'demonstrably awful'.

## Questions
- What role if any should judgments about a patient's quality of life play in decisions about withdrawing or withholding life-sustaining treatment?
- How should quality of life be assessed, and by whom?
- Is it possible to decide whether treatment is 'medically indicated' without reference to the patient's quality of life?

### Sources
Tom L. Beauchamp and James F. Childress, *Principles of Biomedical Ethics*, 138–139. 5th ed., Oxford and New York: Oxford University Press, 2001.

R. A. Hope, K. W. M. Fulford and Anne Yates, *The Oxford Practice Skills Course*, 38–39. Oxford: Oxford University Press, 1996.

Peter Singer, *Practical Ethics*, 203–205. 2nd ed., Cambridge: Cambridge University Press, 1993.

# 3

# PERSONS, BODIES
# AND WHY THEY MATTER

## Introduction

The first two readings in this chapter address in different ways a question that is very frequently asked in bioethical debates: Who, or what, is a person? When philosophers make a distinction between merely 'being alive' bio- logically and 'having a life' that matters morally (cf. chapter 2), they often use the term 'person' to refer to the kind of being who possesses a morally significant life (cf. Harris 1998, 44–46). We have obligations to persons that we do not have to other beings, and there are things which we do to non-persons which we ought never to do to persons.

On this view, most human beings are persons, but the two categories are not identical. There may be human individuals who are not persons (for example, foetuses or permanently comatose patients); there may also be non- human animals that are persons and therefore should be treated as such – a point which will be taken up in chapter 8.

But how do we know a person when we encounter one? In other words, how am I to tell whether this individual before me (perhaps a comatose patient, a foetus or a severely disabled newborn baby) is a person, who as such commands my high moral regard? The significance of this question for bioethics is obvious: if human embryos are persons, embryo experimentation is harder to justify than if they are not; if foetuses are persons, abortion is seriously called into question; if permanently comatose patients have ceased to be persons, euthanasia may be permissible or even desirable; and so on.

Much modern discussion operates on the basis that persons are a class of beings defined by certain properties, capacities or potentialities. Rationality and self-consciousness have been popular criteria in philosophical discussion (e.g. Singer 1993, 85–89), and a similar approach has been adopted by some theologians (e.g. Fletcher 1975).

However, in recent years this emphasis on persons as individual, rational beings has been heavily criticised, and *relationship* stressed as an inescapable aspect of personhood. One influence in this has been the argument of many feminists that the 'rationalist' account outlined above plays down essential human attributes such as caring, mutuality and interdependence (Parsons 1996, 133–147). Another has been the recovery of theological interest in the doctrine of the Trinity (e.g. Zizioulas 1985, Gunton 1997). It is often pointed out that the language of 'person' was taken over from ancient Greek and Latin sources in order to speak of the divine persons of the Trinity, and only later applied to *human* persons in anything like the modern sense (see Habgood 1998 for a helpful introduction to this discussion). Alistair McFadyen is one theologian who has developed a relational account of human persons drawing on some of these influences (McFadyen 1990).

In the first reading in this chapter, Maureen Junker-Kenny explores the implications of debates about personhood for one particular bioethical issue – the moral status of the human embryo. She outlines one example of a 'rationalist' view of personhood (from the philosopher John Harris) and one example of a 'relationalist' view (from the feminist theologian Marjorie Maguire); both these authors use their definitions to deny that embryos and foetuses are persons, thus legitimating embryo experimentation, abortion and other technical medical interventions. Junker-Kenny argues that any definition of personhood is 'caught in a hermeneutical circle'. That is to say, an author's choice of definition is influenced significantly by the conclusions he or she wishes to draw about the status of certain categories of individual (for example, embryos, foetuses or permanently comatose patients). She goes on to explore what it would mean to say that the embryo *is* a person, arguing that some of the apparent difficulties with that view may not in fact be conclusive arguments against it.

Ian McFarland, in the second reading, notes that the question 'who is a person?', in the sense in which it is asked in bioethical debates, is not found in the Bible or early Christian theology. However, he argues that an analogous question can be found in the New Testament, in Luke's Gospel. A lawyer, told by Jesus that one of the two greatest commandments is to love one's neighbour, asks, 'And who is my neighbour?' Jesus responds, not with a straight answer, but with the story of the Good Samaritan (Luke 10:25–37). McFarland concludes that, theologically speaking, the question 'Who is a person?', like the question 'Who is my neighbour?', is the wrong question to ask. Rather, 'the more important ethical question is . . . how I, as one who is treated as a person by Jesus Christ, relate to [others in their particularity] as the person I have been called to be' (p. 82).

A curious feature of the modern discussion of personhood is that it has very often focused on the mind or spirit, and neglected or even demeaned the body. In that respect, it is heir to strands of ancient Greek thought that took a high view of the mind and soul and were suspicious of the body, and to Christian attitudes influenced by such views. Thus there is a long history of body/spirit or body/mind dualism which has been heavily criticised by recent feminist thought, partly on the grounds that it has been used to subjugate those seen as more 'fleshly' and less 'rational' – for example, women. Lisa Sowle Cahill takes up this feminist critique, exploring both older and contemporary dualisms of body and mind/spirit. She argues that a proper appreciation of human life as *embodied* is vital for Christian ethics, particularly sexual and medical ethics. However, she holds that valuing the body is not at odds with the notion that the life of the body must be subjected to a proper *discipline*. A notion of disciplined bodily life can have important and positive consequences for medical ethics, encouraging compassion, solidarity and inclusiveness in the practice of health care.

## References and Further Reading

Joseph Fletcher, 'Four Indicators of Humanhood – The Enquiry Matures', *Hastings Center Report* 4, 4–7 (1975).

Colin E. Gunton, *The Promise of Trinitarian Theology.* 2nd ed., Edinburgh: T & T Clark, 1997.

John Habgood, *Being a Person: Where Faith and Science Meet.* London: Hodder & Stoughton, 1998.

John Harris, 'Experiments on Embryos', in *Clones, Genes and Immortality: Ethics and the Genetic Revolution*, 43–65. Oxford: Oxford University Press, 1998.

Alistair I. McFadyen, *The Call to Personhood: A Christian Theory of the Individual in Social Relationships.* Cambridge: Cambridge University Press, 1990.

Susan Frank Parsons, *Feminism and Christian Ethics.* Cambridge: Cambridge University Press, 1996.

Stanley Rudman, *Concepts of Person and Christian Ethics.* Cambridge: Cambridge University Press, 1997.

John D. Zizioulas, *Being as Communion: Studies in Personhood and the Church.* London: Darton, Longman & Todd, 1985.

# The Moral Status of the Embryo

MAUREEN JUNKER-KENNY

How can one suggest reflection on the moral status of something that is smaller than a speck of dust? For some, the question of moral status would already be answered by this observation, and dismissed as impossible. But it is the different answers to this question which divide the legislation on biomedical matters in different countries. And if there are opposite legal positions, there must be a deeper philosophical controversy about the nature of this entity, its potential, relevant thresholds in its development, and the claims it may pose to society and the law as well as to the woman whose body is its host. What is under debate is whether the embryo can already be called human life, and, more to the point, whether it should be called a person and therefore enjoy the protection which this status accords: the human rights to life and bodily integrity.[1]

I would like to treat this discussion by first analysing two different arguments against ascribing any moral status of its own to the embryo or foetus:
(a) the British philosopher John Harris's thesis of a personhood which is empirically verifiable;
(b) the American feminist theologian Marjorie Maguire's theory of personhood through covenant.

Do they give criteria for personhood? What significance do they attach to terms such as potential, relationality, and to different stages of development?

I shall contrast their theories with the opposing view, which interprets 'potential' as continuity and identity and thus ascribes personhood already to the zygote, i.e. the fertilized egg after the fusion of the nuclei of egg and sperm and before cell division. Here, I shall begin with the insight into the hermeneutical and practical character inherent in all definitions of human life and personhood. I shall then examine from this perspective the objections made against claiming personhood for this stage: the limits of the embryo's potential as shown in the need for implantation into a supporting ecosystem, the mother's womb, the fact that part of what develops from the zygote will be the placenta and not the foetus and the possibility of twinning as an argument against individuation . . .

From Maureen Junker-Kenny and Lisa Sowle Cahill (eds.), *The Ethics of Genetic Engineering: Concilium* 1998/2 pp. 43–53. London: SCM/Maryknoll, NY: Orbis.

## I. The Embryo – Not a Person in its Own Right

### (a) Personhood as an Empirically Verifiable Feature

One position in the present philosophical debate on personhood is that a person can only be someone to whom the empirical traits of persons apply. Only those humans count as persons who are actually and instantly able to give evidence of their capacity for reason and self-consciousness.[2]

In this view, to be a person in the *moral* sense and to be human in the *biological* sense are two independent factors which intersect only partially. 'Not all persons are human, and not all humans are persons.'[3] But is this a correct premise? If this is true, then human embryos, newborn babies and the mentally handicapped or patients in an irreversible coma are humans but not persons. Intelligent animals such as whales, dolphins and chimpanzees have a greater claim to the title of person than these humans.[4] This is indeed the consequence which the Australian philosopher Peter Singer draws. Another representative of this view is the British philosopher John Harris. In his article 'Embryos and hedgehogs: On the moral status of the embryo', he states: 'There are really only two ways in which this question can be approached: one is in terms of the actual moral status of the embryo at any one time, and the other is in terms of the potential of the embryo to acquire a moral status or personhood which it does not at present possess.'[5] Harris goes for the first approach and dismisses the second: 'I argue that the moral status of the embryo and indeed of any individual is determined by its possession of those features which make normal adult human individuals morally more important than sheep or goats or embryos' (79). He declines to name these criteria, but it would be safe to assume that rationality and some kind of self-reflection would belong to them. Without these morally relevant features, however, any being would have no more value than those 'unique, fully formed, sentient' creatures which, as he says, might constitute 'our Sunday roast' (69–70). This may be a needlessly offensive way to put it, but it is certainly clear. Harris might still be able to speak of persons as bearers of unalienable rights, although it is doubtful if there is a basis in Utilitarianism for thinking the term 'unalienable', since there is no concept of the human person as a limit to the desires of the majority, i.e. as someone who should not be instrumentalized. But however these rights are to be described, they do not belong to members of the human species by definition, but only to those actually able to demonstrate their use of reason. And clearly, embryos do not count among them.

### (b) Personhood Through Covenant

A different argument for the same position that embryos have no inherent rights of their own is put forward by the American feminist theologian

Margaret Reiley Maguire. Her theory of covenant is not based on any empirical definition which identifies, as Engelhardt and Harris do, the actual 'performance' of a being with the 'competence' the being has in principle (to use a distinction of Chomsky's). She adopts a 'relational' approach.[6] Her search for 'the precise formal element that constitutes personhood' (103) leads her to the following thesis: 'I would propose that the only person who can be the initiator of covenantal love for prenatal life, bringing that life into the reality of human community and thereby making it a person, is the woman in whose womb the pregnancy' (not the embryo!) 'exists. The personhood begins when the bearer of life, the mother, makes a covenant of life with the developing life within her to bring it to birth . . . The moment which begins personhood, then, is the moment when the mother accepts the pregnancy. At the moment when the mother bonds with the foetus, the foetus becomes a Thou to her rather than an It . . . It is the mother who makes the foetus a person. After that point life is sacred because it is sacred to her' (109–10). If the mother does not consent to the pregnancy, no personhood is established. She concludes: 'The discarding of some of those fertilized ova, and even experimentation on them, is not necessarily immoral if there are no persons floating in petri dishes' (117).

This position is a step beyond the actualistic one, where present command of reason is the defining factor for personhood – as long as it lasts. For Maguire, there is a recognition element to personhood. Her argumentation shows that we can welcome someone who is less than rational into our lives and accord it the status of a 'Thou', instead of the 'It' of the Sunday roast.

However, her theory is based on two explicit presuppositions which are far from evident:

1. 'I believe that no one has a right to life, deserving of full protection of the law, when that life is totally dependent on the body of another human being for its life support' (102). This is a far-reaching claim. Not only when the life of the mother is threatened does a conflict arise between the rights to life of both the embryo and the mother; now the fact of dependence alone is enough to put the embryo's right to life into question. What I find missing here is the recognition that except in cases of rape, pregnancies are the results of the actions of people, and we are responsible for the consequences of our actions. Although degrees of responsibility vary with regard to circumstances, it is not convincing to say that the embryo imposes itself on the life of the mother. If it wasn't for the prior actions of others, the embryo would not be able to make such a claim.

2. The second presupposition already showed up in the line, 'the only person who can be the initiator of covenantal love for prenatal life, *bringing that life into the reality of human community and thereby making it a person*, is the woman'. She states explicitly: 'Sociality is the touchstone of personhood . . . that is why the biological side of personhood is not sufficient

of itself to constitute the formal element of the beginning of personhood' (114). So sociality makes a person? This view plays down the other pole that is decisive: the element of spontaneity, reflexivity, prior familiarity with myself which cannot be explained from intersubjectivity. If this element is not recognized, we would not be able to distinguish between autonomy and heteronomy, authentic selfhood and unquestioning obedience to the rules of convention. But it should be clear that no one becomes a person by virtue of the human community alone.

In summary, the language of covenant barely disguises the feudal relationship proposed here: it is a one-sided power to elect, exercised among humans.

Even with regard to God, the history of theology has witnessed fierce debates on whether election can be squared with the universality of God's love towards humanity. Maguire's interpretation turns pregnancy into a one-sided power-relationship which is asserted and celebrated in a way that denies the 'mutuality' otherwise prominent in feminist ethics. Here this power relationship is asserted and celebrated. Against the absolute power of the electing mother, the embryo has no claim. This is rather like the late mediaeval concept of God's absolute power that led philosophers like Hans Blumenberg to claim that the human subject had to insist on his freedom in order to escape from the arbitrariness of God's unpredictable will.[7]

## II. The Zygote as Person

Before we go on to consider more definitions of potential and personhood from the opposite side, it is time to reflect on the status and implications of this exercise itself.

### (a) The Hermeneutical Circle Inherent in Definitions of Human Personhood

It should have become clear by now that definitions of personhood are not lofty philosophical speculations but have an immediate practical significance. The question of personhood is a philosophical one in which we state our self-understanding as humans. Whom do we accept as a member of our species who is entitled to protection and care?

Any definition of the beginning (and end) of human personhood is caught in a hermeneutical circle. We define its starting point because we want to act in a certain way, and we act according to how we have defined it.[8] If we consider the moment of implantation in the uterus, or the presence of brain activity, or the ability to communicate, as the starting-point for ascribing personhood, we are free to use the embryo prior to this stage in any way we consider useful.

Each definition has a practical intent. Once we ascribe human life and personhood to an entity, we want to protect it. If one wants to give maximum protection, one has to use a minimal definition, such as the new genetic unity created by egg and sperm. A maximal definition of human life, such as the ability to communicate, or to act independently, offers minimal protection to the stages prior to these competencies and after they have been lost. A minimal definition of the beginning of human life that offers maximal protection would be: once there is an auto-reproductive unit in which the nuclei of the sperm and the egg have fused, this new entity should count as having human dignity and human rights to life and the inviolability of its (his or her) body. This unit should be referred to as the 'embryo', not as 'pre-embryo', as it is sometimes done. It should be clear that this usage is already based on the decision that no moral status can be ascribed to the product of conception in the first fourteen days of its existence, and this decision is clothed in the language of science. To call the zygote 'pre-embryo' makes one of many stages in its development, namely implantation, definitive for attributing basic rights to it.[9] In contrast, it makes sense to follow the ethical principle stated by Dietmar Mieth: human life has to be respected and fostered as a fundamental and integral value. 'Integral' means that no lines can be drawn between a stage of no value, where it is at our disposal, and a different stage where it acquires full value.[10]

It is therefore a *practical* decision at what developmental stage we attribute human personhood to the embryo, foetus, or newborn, and it is in the interest of the earliest possible protection of 'the weakest link in the chain of the human species'[11] if one states that this new genetic unity is a person. Let us hear the case of those for whom the unique genetic individuality of the zygote merits its designation as the beginning of 'human personhood' because of the identity and continuity of its development.

### (b) 'Potential' as Identity and Continuity
Schockenhoff insists that the only relevant line that can be drawn is the 'radically new beginning' which happens when the fertilized egg becomes a zygote (307). To those who argue for taking the beginnings of brain formation as the decisive threshold for personhood, he answers: this would be drawing an artificial line in to a continuous process of development. 'The possibility for the later emergence of mind, consciousness and freedom is there in principle from conception onwards; it becomes more probable after implantation and the development of the primitive streak; but the question is whether this probability factor justifies drawing a demarcation to which such a high anthropological relevance and the corresponding normative consequences are attached' (cf. 309–10 n. 41). In Schockenhoff's view, there is one process of development; in principle, all the emergent features are founded on the basic autoreproductive unit of the zygote, and it would be arbitrary to

say any particular stage introduces such a qualitative difference that only from then onwards would there be a sufficient basis for personhood. It is one human being that has all the dispositions for later realizations within itself: it is a potential marked by identity on a genetic basis, and by continuity both temporally and substantially. Therefore formulations such as Harris's, that the embryo is 'potentially a human being; it will eventually become a human being' (312 n. 46) are misleading. Human embryos do not develop *into* humans, but *as* humans. And here, 'the point of the potentiality argument is that what is crucial for being granted a right to life is the capability to become a moral subject, not the feature realized at any actual moment. This potential to become a moral subject does not begin at birth or with coming of age, it unfolds on the basis of the whole natural process of development and is part of a continuous context of human life from the earliest embryonic age onwards. We are asked to respect the future chances for life of an individual at every point of her development in time, even if she does not yet have a reflective concept of the continuity of herself' (313f.).

However, to attribute human personhood to the zygote does not imply that in ethical dilemmas it is always the embryo who 'wins'. It allows one to set up the dilemma and ask whether the right of the embryo to survive is equal, superior or subordinated to the mother's rights to life and self-determination.

## III. Objections
### (a) The Natural Limits of the Embryo's Potential
But what if the 'capability to become a moral subject' presupposes more than the embryo has within itself, namely implantation into the mother's womb? [Baroness] Warnock points to this lack of capacity: 'To say that eggs and sperm cannot by themselves become human, but only if bound together, does not seem to me to differentiate them from the early embryo which by itself will not become human either, but will die unless it is implanted.'[12] True, the only thing an embryo will do by itself is to divide and differentiate its unique genetic combination. If it does not implant *in vivo* or if it is withheld from implantation *in vitro*, it will not develop further.

The counter-argument to this point which identifies 'potential' or 'capacity' with the ability to create one's own conditions for survival, is to highlight that all life needs a supporting eco-system and is inter-dependent: 'Fish need water, humans need air, embryos need wombs' (Janet Soskice). This analogy does not imply that women only count as context for embryos, nor indeed that all embryos need are wombs; it illustrates that the fact that we need supporting conditions to survive and develop does not speak against our personhood.

## (b) Is the Placenta a Person?

Here, the argument is not that there is too little to qualify for personhood, but too much: at this stage, even before the new autoreproductive unit starts reproducing itself through cell division, it is too early to differentiate between what will become the foetus and what will be the placenta.

The trouble with this (and the following) objection is its biological essentialism. To give personhood status to the zygote before the differentiation into the body of the embryo and the placenta occurs does not personalize the placenta. It extends the protection zone of human dignity to the earliest stage when the nuclei of the gametes have fused. The fact that the cells developing from this new genetic unit are totipotent cannot reduce the dignity of the new genetic unit.

## (c) Twinning

It can't be *a* person because it might be *two* persons. Individuation must have occurred for it to be a personal human life, and that only happens by day fourteen (implantation). So this is the earliest time we could speak of personhood.

Again, my point is that if one is aware of the hermeneutical and practical character of one's definition of personhood, one cannot confound the biological and metaphysical levels in such a way as to say that the possibility of twinning speaks against the personhood of the embryo. If one's practical intention is to protect the earliest possible stage of human life against instrumentalization, it does not lessen but rather doubles the dignity of the zygote if it is not one future child, but two who enjoy this protection. We already approach these data from an ethical viewpoint which goes into our definition of what we have before us 'empirically': human tissue, or a bearer of human rights . . .

[Junker-Kenny goes on to discuss the implications of arguments about the status of the embryo for three specific issues, embryo freezing, experimentation and cloning. She concludes:]

It is both exciting and awesome to be at this threshold where new possibilities for curing diseases are beckoning, but where the human person is also being redefined. I hope to have shown why the way in which we define and treat the embryo – as human tissue and raw material for our rational purposes, or at least as human life with a moral claim – says something about how we see ourselves and who we want to be in the future.

## Notes

1. The decisive question is, when does human *personhood* begin? Human *life* clearly begins at fertilization, so it is misleading to say that 'the embryo *becomes* human'.

Genetically, the zygote *is* distinctively human already. But on what level is the decision on human personhood made, and on which criteria is it based?

2. Cf. the discussion in Schockenhoff, *Ethik des Lebens*, Mainz 1993, 45–9, 87–103.

3. Tristram Engelhardt, *The Foundations of Bioethics*, New York and Oxford 1986, 107. See also id., 'Entscheidungsprobleme konkurrierender Interessen von Mutter und Fötus', in V. Braun et al. (ed.), *Ethische und rechtliche Fragen der Gentechnologie und der Reproduktionsmedizin*, Munich 1987, 150–9.

4. Cf. Schockenhoff, *Ethik des Lebens* (n. 2), 45–9.

5. In A. Dyson and J. Harris (eds), *Experiments on Embryos*, London 1990, 65–81. Further page references in text.

6. 'The biological approach (to personhood) never clearly shows why the newly conceived or developing prenatal life should be considered the moral and legal peer of a newborn baby rather than ontologically closer to a separate sperm and egg' ('Personhood, Covenant and Abortion', in P. Jung and T. Shannon [eds], *Abortion and Catholicism*, New York 1988, 100–20: 106). Further page references in the text. She refers to Charles Curran's distinction between 'individual-biological', 'relational', 'multiple' and 'conferred rights' criteria ('Abortion: Ethical Aspects', in *Transition and Tradition in Moral Theology*, Notre Dame 1979, 207–29). Other members of the 'relational' school are the French moral theologians he mentions (228 n. 10) (cf. *Lumière et vie* 21, no. 109, 1972).

7. Hans Blumenberg, *The Legitimacy of the Modern Age* (second revised ed. Cambridge, Mass. 1983).

8. Here I am following the argumentation of Dietmar Mieth, *Geburtenregelung. Ein Konflikt in der katholischen Kirche*, Mainz 1990, 78–82, 95–6. A similar evaluation can be found in Paul Ricoeur's discussion of 'respect for persons at the "beginning of life"'. In Kant's 'bipolar opposition of persons and things, the distinction between mode of beings remained inseparable from practice, that is, from the manner of treating persons and things . . . To be sure, the identification of thresholds and degrees marking the appearance of properties of being is dependent on science alone. But the ontological tenor assigned to the predicate "potential" in the expression "potential human person" is perhaps not separable from the manner of "treating" beings corresponding to these various stages. Manner of being and manner of treating would seem to be mutually determined in the formation of prudential judgments occasioned by each advance in the power that technology confers today on humankind over life in its beginnings' (*Oneself as Another*, Chicago 1992, 270–2).

9. This insight into the inevitable hermeneutical circle between the practical interest of the person defining and the resulting definition is missing in T. Shannon's and A. Wolters' critique of the philosophical essentialism of Vatican statements on this question. Their 'Reflections on the Moral Status of the Pre-Embryo', in T. Shannon (ed.), *Bioethics*, 4th ed., Mahwah, NJ 1994, 36–60, however, seem to replace one essentialism with a different, biological one. The middle route is to take biological observations of stages and thresholds seriously enough to avoid the charge of nominalism, yet see the practical character of any definition of the beginning of human personhood. Ricoeur speaks of the 'complex play between science and wisdom' (272) and rightly analyses any definition as a prudential judgment which has to be all the more cautious in the context of scientific manipulation of embryos (*Oneself*, 272–3).

10. Cf. Mieth, *Geburtenregelung* (n. 8), 95–6.

11. Cf. Dominique Folscheid, 'The Status of the Embryo from a Christian Perspective', in *Studies in Christian Ethics* 9, 1996, 1–21: 21.

12. Quoted in John Harris, 'Embryos and Hedgehogs', 72.

# Who is My Neighbor?
# The Good Samaritan as a Source for
# Theological Anthropology

IAN A. McFARLAND

## I. The Problem of the Person in Biblical Perspective

Given the degree to which the question of who is to be counted as a person has agitated theologians over the past generation, it is rather disquieting to be reminded of the dearth of biblical reflection on what a person is. To be sure, a search through the concordance of some of the major English translations of Scripture may turn up a hundred or more entries for 'person',[1] but one searches in vain for the kind of technical usage that underlies contemporary debates over the status of the severely retarded, the comatose, unborn, or even certain non-human species . . .

The reasons for this lack of reference to the problem of personhood in Scripture are not hard to identify. It was only later that the Greek word *prosopon* (along with its Latin equivalent, *persona*, from which the English word is derived) came to be used in a technical sense to describe a particular kind of being. The watershed event in this development was the formulation of the doctrine of the Trinity, in which those whom the Bible names as Father, Son, and Holy Spirit were distinguished as three persons (*hypostaseis* or *prosopa*) within the one divine essence (*ousia*).[2] Interestingly, within this trinit-arian framework the term 'person' does not name some property common to the Father, Son and Spirit, but rather identifies their difference from each other.[3]

A crucial juncture in the transition from this specifically theological under-standing of 'person' to modernity's characteristically anthropological use of the term was Boethius' definition of a person as 'the individual substance of a rational nature'.[4] Admittedly, Boethius ventured this definition in an effort to explain the theological use of 'person' to a general audience, but the effect was to equate personhood with the possession of a particular property or quality, without any necessary reference to a trinitarian framework. Boe-thius' identification of this crucial property with reason proved enormously influential;[5] but even where some other criterion (relationality, for example) has been proposed, the effect of defining persons as a category of beings has

From *Modern Theology* vol. 17:1, pp. 57–66 (January 2001).

been to cut the term loose from its theological moorings: that which in trinitarian thought identified the Father, Son, and Spirit in their irreducible distinction from one another came to refer anthropologically to some quality or set of qualities that all 'persons' were alleged to hold in common.

This latter way of viewing what it means to be a person entails a particular set of presuppositions and practices. First, it presupposes that an individual's identity as a person can be established by viewing that individual in isolation.[6] If personhood is a matter of possessing certain qualities, then an individual's identity as a person is determined by testing for the presence of those qualities. Second, to the extent that identity as a person is viewed as something worthwhile – specifically, as something which endows an individual with certain rights withheld from non-persons – it becomes important to identify who is included in the category of persons.

Neither of these presuppositions has any place within a trinitarian context. That the Father, Son, and Spirit are persons is not a fact that can be determined by considering them in isolation: since their personhood refers precisely to that which . . . is *not* common to all three, no one of the persons can be identified *as* a person without reference to the other two. This does not mean that divine personhood is in its essence relational, as though the Father, Son, and Spirit's status as persons were the consequence of some capacity, more or less effectively realized, to live in relationship with one another. It is true that the trinitarian persons are *defined* relationally – the Father as the Father of the Son, the Son as the Son of the Father, etc. – but this definition is less reflective of some essence of divine personhood than of our inability to specify any such essence. Because the personal distinctions refer to that which cannot be predicated jointly of the Father, Son, and Spirit, the divine persons' relations to one another do not tell us *what* the Father, Son, and Spirit are, but only provide us a rule for identifying *who* they are. In other words, 'person' refers quite specifically to the Father, Son, and Holy Spirit, and is *not* a genus under which individual beings may be subsumed.

## II. 'Who is My Neighbor?'

Although one searches Scripture in vain for formal discussion of what constitutes personhood, there is nevertheless a clear biblical analogue to the contemporary question 'What is a person?' It comes in Luke 10, in the context of a discussion on the subject of what it is necessary to do in order to inherit eternal life. Under prodding from Jesus, the lawyer who had initially posed the question acknowledges that the requirements are clearly set out in the law as love of God and neighbor (v. 27). The story might well end there (as it does in the Matthean and Markan parallels), but in Luke's version the lawyer asks Jesus a further question: 'And who is my neighbor?' (v. 29).

The fact that this question is put into the mouth of a lawyer highlights its parallelism with modern discussions of personhood which also tend to surface in a legal context. Because persons are understood to have a right to a certain level or quality of treatment – one that would rule out, for example, their being made the objects of medical experimentation without their prior consent – it is necessary to have some criteria for determining who counts as a person. In brief, the fact that I am not allowed to treat persons with the same kind of indifference I might a rock or a tree both confronts me with certain obligations and places definite restrictions on my own freedom of action.

When the matter is put in this way, concern over one's own ethical liability has seemingly eclipsed any genuine interest in the well-being of others. It is therefore not surprising that the lawyer in Luke 10 – who, we are told, asks his question about the identity of his neighbor out of a wish to 'vindicate' or 'justify' (*dikaiosai*) himself – tends to be viewed in a rather unfavorable light. Yet one need not view his question as prompted purely by the selfish desire to avoid censure or minimize responsibility. If nothing less than eternal life hangs on my love of neighbor, then it is only natural that I should want to determine just who my neighbor is. From this perspective, the lawyer's question to Jesus is a sign of no greater presumption or recalcitrance than the ethically serious efforts of participants in contemporary debates over abortion and euthanasia to find a coherent definition of the person.

Whatever the lawyer's motives in asking his question, Jesus responds by telling the parable of the good Samaritan.[7] The story's plot is straightforward enough: a man (presumably Jewish, insofar as his journey begins in Jerusalem) is assaulted on his way to Jericho and left for dead by the roadside. A priest and a Levite, doubtless nervous over the possibility of becoming ritually unclean through contact with a corpse, pass him by. It is a despised Samaritan, evidently unconcerned about any possible effects on his ritual purity,[8] who comes to the victim's aid, tending his wounds, bringing him to a place of shelter, and instructing the innkeeper to spare no expense in his treatment.

Does this story answer the lawyer's question? Considered by itself, the story of the man who fell among thieves might lead the reader (who shares the lawyer's perspective as the one to whom the tale is told) to suppose that the neighbor is the man in need. On this reading, the details of the story are ultimately superfluous, and the parable is only a more or less engaging way of illustrating a fairly straightforward answer to the lawyer's question: your neighbor is anyone who needs your care.

Yet this is not how Jesus himself makes use of the parable. He ends the tale not with a neatly drawn conclusion (e.g., 'Count as your neighbor anyone in need'), but with a question of his own: 'Which of these three seems to you to have been a neighbor to the one who fell among thieves?' (v. 36). If the parable appears at first glance to accept the terms of the lawyer's question (i.e., the problem of identifying who counts as a neighbor), Jesus' counter-question redirects attention from the status of others to that of the lawyer himself. As it turns out, 'neighbor' is not a category that the lawyer is authorized to apply to others; instead, it takes the form of a challenge and recoils back upon him as a moral agent capable either of being or failing to be a neighbor to someone else.[9] In this way, Jesus asks lawyer and reader alike to consider the possibility that the question of their own status as neighbors might be anthropologically prior to any reflection on the status of other people.

Jesus does not so much answer the lawyer's question as turn it around. His counter-question forces the lawyer to apply the term 'neighbor' not to the victim of the assault, but to 'the one who showed . . . compassion to him' (Luke 10:37). This is not to suggest that the effect of Jesus' question is merely to replace one possible definition of the neighbor ('someone in need') with another ('one who meets others' needs'). Indeed, it would be hard to imagine a more serious misinterpretation of the parable than the conclusion that the neighbor is the class of those who show mercy to the afflicted, as though one could be justified in refusing to regard anyone who fails to show mercy as a neighbor.

No, a crucial feature of the parable is precisely the fact that Jesus refrains from offering *any* definition of the neighbor.[10] It is true that the one who showed compassion was a neighbor to the man who fell among thieves, but Jesus' final words to the lawyer are in the imperative rather than the indicative mood: 'You go and do likewise'. The lawyer is not told who his neighbor is.[11] He is simply commanded to imitate the Samaritan's compassion without being given any specific criteria regarding those to whom compassion is owed.[12]

## III. What Is a Person?

If the lawyer's question as to the identity of his neighbor is in some respects functionally similar to more modern discussions of what makes someone a person, Jesus' response seems equally unhelpful in both contexts. Yet in leaving us without a readily applicable criteriology of personhood, the parable of the good Samaritan arguably honors the trinitarian roots of 'person' more effectively than any putative definition of personhood might. As noted above, the term 'person' first acquired a technical sense as a means of referring to the Father, Son, and Spirit. Insofar as the term does not identify a common property that these three share, the only possible 'definition' of a person that might be derived from the doctrine of the Trinity is 'one who participates in the relationships between Father, Son, and Holy Spirit' – which is really to do no more than to identify the Father, Son, and Spirit as what we mean by persons.

At first glance, it might appear that locating the term 'person' in this kind of strictly trinitarian framework simply renders it anthropologically empty. This conclusion, however, is belied by the equally trinitarian confession that one of the three divine persons, the Son, 'became incarnate of the virgin Mary, and was made a human being' named Jesus. It follows that at least *this* human being is a person, since he does 'participate in the relationships between the Father, Son, and Holy Spirit'.[13] Moreover, because the reason for the Son's taking on the human condition was that he might bring the rest of the human family into communion with the triune God, it turns out that the set of human persons is not limited to Jesus alone. On the contrary, as the head of the body into which the rest of us are called (Eph. 1:22–3; 4:15–16; Col. 1:18–2:19), Jesus is the 'first-born of many siblings' (Rom. 8:29); and as members of his body, we share in his status as 'Son' and are thereby empowered to join him in calling God 'Father' (Rom. 8:15; Gal. 4:5–6; cf. Matt. 6:9; Luke 11:2; Eph. 2:18).

Insofar as all human beings are summoned in and through Christ to participate in the relationships between the three divine persons, they, too, are persons. To be sure, . . . they are persons only 'in' Christ; they have no claim to be persons on their own account, by virtue of some particular capacity or quality they possess. They are persons for the sole reason that they are treated *as* persons by God by being called in Christ to participate in the relationships between Father, Son, and Spirit.

Correlating the fact of personhood with membership in the body of Christ might appear to suggest that only baptized Christians should be considered persons. Such a conclusion, however, accords ill with Paul's claim that even those who have received Christ's Spirit in baptism still await their adoption as children of God (Rom. 8:23; cf. v. 19). Paul's point here is certainly not to downplay the significance of church membership, but it does serve as a reminder that no human being's final status with respect to the Trinity is known prior to the Last Day. To the extent that the church acknowledges damnation – eternal exclusion from God's presence – as a conceivable destiny for human beings, it remains possible that not all human beings will turn out to be persons; but the identity of such non-persons is not given to us in the here and now.[14]

Here, too, the rule applies that human personhood cannot be correlated with the possession of a given capacity or property, including the 'property' of having been baptized.[15] Once again, what counts is how we are treated by the divine persons, and here there are simply no prior limits placed on the range of those called through the Son to live as persons with God. On the contrary, Jesus explicitly commands the gospel to be preached to every nation (Matt. 28:19), and, indeed, to every creature (Mark 16:15; Col. 1:23). From this perspective, the measure of personhood is the fact that we are treated as persons by the Son, who invites us to participate in the communion he shares with the Father and the Spirit.[16]

## IV. The Good Samaritan Revisited

Admittedly, the foregoing interpretation of personhood does not seem especially useful for resolving those contemporary ethical dilemmas in which the question of personhood figures prominently. To all appearances, it amounts to a conceptually vacuous latitudinarianism, in which I am obliged to consider every being I encounter as a person until the Last Judgment shows otherwise. In the face of this charge, however, the story of the good Samaritan can serve as steadying theological ballast. As argued above, an important feature of that parable is Jesus' refusal to satisfy the lawyer's desire for a readily applicable anthropology. The neighbor is not defined as the one in need, nor as the one who shows compassion to the needy. Instead, Jesus effectively dismisses the lawyer's question and asks the reader to consider that the crucial anthropological issue is not the status of the other whom I face, but rather who I am.

In working out the implications of this latter point, it is worth recalling that throughout most of the church's history, the parable of the good Samaritan has been interpreted christologically. According to this reading, the man who falls among thieves represents humankind, seemingly dead from its sins; the Samaritan is Jesus, who brings us back to life as the persons we were created to be. If the foregoing analysis of the parable is at all accurate, this traditional interpretation may not be as farfetched as the majority of twentieth-century interpreters suppose.[17] As already noted, the lawyer's question assumes that the status of the other is the crucial theological problem in theological anthropology: love is something he is obliged to show the other – if the other qualifies as a neighbor. But Jesus' counter-question turns things around: it is not the status of the other, but that of the lawyer (and by implication, of the reader) that is at issue.[18]

In this way, the logic of the parable raises the possibility that we first need to be shown compassion by a neighbor as a condition of becoming neighbors ourselves (cf. Eph. 4:32). If a 'neighbor' is the functional equivalent of a 'person', it follows that our status as persons can no more be taken for granted than the recovery of the man set upon by thieves. Rather, our life [as] persons requires a prior act of compassion in which another person treats us as persons. If we adhere to a trinitarian framework in our use of the term 'person', then only the divine persons are capable of showing us this kind of compassion. And since only one of those persons has become flesh and dwelt among us, no human being but Jesus can assume the role of the Samaritan for us. The compassion he shows to us by claiming us as sisters and brothers constitutes us as persons sharing his communion with the Father and the Spirit.

Nor is a christological exegesis of the parable lacking in resources for ethical reflection. An unspoken assumption underlying the lawyer's original question to Jesus is that once the identity of my neighbor has been ascertained, the course of action that follows is clear. In other words, the lawyer seems to have no doubts about what love of neighbor entails, only about the range of its application. The same set of assumptions seems to underlie much of the contemporary quest for a criteriology of personhood. Thus, if the fetus is a person, then I should not abort it; if my comatose aunt is a person, I should not withdraw life support; if monkeys have a claim to personhood, I should not subject them to medical experiments.

Upon further reflection, however, the idea that the range of beings to which love is to be shown is more problematic than the content of love seems a rather odd assumption. Is the status of the other as a person really that crucial to our moral reasoning? After all, though I am quite confident that my wife (for example) is a person, that confidence does not by itself provide me with clear guidelines about how I should behave toward her in any given situation. Indeed, it is precisely in my marriage – arguably the most 'personal' relationship I have with another human being . . . – that I find myself most regularly [having] to ask myself what love requires.

This is not to deny all moral relevance to reflection on the status of the other. If my wife were to become critically ill and unable to make decisions regarding her own care, my understanding of her condition and prognosis would certainly contribute to any decisions I might be asked to make on her behalf. I suspect, however, that my thinking would not turn on the question of whether she still qualified as a person. More importantly, it seems to me that the parable of the good Samaritan provides good theological basis for this suspicion, insofar as this story suggests that the more important ethical question is not whether my wife is a person, but rather how I, as one who is treated as a person by Jesus Christ, relate to my wife (or anyone else) as the person I have been called to be. In other words, the crucial ethical judgment in my behavior toward those I meet on the road is not primarily the determination of the general category under which they fall . . ., but rather the way in which I define my relationship to them in their particularity.[19]

## V. Conclusion

Christian doctrine teaches that there are only three persons in the strict sense of the term: the Father, the Son, and the Holy Spirit. It does not presume to say what it means that these three are persons: the term 'person' is merely a semantic place-holder that marks this threefold distinction within the

Godhead. Strictly speaking, to be a person is simply to be one of these three: the Father, the Son, or the Holy Spirit.

But Christian doctrine also teaches that these three persons have willed to bring others into their fellowship. Those so invited are not persons on their own account, but they are nonetheless persons by virtue of their participation in the life of the Trinity through the Son. They are, so to speak, persons by proxy. Their identity as persons is bound up with their relationship to Jesus, who, as the incarnate Son, is both the model and source of their own personhood.

It follows that Jesus is the proper focus for Christian reflection on what it means to be a person. He assumes this role as the one in whose life is disclosed both the identity of the three divine persons and the form of human personhood they make possible. To know what it means to be a person, one needs to look at Jesus. Because his life is not only the supreme example, but also (and, indeed, primarily) the source of our own identity as persons, it is only on the basis of his prior activity on our behalf that we find ourselves in a position to be challenged by him to 'go and do likewise'.

## Notes

1. For example, the word 'person' occurs 79 times in the NIV, and 129 times in the NASB. Compare the pre-modern KJV, in which the word is used only 56 times.
2. See John D. Zizioulas, *Being As Communion: Studies in Personhood and the Church* (Crestwood, NY: St. Vladimir's Seminary Press, 1997), pp. 36–41.
3. This principle takes classic form in the grammatical rule [that] . . . 'whatever is said of the Son is said also of the Father, except that the Son is the Father'. Bernard Lonergan, *Method in Theology* (New York, NY: Seabury, 1972), p. 307.
4. . . . Boethius, *A Treatise Against Eutyches and Nestorius*, in *The Theological Tractates and The Consolation of Philosophy*, Loeb Classical Library (Cambridge, MA: Harvard University Press, 1973), pp. 84–85.
5. It was endorsed by Thomas Aquinas in the *Summa Theologiae*, 1a qu. 29, art. 1, and would seem to lie behind Locke's definition of a person as 'a thinking intelligent Being, that has reason and reflection, and can consider it self as it self, the same thinking thing in different times and places.' John Locke, *An Essay Concerning Human Understanding*, Book II, ch. 27, §9, ed. Peter H. Nidditch (Oxford: Oxford University Press, 1975), p. 335.
6. Note that this is true even if personhood is defined relationally, insofar as within such a relational model personhood is finally inseparable from one's capacity to participate in relationships of a certain type or quality.
7. Joseph Fitzmyer argues that the practical thrust of the passage makes it less a parable than an *exemplum* or extended simile (Joseph A. Fitzmyer, *The Gospel According to Luke (X–XXIV): Introduction, Translation and Notes* (New York, NY: Doubleday, 1985), p. 883). As the following argument makes clear, I view the story as less straight-forwardly 'practical' and more parabolic than does Fitzmyer. For another argument against the classification of the parable as *exemplum*, see Robert W. Funk, 'The Good Samaritan as Metaphor', in *Semeia* 2 (1974), pp. 75–84.
8. In this context, it is worth pointing out that the Samaritan Pentateuch contained the

same injunctions against contact with the dead as the one the priest and the Levite would have consulted.

9. Cf. J. M. Creed, *The Gospel According to St. Luke: The Greek Text, with Introduction, Notes and Indices* (London: Macmillan, 1930), p. 151.

10. Fitzmyer cites the fact that the parable fails to answer the lawyer's question as evidence that it has been joined to the discussion of eternal life only secondarily (Fitzmyer, *The Gospel According to Luke (X–XXIV)*, p. 883). Without venturing to speculate on the pre-history of the Gospel text, the point can nevertheless be made that Jesus' failure to answer the lawyer's question may itself be of important significance for Luke.

11. Fitzmyer is thus right to conclude that '[n]o definition of "neighbor" emerges from the "example", because such a casuistic question is really out of place'. His judgment here, however, conflicts rather sharply with his earlier statement (on the same page!) that '[t]he point of the story is . . . that a "neighbor" is anyone in need with whom one comes into contact and to whom one can show pity and kindness.' Fitzmyer, *The Gospel According to Luke (X–XXIV)*, p. 884.

12. In this context, Fitzmyer's judgment that '[t]he point of the story . . . is made without the concluding remark of Jesus' is open to question. See Fitzmyer, *The Gospel According to Luke (X–XXIV)*, p. 883.

13. Indeed, it is only by virtue of this incarnation that we are in a position to speak of three persons in God in the first place.

14. And of course, the church has never claimed that baptism constitutes a guarantee of an individual's inclusion or exclusion in the number of the saved.

15. Thus, the church has generally refrained from viewing the fact of baptism as a guarantor of – or its absence an insuperable obstacle to – salvation.

16. A similar argument is made by Thomas Aquinas in the third part of his *Summa Theologiae*. He first argues that because Christ is properly . . . the head only of those united to him in glory (*viz.*, the members of the church triumphant), no human being – Christian or not – is fully incorporated into his body in this life. But he then goes on to argue that Christ is properly considered the head of all human beings insofar as he provides expiation for the sins of the whole world (1 John 2:2) irrespective of present confessional status. It follows that all human beings must be treated as part of his body whether or not they consider themselves to be such. See Thomas Aquinas, *Summa Theologiae*, IIIa. qu. 8, art. 3 (Blackfriars, London: Eyre and Spottiswoode, 1974).

17. Not that modern attempts to affirm a christological interpretation of the parable have been altogether lacking. See, e.g., Jean Daniélou, 'Le bon Samaritain', in *Mélanges bibliques rédigés en l'honneur de Andree Robert* (Paris: Bloud et Gay, 1957), pp. 457–465 and B. Gerhardsson, 'The Good Samaritan – The Good Shepherd?' in *Coniectanea neotestimentica* 16 (1958), pp. 1–31.

18. 'For the question "Which one was neighbour to the man who was waylaid?" requires that the answer be given from the position of the man in trouble; that the lawyer put himself in the place of the waylaid man.' L. P. Trudiger, 'Once Again, Now "Who Is My Neighbour?" ' in the *Evangelical Quarterly* 48 (1976), p. 161. cf. Funk, 'The Good Samaritan as Metaphor', p. 79.

19. This last point is beautifully argued by Stanley Hauerwas in his essay, 'Must a Patient Be a Person to Be a Patient? Or, My Uncle Charlie Is Not Much of a Person But He Is Still My Uncle Charlie', in *Truthfulness and Tragedy: Further Investigations in Christian Ethics* (Notre Dame, IN: University of Notre Dame Press, 1977), pp. 127–131.

# 'Embodiment' and Moral Critique:
# A Christian Social Perspective

LISA SOWLE CAHILL

'Embodiment' is frequently lifted up as central in critiques of the Western moral tradition on both sex and medicine. Yet the prominence of this theme is in some respects puzzling. After all, talk and practice in these two areas could hardly be more explicit about having the 'body' as a key concern. Indeed, ethics as discourse about human relations and practices is always at some level about the body. Consider just war theory and theories of criminal justice as directly affecting human bodies, and government as doing so less directly but nonetheless clearly.

What, then, could be intended by current appeals to recover the significance of the body for moral discourse? Most ethicists use the theme of embodiment to counteract a dualism about body and mind in which the body tends to come off as the inferior partner in an uneasy relationship. Contemporary ethicists, both religious and philosophical, see the integration of body and mind or spirit as a value and a goal. Yet, somewhat paradoxically, choice, consent and autonomy can be so central in (Western) moral and policy discussions that protection of freedom serves to justify almost any medical or technological manipulation of his or her body that an informed moral agent elects. Moreover, liberal moral theory rarely succeeds in integrating the body and the embodied agent or self within their social context. Integration needs to occur not only between body and mind, but also among body, mind, and society. The body is always central in defining the self, while in all cultures, the meaning of the body reflects and augments social relationships. To understand the significance of embodiment for bioethics, it will be useful to set references to the body in sexual and medical ethics against broader discussions of body and society in philosophical, anthropological, and religious discourse. In so doing, it must be noted that society influences and shapes the bodily experience of the self not only in negative, repressive ways, but also in positive, expressive ways.

A thesis I want to develop is that a positive, integrative view of the self as embodied and as intrinsically social does not require the rejection of control

---

From Lisa Sowle Cahill and Margaret A. Farley (eds.), *Embodiment, Morality and Medicine*, pp. 199–215. Dordrecht: Kluwer Academic Publishers, 1995.

of the body in relation to the values of an encompassing social order. To advance this thesis, I will review dualism in the Western tradition, including modern versions of it which focus on autonomy; will examine recent critiques of mind-body dualism; and will examine the proposal, differently elaborated by Michel Foucault and Mary Douglas, that the self-understanding and the social agency of the embodied self reflects and reinforces social organization. Drawing on their work as well as that of Peter Brown, I will use Christian sources to show that the disciplined body can and has functioned as a countersign to hierarchy and domination, and as an inaugural sign of a new social order characterized by solidarity and equality. Consequences for the practice of medicine follow from changed relationships in general, and in particular from Christian symbolization of the new order through the experiences of bodily illness, pain, healing, and death.[1]

## Dualism and Western Tradition

A matter of concern for many [authors] is a body-spirit dualism which pervades Western (North Atlantic) culture, and which was expressed in Christian tradition by a negative view of the body as unruly and in need of control. In contemporary medical practice, we find a different but not un-related objectification of the body as the site of technical intervention, and as the material or even property regarding which autonomous persons exercise free consent . . .

In much of the Western tradition, however, mind and body have often been seen as discrete entities whose conjunction is uncertain, posing a philosophical problem. Modern science builds a strictly material body, and locates the causes of its illness and health in material causes, tending thereby to erode both the interdependence of spiritual and physiological states, and the connectedness of the embodied self with other elements and presences in the cosmos ([17], p. 133). Many place the blame on Descartes, . . . [who] by philosophically privileging thought over physical existence as constitutive of the person, . . . laid the way for later disembodiments and dehistoricizations of subjectivity, and for the body's deprivation of its role in knowledge and in moral valuation.

But Western dualism did not originate in the seventeenth century. While Aristotle cultivated virtue through practical wisdom in daily, bodily, social life, other ancient Greek philosophers deliberated on the distance between the world of lived experience and the world of unmediated truth and goodness. The heights of spiritual and intellectual accomplishment seemed to require escape from the exigencies and tensions of physical function and survival. The Platonists, and to a lesser extent the Stoics, armed their approach to the body with asceticism and rational direction, an approach attractive to many later Christian authors. On the one hand, the problematic body is subject to an impressive number of 'contingencies,' such as the need for food and shelter, and the liability to torture and imprisonment. On the other, when the drive to fulfill its own needs becomes stronger than the rational purposes by which one tries to channel or restrain them, the body seems to have a 'mind of its own' ([12], pp. 130–131). In dualistic views of the body and mind or spirit, body still defines self insofar as the virtues of rationality and asceticism move to center stage precisely in reaction to bodily realities.

## Body and Self in Christianity

One finds, if anything, an anti-dualism about the body in the gospels. God's reign is realized in the life and ministry of a man formed bodily in the womb of a woman, a man who in his very walking, sleeping, eating, drinking, talking, touching, fasting, night-watching, pain and death makes present the compassion of God for human suffering. Human persons are drawn into God's own love and life through the resurrection of their bodies. In earthly existence, the healing of illness is linked to faith, and human beings are called to alleviate the physical hunger, nakedness, and pain of neighbors and enemies alike.

St. Paul may reflect some of the anxieties of the philosophers when he laments that 'I delight in the law of God, in my inmost self, but I see in my members another law at war with the law of my mind and making me captive to the law of sin which dwells in my members' (Rom. 7:22–23). But despite his appreciation of the recalcitrance of the body in conforming to spiritual aims, Paul more generally understands 'flesh' in terms of any sinful turning from God or captivity to the world and its powers. 'Spirit' as flesh's opposite transforms not only the mind but the whole person to a life of righteousness through the indwelling Spirit of God. Certainly, notwithstanding its potentially hierarchical uses, Paul's master metaphor of the Christian community as 'Body of Christ' depends on the literal incorporation of disciples in all their physical reality. In his reaction against prostitution, he insists, 'The body is not meant for immorality, but for the Lord, and the Lord for the body . . . Do you not know that your body is a temple of the Holy Spirit within you . . .? . . . So glorify God in your body' (1 Cor. 6:13–20).

Ambivalence towards the body assumed a higher profile in the tradition, however, as Christians battled and were in the process influenced by, gnostic and other dualistic worldviews. An early example is Origen, who, like Plato, saw the differences among creatures as marks of their deviation from an original unity of being, and was reputed at least to have had himself castrated by a doctor in order to avoid either sexual incontinence or the appearance of immorality in his spiritual relationships with women ([2], p. 168). Augustine is another great thinker whose dualistic inclinations were eventually reconciled to but never eliminated from his defense of the body against Manichean assaults on marriage and childbearing. Though Augustine defined procreation of offspring as a 'good' of marriage (*On the Good of Marriage*, 6–7 . . . ), he was nevertheless able to speculate that in the Garden of Eden conception might have been accomplished by a passionless act of the will (*City of God*, XIV . . . ).

Despite the ultimate victory of the orthodox Christian view that the body is not only essential to the person, but is good as created and redeemed, the uncertainty of much of the tradition's investment in that view led not only to now-incredible theological proposals, but also to much agony of human spirit and body alike. 'The very matter-of-fact manner in which monastic sources report bloody, botched attempts at self-castration by desperate monks shocks us by its lack of surprise' ([2], p. xviii).

## Dualism in Contemporary Views

The 'old' dualism of Western culture, reinforced historically by Christianity, saw the body (especially the sexual body) as the enemy of rational control and requiring subjugation. A 'new' dualism, which sees the body as raw material for choice and intervention, is exercised via the technical and instrumental rationality guiding much of modern science. This attitude is partly responsible for the neglect of the embodied person which [may be detected] in the development of genetic therapies. Defining instrumental reason as the calculation of maximum efficiency in pursuing means to a given end, Charles Taylor notes its evidence 'in the prestige and aura that surround technology,' making us believe that 'we should seek technological solutions even when something very different is called for' ([18], pp. 5–6).

The reign of informed consent in bioethics today is a symptom of technical rationality operating within a lingering body-mind dualism. The self is defined as an autonomous, private, and self-constituting will. After Nuremberg, we may hardly forget that the principle of consent is important to maintain the dignity and inviolability of persons. However, the near absoluteness and self-sufficiency of this criterion in moral decisions about medical care and research reveals a modern version of the idea that the body is inferior and essentially alien to personal freedom. The rhetoric of choice promoting a legal right to physician-assisted suicide or euthanasia is a glaring example, as is the array of 'new reproductive technologies' designed to take advantage of all available means to force the realization of the self's chosen aims. The body relates to the self's freedom primarily as matter to be manipulated, matter which when resistant to the self's elected projects, may and must be overcome or circumvented.

It would be foolish to repudiate all forms of medical resistance to bodily limitations or failures, or to conform the identity of the self to physiological capacities (as do patriarchal definitions of women's roles). The issue is not a choice between bodiliness and freedom, but the appropriate integration of the self *as* body, mind, will, and spirit. The moral exclusions and permissions a wise and practicable integration would entail are no simple matter to define, and no doubt cannot be defined finally or abstractly. Suffice it to say that a naturalist morality of the body, a libertarian morality of the will, a rationalist morality of the intellect, and a fundamentalist morality of divine command all fail to meet the standard of a nuanced and experientially true approach to moral agency. All the constitutive dimensions of the self should be mutually engaged and allowed to carry some normative force.

One dangerous consequence of holding informed consent not only as a necessary but as the sufficient principle of bioethics is that to do so keeps out of our range of vision broader social relations which impinge on the identity of the self and its 'free' choices, including relations and practices focused on the body. Obvious examples are gender, race, and class expectations that make choices less than free, or that create blindnesses and injustices which cannot be redressed by focusing narrowly on providing information and eliciting a decision . . . The informed consent criterion also tends to neglect positive moral experiences and values which may be important to moral identity but which are not captured by the simple ideal of well-informed choice . . .

## Embodiment as a Critical Theme in Sexual and Medical Ethics

It is in sexual ethics that the appeal to embodiment has been most visible. This appeal typically supports a claim that traditional moral norms have been defined in the abstract (with authority attributed to God or nature), and with inadequate attention to the normative value of the actual, embodied experience of sex. For example, to define procreation as the principal purpose of sex is to neglect if not ignore other aspects of sexual experience, such as pleasure, intimacy, and homoeroticism. These aspects might also define goods and values whose claim should be recognized in moral choices. No doubt it *is* actual experience in precisely such dimensions that the experientially incommensurate norms are intended to control. In this sense, they do address sexual reality, even if only to assert a norm over against it. But this fact only verifies the critique: received sexual norms themselves do not build constructively on the embodied experience of the persons they are aimed to address. As far as sex is concerned, then, the corrective advanced via 'embodiment' is the counteraction of repressive attitudes toward the body with a more positive attitude toward the fullness of its capacities, an important feature of which is the potential of the sexual body for intimacy and pleasure as well as for procreation.

Because it is derived from biological sex as its social interpretation, gender also enters into the positive reconstrual of the body. Specifically, women's bodies are affirmed as constituting selves who are equal to men in moral agency and moral value. Women's reproductive capacities in no way signal lesser rational and volitional abilities, nor should women's roles be constrained or accorded lesser value on account of women's distinctive reproductive contributions. Women's bodies are a source of moral knowledge equal to, if somewhat different from, that yielded by the male embodied experience.

In medicine, the point commonly advanced by means of the theme of embodiment is that the 'patient' whose body is manipulated is also a 'person' who is embodied. The self is constituted by the person's materiality as much as by his or her intellectual, spiritual, and psychological dimensions. The body enters into the subjectivity of the person, mediates that subjectivity to the world, and is a medium through which the world and other persons interact with the subject as embodied self. In the words of Merleau-Ponty, 'the body expresses total existence, not because it is an external accompaniment to that existence, but because existence comes into its own in the body'([13], p. 166). Bodies are not just living organisms which as such become the objects of scientific, technical intervention. Bodies are the spatiality and temporality of selves, and it is to persons – not only to bodies – that medical professionals must respond. In medicine, the corrective which 'embodiment' brings is a holistic view of the person. In addition to the unity of self and body, this holism extends to a unity of all the physical parts and processes of the body in their personal and social meanings.

It is just this emphasis on holism that often brings sexual discourse into conjunction with biomedical talk of the significance of the body, especially in the case of the medical relevance of biological sex socially mediated as gender. The self as embodied is quite strongly constituted by the social significance of gender as an elaboration of maleness or femaleness. Medical practice can become oppressive to women to the extent that it incorporates patriarchal gender models in its approach to women's health. A revealing treatment of the practical interpenetration of sexual and medical discourses is Emily Martin's *The Woman in the Body* ([11]). In the medicalization of women's reproductive processes, the female body is often objectified in a way reflecting cultural views of women's passivity and inferiority. The obstetrician, for instance, often assumes the role of 'supervisor or foreman' of a labor process in which two images compete: 'the uterus as a machine that produces a baby and the woman as laborer who produces the baby' ([11], p. 63). If Gerda Lerner is right that patriarchy is the first and paradigm case of oppression ([10]) then we will not be surprised to see further objectification of the bodies of those in 'lower' racial, ethnic, and class groups, all of which are compounded when the medical subject/object is a woman.

In overview, Western authors writing today ... are almost unanimously inclined to see dualism as bad and integration as a value, and to affirm that the body's contribution to selfhood is not only essential but is a component of the highest levels of human value and accomplishment, such as love, friendship, moral insight, and art. Contemporary Western affirmations of embodiment as a value may be seen to address three axes along which the body is understood, each structured by an internal polarity. Affirmations of embodiment are generally intended to move perception and practice away from the first pole in each set, and toward the second. These axes are *dualism – integration* (of body and mind, reason or spirit); *denigration – affirmation* (of the body as part of the person); and *control – freedom* (presence or absence of a definite social ordering of the parts and processes of one's own body, as well as of one's own person in relation to the bodies of others). The third move in combination with the first two has a somewhat paradoxical effect at the level of moral practice and public policy. There we find a cultural and philosophical insistence on the freedom to control, reshape, or even kill the body as a prerequisite of genuine moral agency and as a form of resistance to the heteronomous control of social institutions which serve the vested interests of some groups of individuals in control over the bodies of others.

We find examples in the phrasing of the morality of avoiding or under-taking parenthood as a matter of reproductive choice, and when sexual morality is phrased as a matter of creating or constructing one's own sexual identity. The merits of both agendas lie in their unmasking definitions of the body's moral significance which employ a rhetoric of the biologically natural to disguise social power relationships. However, such critiques would be strengthened by the development of positive alternative ways to bring freedom back into interdependence with the body, and with other material and social conditions of freedom. Charles Taylor instructs us that any non-trivial 'choice' reflects a set of value priorities which at the very least highlight the realms of moral conduct which are of the highest importance, and which reflect a dialogical community of other moral agents ([18], p. 39).[2] Freedom as a moral value makes no sense without a material and social context.

## The Body as a Symbol of Social Organization

A lesson that we learn in different ways from Mary Douglas and Michel Foucault is that the individual body is always interpreted and ordered to reflect social relationships. It is both a symbol of those relationships and a medium through which they are realized, realigned or replaced. Conceptions of the individual body and of the social body are interdependent. Interest-ingly, writers who explore the social history behind the early Christian religious world often draw on Mary Douglas and, less centrally, on Foucault. (Peter Brown [2] cites both in his bibliography; see John Dominic Crossan

([5], p. 77) for a discussion of Mary Douglas.)[3] A counterpoint to the social interpretation of the body is the fact that the body is to some extent a biological given. Presumed 'universals' of human embodiment run through [the literature in this area]: need for food and shelter, sexuality and reproduction, pain and pleasure, health and disease, aging and death. At the same time, [many authors] focus . . . on the variety of ways in which such embodied experiences as these have been understood, and especially on how religious understandings of embodiment have changed or remain in need of change.

Foucault writes precisely to resist the 'universals' of reason and nature by showing that experience and knowledge are thoroughly historical. He argues that our self-consciousness, our freedom, our values, and our very construal of what is central in our own experience are created by social practices which represent and perpetuate power relationships. Part of the originality of his contribution lies in his demonstration that in order to shape the self at its deepest levels, power does not need to coerce consciousness or behavior directly. Power determines consciousness through a comprehensive set of strategies which focus on the body (whether through hospitals, prisons, insane asylums, education, theories of sex, and – across all of these – modern medicine), and which determines the parameters within which we imagine our identity and our options. Foucault convincingly displays the ways in which power 'controls' bodies as a positive and constructive force, not just by repression and constraint. He writes of 'deployment' of discourses or 'regimes' of knowledge and power which induce people to construct reality on their terms. He regards the whole notion of 'sexuality' as such a discourse ([8]). He illustrates how Christian confessional practice and medical-psychiatric discourses about sex, supposedly responsible for repression, have actually resulted in endlessly proliferating talk about sex and in our conviction that the secret and truth of our very being lie in our sexual identity and behavior.[4] Our present quest for sexual 'liberation' is no more than the ultimate victory of a discourse of sexuality which procures our consent to our own domination by means of a discipline of the body which we all too readily embrace ([8], pp. 151–159). While Foucault resists describing power as the 'power of' any distinct social group by which it is consciously and purposively exercised, he often portrays medical science as facilitating the control both of individuals and of whole populations by its socially aggressive definitions of the body's significance.

Mary Douglas also sees the meaning of the body as culturally determined to a large extent. She finds in all cultures a human 'drive to achieve consonance between social and physical and emotional experience' which finds expression in the use of the body as a natural symbol of the social order. The symbolic potentials of the body are in some way culturally constant. To present the front rather than the back of one's body signifies respect; physical closeness signifies intimacy; the casting-off of physical waste products (spitting, urinating) is incompatible with formal discourse and may be used to interrupt it; and the more strongly classified and controlled is the social hierarchy, the more controlled the individual's bodily movements will be, even to the point of 'etherealization' or the relative disembodiment of personal interactions ([6], pp. 100–101).

In cultures where there is a strongly defined structuring of the roles of individuals and groups, controlled and formal behavior will also be highly valued ([6], p. 99). Conversely, in societies in which individuality and freedom are prized over and above social expectations, freedom of physical movement and expression – the individual's 'control' over his or her own body – will also be accepted and valued. It is important to make explicit the implication, however, that even in ostensibly unrestricted societies, the significance of the body and its movements still follow social norms, are still ordered and even in a sense controlled by the social ethos.

Douglas discerns a movement in Western societies away from systems characterized by a high respect for social roles and structures, and the duties they present for individuals, to systems in which the sincerity and authenticity of the subject become more important than structures, and in which personal success eventually overrides respect for roles and duties ([6], p. 50). The latter sort of society, to which Douglas says 'we' now belong, sees a demise of ritualism in public and private ('the celebration of Sunday dinner'), and a great informality of social and family life (the disappearance of rank according to age and sex, as reflected in the arrangement of living room chairs) ([6], p. 55). Children are educated to be interested in their own internal states and the feelings of others. But the 'seeds of alienation' ([6], p. 190) are contained in the relocation of control to the personal system, and the lack of integration of the individual with the social body. We may infer that alienation from the social significance of one's own body will also result, so that individuals neither realize the social shaping of their embodied behavior nor take into account the social effects of their choices to execute their sincere and 'autonomous' life-plans by means of embodied relationships. They may even see the body as, in Douglas's phrase, an 'alien husk' from which to escape ([6], p. 191).

Despite a common emphasis on socialization of the body, Douglas and Foucault obviously differ in significant ways. First, Douglas sees the body in its physicality as in some sense a universal which is socially interpreted ([6], p. ix), while Foucault edges towards the claim that the body is itself a construction. Second, Douglas avoids Foucault's heavy, even cynical, association of social control with domination, leaving open in her cross-cultural studies the possibility that the body and its parts can be ordered to reinforce social relationships which are not necessarily repressive, or which are at least characterized by a solidarity in which the embodied individual immediately participates.

In her study of trance states ([6], pp. 104–110), Mary Douglas also paves the way to a recognition, fully achieved for instance in the work of Caroline Walker Bynum ([4], [3]), that Christianity, along with most or all other societies, sees the body (not only the spirit) as an avenue of transcendence and even of union with the divine. 'Control, discipline, even torture of the flesh is, in medieval devotion, not so much the rejection of physicality as the elevation of it – a horrible yet delicious elevation – into a means of access to the divine' ([3], p. 182). Among the most universal bodily routes to the divinity are sex, food, and death, along with death's foretastes, pain and illness. Christianity has used all three.

## The Body and Christian Society

While positive construals of the religious significance of sexual activity may have been scarce in Christian culture until the modern period,[5] permanent virginity as a religiously dedicated and ideal sexual identity was a distinctive contribution of early Christianity (1 Cor. 7:8; this is Peter Brown's thesis [2]). Moreover, Bynum illustrates that the self-expressions of many mystics have strongly physical and indirectly sexual overtones ([4], p. 248; [3], p. 133). Food becomes a physical sharing in the divine life in the eucharistic meal ([4], pp. 252–253); in the sharing of food with the poor in imitation of God's mercy (Luke 6:36; Acts 6:1–6); in mystical and symbolic experiences of giving and receiving nurturance through feeding, even nursing ([4], pp. 269–276; [3], p. 133); and in the renunciation of food by fasting, complemented by the feast in celebration of divine grace and presence ([4], p. 250).

Likewise, Christianity is hardly alone among the world's religions in seeing death as a point of entry into a transcendent realm and of approach to God. Christians elaborate the religious significance of death in terms of last rites for the dying, funerary and burial practices, veneration of the dead and of their relics, martyrdom, resurrection, eternal life, eternal reward and punishment, and God's sharing in human death through the Cross of Christ. Anticipations of death in this life, often called 'mortifications' of the body, include ascetic deprivation of the body and deliberate infliction of pain on it (including fasting); religious interpretations of illness as a trial, a gift, or a sign of sanctity; healing of illness, including New Testament healing miracles and the religious ministries of healing which have existed throughout Christian tradition; and the actual bodily manifestation of the wounds which caused Christ's death (stigmata). Mystical experience also can include sensations of pain and of dying or of being near death or of passing through it . . .

These examples serve to demonstrate that Christianity has been neither intransigently dualistic nor negative about the body. They also indicate that a positive, integrated approach to the body and soul, or body and mind, need not exclude – indeed may depend upon – an ordering of the body in relation to a social vision. But where Foucault tends to portray social forces which determine the significance of the body as discourses of power-knowledge which serve regimes of domination, Douglas permits us to see that the background of social conditions within which we are embodied provides us with a framework for channeling, shaping, and disciplining our embodied experiences. Freedom never exists outside of some social vision; the communal vision which shapes bodily experience also brings the self's embodiment to consciousness, to expression, and to social agency.

Like other societies, Christianity both channels a social vision through the body, and defines community partly in terms of bodily experiences and roles. As current scholarship attests, the biblically authentic Christian social vision is characterized by inclusiveness and solidarity, especially toward enemies and toward marginalized and outcast persons and groups. The solidarity of the New Testament communities challenged social relations built on status, power, and economic dependency, even if it did not completely overturn them.[6] Inclusive solidarity as a defining feature of Jesus' kingdom preaching is familiar in the Sermon on the Mount's Beatitudes (Matt. 5:1–12), and in Jesus' instruction to 'love your enemies, do good to those who hate you' (Luke 6:27); in the parable of the Good Samaritan (Luke 10:30–37); in Jesus' association with sinners and outcasts; in his approach to women; in his sacrificial death. A representative restatement of the cultural challenge presented by Jesus and his first followers is offered by John Dominic Crossan. In Jesus' teaching, life, and death,

> the Kingdom of God is a community of radical or unbrokered equality in which individuals are in direct contact with one another and with God, unmediated by any established brokers or fixed locations ([5], p. 101).

Crossan uses Mary Douglas on the body as a microcosm of the social order to show how Jesus manifested social equality through practices of table fellowship, itinerancy, healing, the raising of Lazarus, and exorcisms. Jesus' healing miracles are of special relevance to medical practice. For Crossan, their significance does not consist in any intervention into the natural, physical order of 'disease' but into the social world of 'illness,' in which disease often meant ritual uncleanness and social ostracization. Jesus' violation of the purity code by contact with a leper challenged both the body politic and the priestly authorities, impugning 'the rights and prerogatives of society's boundary keepers and controllers' ([5], p. 82). Jesus' healing miracles are important for their social significance, for their relevance to the new kingdom which includes the 'marginalized and disenfranchized' ([5], p. 83), and refuses the traditional boundaries of order and exclusion symbolized in the disordered and thus excluded body of the sick. The Christian transformation of the social significance of the diseased body both symbol-izes, and advances at the practical level, an inclusive community in which traditional hierarchies are overturned. A particularly good example is Jesus' healing of the woman who had had a 'flow of blood' for twelve years (Mark 5:25–34), since she was not only sick but female. She would have been especially stigmatized if the hemorrhage from which she suffered involved menstrual blood, making her ritually impure.

Peter Brown illumines ways in which the early churches shaped the sexual body to advance this same vision. Especially in its implications for gender relations and for social relations of unequal power in general, this reshaping too is relevant to medical practice. Brown contrasts the hierarchical household of the ancient world with egalitarian Christian communities which threatened the social order. Celibacy was sometimes practiced in the ancient world, but it never replaced marriage as the general ideal and cornerstone of the social welfare. When undertaken, it was often temporary (as in the case of the Vestal Virgins). In Roman society, the sexual act, the relation of husband and wife, their marriage, the hierarchy of the household, and the government of the state, were not only analogous as concentric circles of order, but were dependent on one another for their existence . . .

Against this environment, Christian sexual renunciation may be seen, not as a mere repression of the body under the influence of dualistic philosophical and religious currents, but as a form of resistance to the hierarchical social order maintained through the reality and the symbolism of sex, marriage, and family. Perpetual virginity transformed the bodies of both men and women in their social significance, and enabled Christians (perhaps most especially women) 'to break with the discreet discipline of the ancient city' [2], p. 31). And beyond transforming the orders of personal relationships taken for granted in the ethos of the age, continence also broke with the continuity of history and of generations, announcing the eschatological advent of the kingdom of God, and a 'new creation' ([2], pp. 32, 64, 435).

Paul had a distinctive way of refracting Christian social cohesiveness through the body. The body is sanctified and an inauguration of the new age insofar as it is a 'temple of the Holy Spirit' (1 Cor. 6:19). The community of disciples as a whole is the material and historical presence of the body of Christ. The body of the believer participates in this communal identity to so great an extent that an act of sexual immorality will contaminate the very body of Christ (1 Cor. 7:15). Corinth was a place where division built on status had fractured the community and introduced disorder into this transformed community. Some at Corinth apparently had taken the solution of embracing celibacy and totally dissolving the household. Paul himself recognized the radical effects of Christian baptism as an induction into a new social order (Gal. 3:28). However, he resisted complete separatism from the pagan world, and emphasized the continuing validity of social bonds, including marriage and slavery.

While Paul's preference for celibacy may reflect a Stoic dualism of reason and passion to some extent, it also signifies a radical social critique of the social order in which hierarchy reigned. His stated reasons for the preference are a suspicion neither of women (for he addresses both the wife and the husband) nor of the body, nor of sex itself.[7] Marriage should be avoided specifically to avoid 'anxiety about worldly affairs' – the business and ordering of the household. Paul desires 'to promote good order' instead, that is, 'to secure your undivided devotion to the Lord' (1 Cor. 7:32–35). In other words, celibacy is for the sake of the transformed and transforming social order of the eschatological community, of which the body is a symbol.

Even in preferring celibacy ('I wish that all were as I myself am,' 1 Cor. 7:7), Paul does not make this sign of the new order into an entrance requirement ('But each has his own special gift from God, one of one kind and one of another,' 1 Cor. 7:7). The egalitarian solidarity of discipleship can also be at least partially reflected in marriage, even though Paul anticipates that it will in that state be more difficult to maintain. For instance, wife and husband 'rule' over each other's bodies (1 Cor. 7:4); neither partner is to divorce an unbelieving spouse who is willing to continue the relationship, though either may do so if the spouse is not (1 Cor. 7:12–16); and Christians are exhorted to enact the transformative effects of mutual love even within the hierarchical household (Eph. 5:21–6:9).[8]

Yet, as we have seen, Paul specifically contrasts the social ordering celibacy symbolizes to the social order of that household. In later Christianity, celibacy became an instrument of hierarchical control over believers, especially clergy and religious. Yet, following Brown's lead, we may say that permanent virginity for the early Christian signs, not merely or simply the evils of the sexual body, but the solidarity of the kingdom which is radical and total. Involvement with sex, even sex 'well-ordered' from a cultural point of view, will involve the disciple with a set of social relationships (organized around sex, gender, procreation, and family) in which it will be difficult to live out fully the equality, solidarity, compassion and mercy among men and women, slave and free, and finally Jew and gentile (Gal. 3:28) in which the kingdom of God is present.

Paul's representation of the sexual body as not fundamentally compliant with the norms of the social order is carried out in the early Christians' presentation of the body and its functions as in other ways subversive of power and hierarchy. Many disciplines of the Christian body have to do with eating or feeding in a way which symbolizes the unity of the community. For instance, Paul accuses those who maintain distinctions among rich and poor at the eucharistic table, by providing sumptuously for themselves while others go hungry, of 'profaning the body and blood of the Lord' (1 Cor.

11:27). Ministers to the needy were appointed in the community, and were charged with such duties as distribution of food to widows. Whether Jewish or Greek, the widows should be treated similarly (Acts 6:1–6). Concerning whether Christians should partake of meat that had been offered to idols, Paul acknowledges that idols have no real existence (1 Cor. 8:4), and that food in and of itself does not establish one's relationship with God (1 Cor. 8:8). Nonetheless, each should be concerned for the consciences of others in the community, and should not cause scandal to 'weaker' members who may not yet have reached the same freeing knowledge (1 Cor. 8:7; 10:28–29). ' "Knowledge" puffs up, but love builds up' (1 Cor. 8:1). Love as solidarity in community is symbolized by a control of the body which denies that the knowledgeable are 'superior.'

Symbolizations of the new order by means of bodily suffering and death pervade gospels and epistles, and center on the death and resurrection of Jesus. We may add just a few examples of the appropriation of this unifying death in the Christian life. Paul, whom later sources attest was eventually martyred, sees his own imprisonments as a confirmation of his defense of the gospel and as a means of strengthening other members of Christ's body in their commitment to the faith (Phil. 1:7, 14; see also Col. 4:10; Eph. 3:1, 4:1, 6:20). In his own name as 'a prisoner for the Lord,' Paul implores the church at Ephesus 'to lead a life worthy of the calling to which you have been called, with all lowliness and meekness, with patience, forbearing one another in love, eager to maintain the unity of the Spirit in the bond of peace' (Eph. 4:1–3). Paul rejects the bodily mark of circumcision because it is used to distinguish higher religious status, to set off the 'glory' of those who belong from those who do not (Gal. 6:12–15). Instead, he says, he bears on his own body 'the marks of Jesus,' possibly a reference to his having been beaten (Gal. 6:17). Although Paul's death is not recounted in the New Testament, the Acts of the Apostles tells other martyrdoms, including the stoning of Stephen (Acts 7:57–60), and the death of James at the hands of Herod (Acts 12:1–2). Stephen, like Jesus, died praying for the forgiveness of his persecutors (Acts 7:60).

## Overview and Recommendations

Certainly in the tradition, perhaps most of all in Augustine's writings, Christian control of the sexual body has come into alignment with dualistic and negative currents, leading Christians to see the body preeminently as a temptation to sin. This negativity is not only not required by, but is inconsistent with, New Testament symbolization of the body, especially the presence of God's reign in Jesus' birth, life, death, and resurrection; the Christian community as inclusive Body of Christ; the resurrection of the body as the full incorporation of the whole person into God's kingdom.

As we bring Christian views of the body toward medical practice, what perhaps is in most need of emphasis is the positive *social* significance of those views. A first significance of embodiment for a Christian ethics of medicine and healing is the importance of a stance of compassion toward the sick on the part of care-givers. The point is not pity, but an empathic identification with the suffering of the other, which, to the extent humanly possible, reaches through boundaries of race, gender, class, and economic status. Only then can one serve, as did the Good Samaritan, as a 'neighbor' to those who are injured and vulnerable.

A second significance proceeds partly from that identification; it is the realization that we too suffer and die, whether pain and mortality mark us already in profound ways or in temporarily subtle ones. With that realization comes the recognition of the vulnerability of every human being, and the need of every one for redemptive inclusion in the unity of all being which the Christian eucharist signifies and of which the mystics of all religions have had a premonition. Doctors and patients are but provisionally set apart by the pain and supplication of the latter. A third significance proceeds both from compassion and from the universality of disease and death. That is the moral importance of a genuinely inclusive social practice of health care, which alleviates suffering, even while acknowledging the inevitability of death and the interdependence of health and bodily life with other social, personal, and spiritual goods.

The social significance of embodiment for a Christian bioethics is neither a knowing priesthood of the medical professions, nor a resignation to human suffering as 'God's will,' nor an absolutization of the individual's 'right to life,' nor even the cultivation of altruistic virtues by members of care-giving professions. It is the challenge to create a community of solidarity in which suffering and death are healed and avoided where possible, and are recognized as constitutive of human selfhood even after they are not. In such a community, the suffering and dying self would not experience dependency as defilement, but as an extenuation and deepening of the self's social destiny. All persons in such a community might learn to take their own bodily vulnerability as an occasion for self-transcendence through compassion for the vulnerability of others and in openness to the sustaining communion of being which Christians symbolize as 'resurrection life.'

## Bibliography

1. Ames, R. T.: 'The Meaning of the Body in Classic Chinese Philosophy', in T. P. Kasulis *et al.* (eds.), *Self as Body in Asian Theory and Practice*, State University of New York Press, Albany, pp. 157–177.
2. Brown, P.: 1988, *The Body and Society: Men, Women and Sexual Renunciation in Early Christianity*, Columbia University Press, New York.

3. Bynum, C. W.: 1991, *Fragmentation and Redemption: Essays on Gender and the Human Body in Medieval Religion*, Zone Books, New York.
4. Bynum, C. W.: 1987, *Holy Feast and Holy Fast: The Religious Significance of Food to Medieval Women*, University of California Press, Berkeley, Los Angeles and London.
5. Crossan, J. D.: 1993, *Jesus: A Revolutionary Biography*, HarperCollins Publishers, New York.
6. Douglas, M.: 1973, *Natural Symbols: Explorations in Cosmology*, Barrie and Jenkins, London.
7. Finley, M. I.: 1973, *The Ancient Economy*, University of California Press, Berkeley and Los Angeles.
8. Foucault, M.: 1978, *The History of Sexuality, Vol. 1: An Introduction*, R. Hurley (trans.), Random House, New York.
9. Kasulis, T. P.: 1993, 'Introduction', in T. P. Kasulis *et al.* (eds.), *Self as Body in Asian Theory and Practice*, State University of New York Press, Albany, pp. ix–xx.
10. Lerner, G.: 1986, *The Creation of Patriarchy*, Oxford University Press, New York and Oxford.
11. Martin, E.: 1987, *The Woman in the Body: A Cultural Analysis of Reproduction*, Beacon Press, Boston.
12. Meeks, W. A.: 1993, *The Origins of Christian Morality: The First Two Centuries*, Yale University Press, New Haven and London.
13. Merleau-Ponty, M.: 1962, *Phenomenology of Perception*, C. Smith (trans.), Routledge and Kegan Paul, London and Henley, NJ.
14. Moxnes, H.: 1988, *The Economy of the Kingdom: Social Conflict and Economic Relations in Luke's Gospel*, Fortress Press, Philadelphia.
15. Schüssler Fiorenza, E.: 1983, *In Memory of Her: A Feminist Theological Reconstruction of Christian Origins*, Crossroad Publishing Company, New York.
16. Sheets-Johnstone, M. (ed.): 1993, *Giving the Body Its Due*, State University of New York Press, Albany.
17. Sheets-Johnstone, M.: 1993, 'The Materialization of the Body: A History of Western Medicine, A History in Progress', in M. Sheets-Johnstone (ed.): 1993, *Giving the Body Its Due*, State University of New York Press, Albany, pp. 132–158.
18. Taylor, C.: 1991, *The Ethics of Authenticity*, Harvard University Press, Cambridge, MA and London.
19. Turner, B. S.: 1984, *The Body and Society: Explorations in Social Theory*, Basil Blackwell, Oxford and New York.

## Notes

1. Thanks to Francis Elvey, S.J., Margaret Farley, Karen Lebacqz, Therese Lysaught, and James Nelson for very helpful critical comments on a first version of this essay.
2. Taylor perceptively explains why 'authenticity' as 'self-determining freedom' has to depend on 'the understanding that independent of my will there is something noble, courageous, and hence significant in giving shape to my own life.' Within the horizon of values against which moral authenticity takes place, some issues and values are more important than others, or 'the very idea of self-choice falls into triviality and hence incoherence' ([18], p. 39).
3. I am grateful to Francis Elvey, S.J., for sharing with me his work in progress on the relevance of Foucault and Douglas to Christian conceptions of the body, which he applies to Thomas Aquinas's use of the body as a metaphor for society.
4. As Michel Foucault shows so well, a 'controlling' discourse about sex all the better serves to accentuate it, to elevate sex as the secret of the self's identity, so that the

long run effect is guilty fascination or confessional self-display, rather than repression. Perhaps a Christian dualism about sex has ensured the repetition of social situations in which a normative discourse of strict sexual control has been accompanied by or broken out into anarchic practices of sexual perversion, especially by those in power – including the age-old rape and prostitution of women and sexual exploitation of children, the Victorian 'double standard,' and sexual abuse by clergy.

5. Take possibly Ephesians 5:23–32 on husbands and wives, and recall the sacramental status of marriage in at least some Christian communities, e.g., the Roman Catholic.

6. Several authors have recently made this argument, based on a social history approach to the distribution of power and status in the communities in which Christianity first arose. An example is Halvor Moxnes ([14]). This literature commonly draws on Moses Finley's description of client-patron relationships in first-century society ([7]).

7. Scholars widely agree that 1 Cor. 7:1 ('It is well for a man not to touch a woman') is Paul's restatement of his opponents' position, to which he is about to reply.

8. The critical question is whether a transformation which still leaves the essential hierarchical structure intact is an adequate social adaptation or a betrayal of Kingdom solidarity ([15]).

# CASE STUDY:
## A Dilemma about Abortion

Mary and David are a married couple with one school-age daughter. They both have challenging and enjoyable jobs and are active in their local church. Much to their surprise, they recently discovered that Mary was pregnant again, and though the pregnancy was unplanned, they were initially delighted at the prospect of having another child. However, a history of fragile X syndrome had recently come to light in Mary's family. Fragile X is an inherited disease which can cause mild to severe learning disability and behavioural problems. Because of this family history Mary was advised to have a prenatal test for fragile X. She and David were devastated when the test indicated that the child would have this condition. The question of terminating the pregnancy has been raised with them: they have serious doubts about the morality of this, but at the same time they are fearful of having a child severely affected by this condition.

## Questions
- What light, if any, can discussions of personhood and embodiment shed upon arguments about abortion?
- Under what circumstances, if any, would you consider abortion morally justified, and why?
- If Mary and David asked you for advice, how would you advise them, and why?

# 4

# HEALTH, DISEASE AND WHOLENESS

## Introduction

If human persons are to be regarded in an integrated way as embodied, mental, spiritual and relational creatures, what does it mean to describe them as healthy or diseased? This question is clearly important for the health care professions. If they are called to care for and heal the sick, and to protect and promote health, then an understanding of what their roles and responsibilities entail must depend on some account of what is meant by health and its opposites, disease, illness and sickness.[1]

Definitions of health range from the minimal to the maximal. Near the minimal end of the scale lies the so-called 'medical model' (Pattison 1989, 22ff.): the body is regarded as a machine which is healthy insofar as it functions normally and diseased insofar as it malfunctions. Near the other end of the scale is the well-known definition adopted by the World Health Organisation (WHO) in the Preamble to its Constitution of 1948:

> Health is a state of complete physical, mental and social well-being, and not merely the absence of disease or infirmity. (cited in Wilkinson 1998, 13)

The WHO definition has proved attractive to many Christian writers who wish to identify health with biblical notions of *shalom* or wholeness; indeed, some would argue that it is not sufficiently all-embracing, and should include reference to spiritual well-being and right relationship with the natural environment (Wilkinson 1998, 19). However, it has been heavily criticised by others, not least because it tends to subsume all human well-being under the

category of health, and so to hand over all authority and responsibility for
our well-being to the health care professions (Callahan 1973).

Some definitions of health and disease are attempts to understand the
concept in purely objective, value-free terms. The 'medical model', understanding disease in mechanistic terms as a deviation from the normal
functioning of the body, is a case in point. However, critics of this understanding argue that we cannot avoid value-judgments in talking about health
and disease. As the philosopher Richard Hare puts it, 'what makes us classify
conditions as diseases is that *in general* . . . they are *bad* things for the patient
to have' (Hare 1986, 178; italics original). If this is true, it raises further
questions: where do the values embedded in our understandings of health
and disease come from, and how adequate are they? The theologian Jürgen
Moltmann acknowledges that the understanding of health in a given society
will reflect that society's system of 'received values' – but, he cautions,
'this does not mean that these ideas of "health" are necessarily healthy in
themselves' (Moltmann 1985, 270–271). One need only think of the popularity
of 'eugenic' ideas – that the 'fit' should be encouraged to reproduce and the
'unfit' discouraged or prevented – in many countries early in the twentieth
century to appreciate the force of Moltmann's warning.

The first reading in this chapter is a classic theological account of health
and disease by the influential Protestant theologian Karl Barth, who locates
his discussion in the context of 'the command of God the Creator'. God calls
us, first, into relationship with himself, and second, into relationship with
our fellow human beings; but there is also a necessary 'third dimension' to
God's command: 'simply . . . to exist as a living being of this particular, i.e.
human, structure' (*Church Dogmatics* III/4, p. 324). Barth defines health as
'the strength for human life' (p. 107) – in other words, the strength that God
himself gives us to obey his command and live a human life. He understands
disease or sickness[2] in negative terms, as 'the weakness opposed to this
strength' (p. 110) – but although defined negatively in relation to health,
disease is nonetheless real and important.

Barth says two things about disease that at first sight appear to be contra-
dictory. First, it is part of the disorder of a world in rebellion against God,
and therefore also a sign of God's judgement on such a world.[3] The good
news in this understanding lies in the knowledge that God in Christ has
acted to overcome the forces of evil and chaos in the world, and our proper
response must be to resist disease and exercise the 'will to be healthy', as far
as it lies in our power. But second, disease can be a reminder that our
present life and health are limited by our mortality, and that God's love and
faithfulness towards us are not only concerned with this present life, but
with our eternal life.

By holding in tension these two understandings of disease, Barth does
justice to the paradoxical witness of the New Testament, expressed on the

one hand by the healing miracles of Jesus, and on the other by Paul's 'thorn in the flesh' (2 Cor. 12:1–10), a weakness which remained with him despite his prayers, but through which he was able to discover the strength of Christ. Perhaps Barth also offers us a way of understanding our own equally paradoxical experience of disease.

The second reading approaches these questions in a very different way: John Hull gives a blind person's reflections on some biblical texts that relate to sight, blindness and healing. In some passages he finds an 'inferior' theology of competition between gods, where the God of Israel proves his superiority by his ability to restore sight to the blind. In others, however, God's people are called to be a covenant community in which all kinds of people, including blind people, are welcomed and included as they are. Some texts go further, so that blind people become models of faithfulness and trust in God. Hull argues that passages which do promise restoration of sight to the blind are first and foremost concerned with justice for the oppressed, not with spectacular miracles of healing.

This raises radical questions about disease and diversity. Blindness is often regarded as a medical problem, for which we should seek a medical cure or, failing that, pray for a miracle. But perhaps the more pressing problem is that the world is organised to suit sighted people, and a higher priority should be the creation of structures and conditions that do not disadvantage blind people. What is the proper balance between 'medical' and 'social' approaches to disabilities? These questions are raised once again by the case study at the end of this chapter.

### References and Further Reading

Daniel Callahan, 'The WHO Definition of "Health" ', *Hastings Center Studies* 1.3, 77–87 (1973). Reprinted in Stephen E. Lammers and Allen Verhey (eds.), *On Moral Medicine: Theological Perspectives in Medical Ethics*, 253–261. 2nd ed., Grand Rapids: Eerdmans, 1998.

Nancy Eisland, *The Disabled God*. Nashville: Abingdon Press, 1994.

Andrew Fergusson (ed.), *Health: The Strength to be Human*. Leicester: IVP, 1993.

Bernard Häring, *Medical Ethics*. 3rd ed., Slough: St Paul's, 1991.

Richard M. Hare, 'Health'. *Journal of Medical Ethics* 12, 174–181, 1986.

Stanley Hauerwas, *Suffering Presence: Theological Reflections on Medicine, the Mentally Handicapped, and the Church*. Notre Dame: University of Notre Dame Press, 1986/ Edinburgh: T & T Clark, 1988.

Ivan Illich, *Limits to Medicine: Medical Nemesis – the Expropriation of Health*. London: Marion Boyars, 1995.

Jürgen Moltmann, *God in Creation: An Ecological Doctrine of Creation*, trans. Margaret Kohl. London: SCM, 1985.

Stephen Pattison, *Alive and Kicking: Towards a Practical Theology of Illness and Healing*. London: SCM, 1989.

John Wilkinson, *The Bible and Healing: A Medical and Theological Commentary*. Edinburgh: Handsel Press/Grand Rapids: Eerdmans, 1998.

**Notes**
1. A distinction is often made, particularly in the social scientific literature, between disease (a clinically diagnosed condition or set of symptoms), illness (the condition subjectively experienced by the patient, which may correspond to a greater or lesser extent to his or her clinically diagnosed condition) and sickness (a sociological phenomenon whereby a person who develops a disease or illness takes on a particular social role, the 'sick role', which carries altered responsibilities and expectations). See Pattison 1989.
2. Barth does not distinguish between these terms in the way described in note 1.
3. As I understand him, Barth does *not* mean that diseases are to be understood as God's punishment of individuals for specific sins.

# The Strength for Human Life

KARL BARTH

We now [turn] to the question of respect for life in the human sphere. In its form as the will to live, it also includes the will to be healthy. The satisfaction of the needs of the impulses corresponding to man's vegetative and animal nature is one thing, but health, although connected with it, is quite another. Health means capability, vigour and freedom. It is strength for human life. It is the integration of the organs for the exercise of psycho-physical functions . . .

If man may and should will to live, then obviously he may and should also will to be healthy and therefore to be in possession of this strength too. But the concept of this volition is problematical for many reasons and requires elucidation. For somehow it seems to be part of the nature of health that he who possesses it is not conscious of it nor preoccupied with it, but hardly ever thinks about it and cannot therefore be in any position to will it . . .

If this is so, we must ask whether a special will for health is not a symptom of deficient health which can only magnify the deficiency by confirming it. And a further question which might be raised with reference to this will is whether we can reasonably affirm and seek health independently, or otherwise than in connexion with specific material aims and purposes . . .

Yet included in the will to live there is a will to be healthy which is not affected by these legitimate questions but which, like the will to live, is demanded by God and is to be seriously achieved in obedience to this demand. By health we are not to think merely of a particular physical or psychical something of great value that can be considered and possessed by itself and therefore can and must be the object of special attention, search and effort. Health is the strength to be as man. It serves human existence in the form of the capacity, vitality and freedom to exercise the psychical and physical functions, just as these themselves are only functions of human existence. We can and should will it as this strength when we will not merely to be healthy in body and soul but to be man at all: man and not animal or plant, man and not wood or stone, man and not a thing or the exponent of an idea, man in his determination for work and knowledge, and above all

From *Church Dogmatics*, vol. III/4, §55.1, pp. 356–374, trans. A. T. MacKay et al. Edinburgh: T & T Clark, 1961.

in his relation to God and his fellow-men in the proffered act of freedom. We can and should will this, and therefore we can and should will to be healthy. For how can we will, understand or desire the strength for all this unless in willing we put it into operation in the smaller or greater measure in which we have it? And in willing to be man, how can we put it into operation unless we also will and seek and desire it? We gain it as we practise it. This is what is demanded of man in this respect.

Though we cannot deny the antithesis between health and sickness when we view the problem in this way, we must understand it in its relativity. Sickness is obviously negative in relation to health. It is partial impotence to exercise these functions. It hinders man in his exercise of them by burdening, hindering, troubling and threatening him, and causing him pain. But sickness as such is not necessarily impotence to be as man. The strength to be this, so long as one is still alive, can also be the strength and therefore the health of the sick person. And if health is the strength for human existence, even those who are seriously ill can will to be healthy without any optimism or illusions regarding their condition. They, too, are commanded, and it is not too much to ask, that so long as they are alive they should will this, i.e., exercise the power which remains to them, in spite of every obstacle. Hence it seems to be a fundamental demand of the ethics of the sick bed that the sick person should not cease to let himself be addressed, and to address himself, in terms of health and the will which it requires rather than sickness, and above all to see to it that he is in an environment of health. From the same standpoint we cannot count on conditions of absolute and total health, and therefore on the existence of men who are already healthy and do not need the command to will to be so. Even healthy people have great need of the will for health, though perhaps not of the doctor. Conditions of relative and subjectively total ease in relation to the psycho-physical functions of life may well exist. But whether the man who can enjoy such ease is healthy, i.e., a man who lives in the power to be as man, is quite another question which we need only ask, and we must immediately answer that in reality he may be severely handicapped in the exercise of this power, and therefore sick, long before this makes itself felt in the deterioration of his organs or their functional disturbance, so that he perhaps stands in greater need of the summons that he should be healthy than someone who already suffers from such deterioration and disturbance and is therefore regarded as sick in soul or body or perhaps both. And who of us has not constantly to win and possess this strength? A fundamental demand of ethics, even for the man who seems to be and to a large extent really is 'healthy in body and soul,' is thus that he should not try to evade the summons to be healthy in the true sense of the term.

On the same presupposition it will also be understood that in the question of health we must differentiate between soul and body but not on any account separate the two. The healthy man, and also the sick, is both. He is the soul of his body, the rational soul of his vegetative and animal body, the ruling soul of his serving body. But he is one and the same man in both, and not two. Health and sickness in the two do not constitute two divided realms, but are always a single whole. It is always a matter of the man himself, of his greater or lesser strength, and the more or less serious threat and even increasing impotence . . . [He] lives the healthy or sick life of his body together with that of his soul, and again in both cases, and in their mutual relationship, it is a matter of his life's history, his own history, and therefore himself. And the will for health as the strength to be as man is obviously quite simply, and without duplication in a psychical and physical sphere, the will to continue this history in its unity and totality. A man can, of course, orient himself seriously, but only secondarily, on this or that psychical or physical element of health in contrast to sickness. But primarily he will always orientate himself in this contrast on his own being as man, on his assertion, preservation and renewal (and all this in the form of activity) as a subject. In all his particular decisions and measures, if they are to be meaningful, he must have a primary concern to confirm his power to be as man and to deny the lack of power to be this. In all stages of that history the question to be answered is: 'Wilt thou be made whole?' (John 5:6), and not: 'Wilt thou have healthy limbs or be free of their sickness?' The command which we must always obey is the command to stand upright and not to fall.

From exactly the same standpoint again there can be no indifference to the concrete problems of getting and remaining well. If in the question of health we were concerned with a specific psychical or physical quantity, we might be interested at a distance in the one or the other, and seek health and satisfaction first in psychology and then in a somatic form of healing, only to tire no less arbitrarily of one or the other or perhaps both, and to let things take their course. But if on both sides it is a matter of the strength to be as man, on both sides we are free from the anxious or fanatical expectation that real decisions can and must be made, but also free to give to the psychical and physical spheres the attention due to them in this respect because they are the field on which the true decisions of the will for health must be worked out. It is precisely in the continuation of his life of soul and body that the history of man must continue in the strength to be as man. What he *can* do for the continuation and therefore against every restriction of his life of soul and body, he ought to *will* to do if he is to proceed in the strength of his being as man. In order that this strength may not degenerate into a process in which he is only driven as an object and is therefore no longer man, in order that he may remain its subject and therefore man, he must be on the watch and active for the continuation and against the constriction of his psychical and physical life. The fact that he wills to rise up and stand in this power, and not to fall into weakness is not in the least decided by the various measures which he might adopt to maintain and protect his psychical and physical powers. He could adopt a thousand measures of this kind with full zeal and skill, and yet not possess the will to maintain this strength, thus lacking the will for health and falling in spite of all his efforts. But if he possesses the will to win and maintain this strength, it is natural that he should be incidentally concerned to take the necessary precautions to preserve and protect his psychical and physical powers, and this in a responsible and energetic way in which the smallest thing is not too small for him nor the greatest too great . . .

But we have now to answer the two most difficult questions in this sphere. We have so far accepted the fact that man has the strength to be as man, that he can will and affirm it as such, and that he can therefore will and adopt the corresponding measures of this will in the sphere of his vital functions of soul and body. We have understood disease as merely the weakness opposed to this strength, as that which is not to be willed but contested in the will to live, as the shadow which recedes as it were before health and the will for health. This is one aspect of the matter. But there are two very different aspects, and we must now try to explain what the will to be healthy is in relation to them. We may begin by saying generally that sickness is not an illusion, even though there is such a thing as illusory sickness and therefore those who are ill only in their imagination . . .

[Barth attacks the notion that all sickness is illusory, particularly with reference to the writings of Mary Baker Eddy, founder of 'Christian Science', and continues . . .]

Sickness is real. Certainly, as an encroachment on the life which God has created, it is not real in the same way as God is. In what sense, then, is it real? We shall take up this point in a moment, but we may begin by observing that if man, even the sick man, is really healthy in the strength which he still has and can exert to be as man, then the weakness which opposes this strength is not as such an appearance but is effective and real, so that his will for health already meets a hard 'object' in this primary and essential sense . . . [The] will to live as the will for health is a serious act of obedience to a serious command of God because man is not dealing with a fake or imaginary opponent but with an enemy which is in some sense real. Yet the question arises what kind of reality this is. And we must try to explain this if we are to understand more deeply and seriously what the will to be healthy really means and does not mean. Again, however, two different aspects open up before us.

The one aspect which dominates the field in the Old and New Testament Scriptures, and which has always to be remembered first materially, is the one in which sickness is a forerunner and messenger of death, and indeed of death as the judgment of God and the merited subjection of man to the power of nothingness in virtue of his sin. From this standpoint, sickness like death itself is unnatural and disorderly. It is an element in the rebellion of chaos against God's creation. It is an act and declaration of the devil and demons. To be sure, it is no less bound to God and dependent on Him than the creature which He created. Indeed, it is impotent in relation to him in a double way. For like sin and death it is neither good nor is it willed and created by God at all, but is real, effective, powerful and menacing only as part of that which He has negated, of His kingdom on the left hand, and therefore with its nullity. But in accordance with the will of God and under His reign it is necessarily dangerous – as the forerunner and messenger of death, the executor of God's final sentence – to the man who has fallen from God and become His enemy.

What does health mean as the power to be as man, and what do the vital functions of soul and body mean as the sphere for the exercise of this strength, if sickness is this reality, if it is an element and sign of the power of the chaos threatening creation on the one hand, and on the other an element and sign of God's righteous wrath and judgment, in short, an element and sign of the objective corruption which is related and corresponds to human sin and from which there is no deliverance apart from the mercy of God in Jesus Christ? . . .

What does health mean from this standpoint, and what is the meaning of the will to be healthy in the primary and secondary senses in which we have hitherto understood it?

The following consideration suggests itself. When seen in this way, sickness is a superior power in relation to which there can be no question at all of health or the will to be healthy. What is man with his health and will for health in face of the invasion of the realm of death to which he has deliberately opened the defences? What is he in the face of the divine judgment by which he is overtaken in this assault? What can he do in this situation? What can the whole field of ethics tell him in these circumstances? What is there left to will? Strength to be as man? Psycho-physical powers? Is it not almost grotesque from this standpoint to try even to think of a human determination, let alone of human measures, along the lines considered? Are not faith and prayer the only real possibilities in the face of this reality of sickness?

But this whole consideration is only defeatist thinking, and not at all Christian. It overlooks the fact that the command of God is not withdrawn but still in force, namely, that man must will to live and not die, to be healthy and not to be sick, and to exercise and not neglect his strength to be as man and the remaining psycho-physical forces which he has for this purpose, and thus to maintain himself. This command has not been revoked even for sinful man forfeited to the judgment of God, and it is not for him to counter God with speculations whether obedience to it is possible or offers any prospects. Unquestioning obedience is his only option if he is not to bring himself into even greater condemnation. Again, this consideration overlooks the fact that the realm of death which afflicts man in the form of sickness, although God has given it power and it serves as an instrument of His righteous judgment, is opposed to His good will as Creator and has existence and power only under His mighty No. To capitulate before it, to allow it to take its course, can never be obedience but only disobedience towards God. In harmony with the will of God, what man ought to will in face of this whole realm on the left hand, and therefore in face of sickness, can only be final resistance. Again and supremely, this consideration overlooks the fact that God Himself is not only Judge but faithful, gracious and patient in His righteous judgment, that He Himself has already marched against that realm on the left, and that he has overcome and bound its forces and therefore those of sickness in Jesus Christ and His sacrifice, by which the destroyer was himself brought to destruction. Those who know this, and therefore that they are already helped in this matter, can only reply to the faithfulness of God with a new unfaithfulness if they try to fold their hands and sigh and ask what help there is or what more they can will. Within the modest limits in which this is still possible they must will what God has already willed and indeed definitely fulfilled in Jesus Christ concerning sickness and that whole kingdom on the left hand. With God they must say No to it without asking what the result will be or how much or little it will help themselves or others, without enquiring whether it is not rather feeble and even ridiculous to march into action in accordance with this No. A little resolution, will and action in the face of that realm and therefore against sickness is better than a whole ocean of pretended Christian humility which is really perhaps the mistaken and perverted humility of the devil and demons.

There is, of course, a right deduction to be drawn from the fact that sickness is real in this sense, i.e., as an element and sign of the power of chaos and nothingness, and therefore as an element and sign of the judgment of God falling on man. The right deduction is that all resistance to sickness, all human willing of the strength to be as man, all human affirmation, cultivation and promotion of the vital forces of body and soul, is necessarily in vain if God is not God; if He does not live, speak, act and make Himself responsible for man; if this whole cause is not first and supremely His own cause; if His is not the judgment on man from which we cannot escape; if His is not the grace which is the meaning of this judgment; and above all if His is not the judgment on the destroyer and destruction itself which by reason of man's sin can have a little space, but which can have only the space allowed and allotted by God, and in relation to which God is absolute Lord and conclusive Victor. Without or even against God there is, of course, nothing that man can will in this matter. And if faith in Him and prayer to Him cannot be a refuge for weak-willed and defeatist Christians who are lazy, cowardly and resigned in the face of His and their enemy, we must also say with the same certainty that if the conflict enjoined upon man in this matter is to be meaningful, faith in Him and prayer to Him must never be lost sight of as its *conditio sine qua non*, but continually realised as the true power of the will required of man in this affair. They cannot replace what is to be modestly, soberly and circumspectly, but energetically, willed and done by man. They cannot replace his determination to exercise his little strength to be as man, and thereby to maintain himself. They cannot replace hygiene, sport and medicine, or the social struggle for better living conditions for all. But in all these things they must be the orientation on the command of God which summons man inexorably, and with no possible conditions, to will and action. They must be the orientation on the righteous judgment of God in recognition of which man constantly discovers, and again without murmuring or surrender, the limitation of his willing and doing and its consequences. Above all, they must be the orientation on the inexhaustible consolation of the promise, on true and effective encouragement by the One who as the Creator of life primarily espouses this as His own cause, and fights and has already conquered for us in the whole glory of His mercy and omnipotence. It is true that without Him, without the orientation on Him, all ethics, all human willing and doing, can only be futile and impotent in relation to the superiority of evil which opposes us also in the form of sickness; and worse still, that it can only be rebellion against the judgment of God and therefore increase its severity. But it is also true, and even more so, that human willing and acting with God, and in orientation on Him, and with faith and prayer to Him, whatever the outcome, has the promise which man cannot lack, and the fulfilment of which he will soon see, if he will simply obey without speculation. Those who take up this struggle obediently are already healthy in the fact that they do so, and theirs is no empty desire when they will to maintain or regain their health . . .

But the fact is undeniable that sickness also has another aspect. For health, like life in general, is not an eternal but a temporal and therefore a limited possession. It is entrusted to man, but it does not belong to him. It is to be affirmed and willed by man as a gift from God, yet not in itself and absolutely, but in the manner and compass in which He gives it.

We have defined health as the power to be as man exercised in the powers of the vital functions of soul and body. And we have defined sickness as the impairing of this power, as crippling and hampering weakness. We have seen that in the antithesis, contrast and conflict of these two determinations of human life we have to do with a real event in the existence of the real man. And we have first attempted to evaluate this event from the angle from which it presents itself as the collision of normal being, as willed, created and ordered by God, with its negation, so that it is brought under the threat of abnormality and even destruction. On this view it can be understood only as man's encounter with the realm of death and therefore the experience of God's judgment. We have been able to describe the required human attitude, the will to live and to be healthy, only in terms of the resistance and conflict of faith and prayer appealing to the grace and gracious power of God. And if we have now to draw attention to another aspect of the same matter, there can be no question – we are irresistibly prevented by the biblical witness concerning health and sickness – of looking away from this first aspect or even trying to relativise or weaken it. Sickness is one of the elements in the situation of man as he has fallen victim to nothingness through his transgression, as he is thus referred wholly to the mercy of God, but as he is summoned by this reference to hope and courage and conflict. Not a single word of what we have said in this connexion can be retracted or even limited. It must not be lost sight of or forgotten in whatever we have to add.

What is there to add? Simply that, quite apart from his transgression, quite apart from his abandonment to the power of nothingness, and quite apart from the consequent visitation of God's judgment upon him, the life of man, and therefore his health as the strength to be as man in the exercise of the powers of all his vital functions of life, is a life which even according to God's good will as Creator, and therefore normally and naturally, begins and ends and is therefore limited. Man does not possess the power to be as man in the same way as God has His power to be as God, nor does he have power over his vital functions as God has His power as Creator, Ruler and merciful Deliverer of His creature. Rather, he may see the goodness of God the Creator in the fact that to his life and strength and powers a specific space is allotted, i.e., a limited span. He may and should exercise them in it and not in the field of the unlimited. They are adapted for it, for development and application within it. Within its confines he may and should be as man in their possession and exercise. Within its confines he stands before God, and at the limit of this span God is mightily for him and is his hope. Just because it is limited, it is a kind of natural and normal confirmation of the fact that by God's free grace man may live through Him and for Him, with the commission to be as man in accordance with the measure of his strength and powers, but not under the intolerable destiny of having to give sense, duration and completeness to his existence by his own exertions and achievements, and therefore in obvious exclusion of the view that he must and may and can by his own strength and powers eternally maintain, assert and confirm himself, attaining for himself his own dignity and honour. The eternal God Himself guarantees all this, and tells him that He does so by giving him a life that is temporal and therefore limited. In this way it always remains in His hand both in its majesty and in its littleness. In itself and as such this fact cannot be an object of complaint, protest or rebellion, nor can the fact that man must make the concrete discovery that his life and therefore his health and strength and powers are not an unlimited reality, but that he is impeded in their possession and exercise, that weakness is real as well as strength, that there is destruction as well as construction, obstruction as well as development. This is all the more terrible because it is just from this direction that we find ourselves threatened by death and judgment. But is it really surprising and shocking in itself? The life of man, his commission, and his strength to fulfil it, are not limited accidentally but by God, and therefore not to his destruction but to his salvation. Inevitably, then, he always in some way comes up concretely against this boundary of his life. Inevitably he must grow old and decline. Inevitably he must concretely encounter his Creator and Lord and therefore God's omnipotence and mercy. But is it merely a question of necessity? In the correct sense, is it not true to say that, no less than in his unimpeded movement within these confines, this is also a possibility? May it not be that genuine freedom to live can and must be concretely realised in the fact that in the impending and impairing of his life he is shown that neither his life nor he himself is in his own hand, but that he is in God's hand, that he is surrounded by Him on all sides, that he is referred wholly to Him, but also that he is reliably upheld by Him? Does not this freedom begin at the very point where we are confronted by the hard actuality of the insight that 'Christ will be our consolation'? But what if sickness as the concrete form of weakness, of destruction, of the impairing of his strength and powers, of growing old and declining, is the hard actuality which ushers in this genuinely liberating insight? What if it is not only the forerunner and messenger of death and judgment, but also, concealed under this form, the witness of God's creative goodness, the forerunner and messenger of the eternal life which God has allotted and promised to the man who is graciously preserved and guided by Him within the confines of his time? . . .

It is surely clear that there can be no question of anything but a bold penetration beyond the form of death and judgment, when we maintain that what we know as sickness has in deep concealment another form, in which it reflects not only the power of the devil or even the wrath of God but also the divine benevolence. We surely cannot think and speak of this lightly, nor can it be meant as an alternative to the first view of sickness. All that can be meant is that when the hard and bitter shell of the first aspect is broken, when therefore the fight of faith and prayer and action is manfully and with God's help victoriously fought against sickness, it finally contains and reveals this kernel, namely, that it is good for man to live a limited and impeded life, and to be aware of the fact that, when he has exercised and used his strength and powers in obedience, he must return them to the One who has lent them to him. There is still no question of capitulation to sickness, far less to the realm of death manifested in it. But there is certainly capitulation to God who is the Lord even of sickness and the realm of death, and who is gracious to man even in the fact that He permits him to fall sick, to be sick and perhaps even to die of sickness. Again, there is no question of being no longer terrified at death or of taking lightly the judgment of God revealed in it. But there is certainly a recognition and apprehension in suffering and dying as such of a natural happening now necessarily concealed by death and judgment, of a form of the creative goodness of God beyond death and judgment, of the objectively near promise of His free grace. Again, there is no question of giving up the will for health and the fight against sickness. But there is certainly a full and true readiness to become and be well exclusively through and for God, which must necessarily consist in quiet endurance of the present and perhaps triumphant sickness. Strictly speaking, therefore, the necessary augmentation of what we have already said can consist only in the recollection that, if this fight is to be fought rightly and finally, it will not exclude but include patience. Sickness in so far as it is still present, the impairing, disturbing and destroying of life in so far as these are an event and cannot be removed by faith and prayer and the most manful fighting, have therefore to be 'borne' in the sense that they are drawn by God – who is present in this way, too, as Lord and Victor – into what He wills from and with man, and what in its entirety, because it comes from Him, cannot be evil but only good, and cannot finally be pain but only joy.

# A Blind Person's Conversations with the Bible

JOHN M. HULL

## To Heal or to Transform Through Acceptance

> Care for the injured and weak, do not ridicule the lame, protect the maimed, and let the blind have a vision of my splendour. Protect the old and the young within your walls. (II. Esd. 2:21f.)

> They [the idols of the heathen] cannot save anyone from death or rescue the weak from the strong. They cannot restore sight to the blind; they cannot rescue one who is in distress. (The Letter of Jeremiah (Baruch) 6:36f.)

These passages present contrasting theologies of disability. The first, from II Esdras, is a beautiful passage in which the people are called upon to renew their covenant with God in justice, mercy and peace. The community is to be transformed through acceptance and inclusion. Differences between people are not to be greeted with ridicule but to be accepted peacefully. Whereas quite often in the Bible one gets the impression that blind people have somehow failed to meet the standard of a perfect creation and are thus excluded from intimacy with God, in this remarkable passage the religious equality of blind people is affirmed. Without ceasing to be genuinely blind, visually impaired people can nevertheless have a vision of the divine splendour. Blindness is not an impediment in the holy place where God's glory is to be seen.

The passage from the Letter of Jeremiah[1] represents an inferior theology. We are now in the atmosphere of a crude competition between the true and the false gods, and a simple list of criteria is offered to tell the difference. A characteristic of the false gods is that they are unable to restore the sight of blind people. The consequence of this crude theology of intervention is that blind people who remain in their blindness, and may even behold a vision of the divine splendour, are regarded as being under the power of an idol or demon simply because they continue to be blind. It is the survival of this approach to blindness, often reinforced by the healing miracles in the

From *In the Beginning There Was Darkness: A Blind Person's Conversations with the Bible*, pp. 107–113. London: SCM, 2001.

Gospels, which makes some sighted Christians feel uncomfortable in the presence of blind Christians.

In September 1996, when I was lecturing in Seoul, I was invited to speak at a church for disabled people. This was a remarkable experience for me, There were about twenty or twenty-five there. Some were lame or had lost part of a limb. Some were in wheelchairs, others were deaf or had speech defects. Others, like myself, were blind or partially sighted. I asked them why it was necessary for them to have their own special church. 'Oh,' they replied, 'it's because the people in the ordinary churches say that we make them feel uncomfortable.' I spoke to them about the disabled persons' God, and then we held hands (if we had any) and sang until the tears ran down our cheeks. On the way back in the car, my host said, 'Now you have experienced *enyuan*.' This is a Confucian concept and refers to the joyful solidarity which is experienced by the oppressed when they encounter deliverance. 'When the Lord restored the fortunes of Zion, we were like those who dream. Then our mouth was filled with laughter, and our tongue with shouts of joy' (Ps. 126:1f.) It was sad that the people in ordinary churches, controlled by their rigid view of perfection and their competitive God, could not share in that joy.

## Restoring or Accepting: Two Policies Towards Blindness

> I will lead the blind by a road they do not know, by paths they have not known I will guide them. I will turn the darkness before them into light, the rough places into level ground. These are the things I will do, and I will not forsake them. (Isa. 42:16)

Restoration of sight is a distinctive feature of the activity of God as Saviour and Redeemer in the Bible. In Psalm 146:8 we read, 'the Lord opens the eyes of the blind, the Lord lifts up those who are bowed down'. This is a particular feature of the coming reign of God. When Isaiah is describing the Messianic age, he says, 'Then the eyes of the blind shall be opened, and the ears of the deaf unstopped; then the lame shall leap like a deer, and the tongue of the speechless sing for joy' (Isa. 35:5f.). This is to be one of the characteristics of the work of the Servant of the Lord, whose mission is described in the famous series of psalms which begin in Isaiah 42.

> I am the Lord, I have called you in righteousness,
> 　　I have taken you by the hand and kept you;
> I have given you as a covenant to the people,
> 　　　a light to the nations,
> 　　　to open the eyes that are blind,

to bring out the prisoners from the dungeon,
>    from the prison those who sit in darkness.
>                                    (Isa. 42:6f.)

It is all the more remarkable, in view of the popularity of the idea that God would open the eyes of the blind, to find in the passage quoted at the heading of this section, no such thing takes place. Blind people are not changed, restored or miraculously healed. They are accepted and the behaviour of others around them is modified to give them equal opportunities.

To blind people, familiarity is all important. When I am walking on one of my familiar paths, I need no assistance. It is when I venture into the unknown that I become hesitant. The opening up of a new route is as much an adventure as blazing a new trail through the wilderness. It is almost imposs-ible to do this when sighted people are around, because one inevitably gives the impression of being lost. To sighted people, the behaviour of an exploring blind person cannot be distinguished from the behaviour of a lost blind person. When you are lost, you are not exploring the unknown, because you do not know whether the place you are at is known or not. You have become disorientated. When you are exploring a new route, you are oriented towards the direction of the route. However, this necessarily involves exploring peri-meters, going around all four corners of a square, tracing the lawn right around the quadrangle in order to find where it goes. To sighted people watching, the desire to help is irresistible, and very understandable and forgivable. It is self-defeating, however, for when a blind person is being helped it is more difficult for him or her to learn independence on the new route.

In the situation where you do not have to learn a route but simply need to get somewhere, then a guide is important. There is no point in learning the route, since you probably will not come that way again. So we see that the words in Isa. 42:16 are most appropriate, 'I will lead the blind by a road they do not know'. In other words, because they are passing through a strange territory, I will be their guide. There is no need for them to learn the route because they are being led into a new land. Therefore the Lord will lead us in paths which we have not known. It does not mean that God will deliberately lead us into places we do not know; it means that because we do not know the way, God will lead us. By this process of guidance, the darkness in front of us will be turned into light. When I am touching the elbow of an experienced and trusted guide, I do not have to worry about falling into a trench or stumbling down some stairs. It is as if the rough places were turned into level ground – not that rough places present a particular difficulty to blind people, but unexpected ledges and unpredictable rough places are a bit of a problem. God as the guide understands all these techniques. Where would I be now if my guide should suddenly desert me?

Would I be able to find my way out, or back? Such questions need not trouble us, because our guide says, 'I will not forsake them'.

Why does God not save all this trouble by simply restoring our sight? Then God would not have to guide us. Well, it looks as if God likes us the way we are. God enjoys guiding us and likes us to trust God's expert assistance. God does not patronize us but simply gets on with the job, giving us a sense of confidence as we walk. After all, as we allow God to lead us in this way, we are like God's chosen servant. Although sometimes God's servant is described as opening the eyes of the blind, at other times the servant himself is blind. Sometimes this is said ironically, because the servant himself does not seem to understand the high calling of God.

> Listen, you that are deaf;
> > and you that are blind, look up and see!
> Who is blind but my servant,
> > or deaf like my messenger whom I send?
> Who is blind like my dedicated one,
> > or blind like the servant of the Lord?
> He sees many things, but does not observe them;
> > his ears are open, but he does not hear.
> > > (Isa. 42:18f.)

The blindness and deafness of the servant, who represents the chosen, suffering people of God, is a metaphor for the failure of the people to interpret their mission, but in Isa. 50:10 the tone is quite different. 'Who among you fears the Lord and obeys the voice of his servant, who walks in darkness and has no light, yet trusts in the name of the Lord and relies on his God?' In this verse, the model of the blind person who with calm assurance allows God to be the guide is applied to the relationship between God and God's special servant. The trustfulness of the servant who walks calmly forward in the darkness, depending upon God, is a challenge to all who witness it. It is not so much that they look but do not perceive; it is a question of whether they have sufficient faith to follow the example of blind people. Far from having their sight miraculously restored, blind people become a model of faithfulness in their very blindness. A similar ideal is offered by Jeremiah, when he is describing the return of the exiled people to their promised homeland:

> See, I am going to ring them from the land of the north,
> > and gather them from the farthest parts of the earth,
> among them the blind and lame,
> > those with child and those in labour, together;
> > a great company, they shall return here.

With weeping child they shall come,
    and with consolations I will lead them back.
                                                (Jer. 31:8f.)

The wonderful thing about this passage is that it does not entice or insult disabled people by amazing promises. It simply says that they will be included along with everyone else in the joyful repatriation. Indeed, they will have as natural a part in the crowd as expectant mothers, for pregnancy is not a disease or deficiency. Moreover, no matter how great the crisis into which their disability plunges them, they, like the women who are actually in childbirth, will be accepted and assisted in their crisis, and normalized within the community.

An even more dramatic thought is found in Micah, who suggests that disabled people will not only be included in the community of the returning exiles; they will be the very heart and soul of that community.

In that day, says the Lord,
    I will assemble the lame
and gather those who have been driven away,
    and those whom I have afflicted.
The lame I will make the remnant,
    and those who were cast off, a strong nation;
and the Lord will reign over them in Mount Zion
    now and evermore.
                                                (Mic. 4:6f.)

To some extent, the idea is that there is no limit to God's restoring power. Perhaps the able-bodied people were a bit bothered about the long return journey, but Micah says that even if they were disabled, God would bring them back. Indeed, God prefers the lame and other people who in weakness and disability have been driven out, because in a very special way they symbolize the alienated and oppressed people whom God delights to deliver. We notice also that they are delivered not by being saved from their disabilities, in a series of healing miracles, but by becoming the people of God. Their delight is not in ceasing to be disabled but in having God as their Redeemer and King.

Now we can return to the passages where the restoration of sight is promised. It is important to realize that this is not offered as a wonderful miracle, of the kind that would startle the medical profession, as is claimed in so many modern healing crusades. Rather, it is almost always in the context of the restoration of an oppression, the setting right of an injustice. We referred to Psalm 146, where it says that the Lord opens the eyes of the blind and lifts up those who are bowed down. It is time now to consider the context of these promises. In verse 7, God is described as one who 'executes justice for the oppressed; who gives food to the hungry. The Lord sets the prisoners free', and then we have (v. 8), 'The Lord opens the eyes of the blind'. This is the first place (not necessarily the oldest) in the Bible where opening of the eyes of the blind is mentioned, and we fail to understand this unless we recognize that it is the context not of medical miracle but of the determination of God to rectify injustice. Those who remove miracles of healing from this justice context are not faithful to the spirit of scripture. Too often, they literalize the illustration and forget the context. Their hearts are set on the sensationalism of the miracle rather than on the social and political calling to alleviate the oppressed.

**Notes**
1. Sometimes printed as chapter 6 of Baruch.

# CASE STUDY:
## Cochlear Implants for Deaf Children

Cochlear implants are electronic devices which can be inserted into the inner ears of totally deaf people to enable them to perceive sound. Sound is picked up by an external microphone and converted into an electric stimulus to the auditory nerve, which transmits signals from the ear to the brain. It is widely agreed that implants can benefit adults who have become profoundly deaf after acquiring speech and language. There is more controversy over cochlear implantation in young children who have been born profoundly deaf. Medical studies suggest that many children who receive implants around the age of two can acquire some intelligible speech and be educated in mainstream schools. However, the British Deaf Association (BDA) opposes cochlear implantation in young children, arguing that this treatment assumes a 'medical model' of deafness as a defect that must be corrected. The BDA argues instead for a 'social model' in which the Deaf community is regarded as a linguistic minority whose first language is sign language. On this view, giving children limited hearing and speech by means of cochlear implantation may cut them off from the vibrant culture of the Deaf community without enabling them to be fully integrated into the hearing world.

## Questions
- Is it possible to make a distinction between disease and human diversity, and how can we discern which is which?
- Which model or models are most helpful for understanding deafness: medical, social or other models, or some combination of them?
- If you had to take part in a decision about giving a cochlear implant to a profoundly deaf young child, what would guide your decision?

## Sources
Richard Ramsden and John Graham, 'Cochlear Implantation', *British Medical Journal* 311, 1588 (1995).
British Deaf Association, *The British Deaf Association Policy on Cochlear Implants*, www.britishdeafassociation.org.uk/cochlearpolicyfull.html (accessed 15 February 2002).

# 5

# DEATH

## Introduction

It is often said that modern medicine has raised many new problems and conundrums about death. For example, it is possible to treat many conditions that in earlier generations would have proved fatal – but is it always right to do so? How aggressively should antibiotics be used, for example, to treat infections such as pneumonia in patients who are in any case near the end of their lives? Judgements as to when to intervene and when to refrain can be difficult and finely balanced. In this context, the further questions of active euthanasia and physician-assisted suicide arise: is it ever right to kill patients who may be terminally ill and suffering terrible pain, or to help them kill themselves? In recent years, well-publicised court cases have placed these issues firmly on the agenda of public debate.

Further difficult questions arise in cases where medical devices can keep a patient's body functioning for a time even when the brain is so severely damaged that its functions are irreversibly lost. This has given rise to the concepts of 'brain death' and 'brain stem death'. 'Brain death' refers to the irreversible loss of at least the higher centres of the brain, while 'brain stem death' refers to the irreversible loss of the part of the brain which maintains the body's vital functions (Vere 1995). These concepts can seem paradoxical, since a patient can be declared dead while her heart, aided by life support machinery, is still beating. Gregory Rutecki points out that it may not be as odd as it seems: death in these circumstances is inevitable, since without a functioning brain stem, the heart, lungs and other vital organs will inevitably cease to function within a few days despite artificial life support (Rutecki 1995, 286). However, as Stanley Hauerwas cautions in the first reading of this chapter, we should not confuse criteria for establishing that death has occurred with an account of the meaning of death.

Pragmatically, irreversible loss of brain function may be a reliable indicator that death has occurred, but to say this is not to say that death simply *means* the irreversible loss of consciousness and other brain functions.

More difficult still are conditions such as persistent vegetative state (PVS), in which the brain stem remains alive, and capable of sustaining vital functions, but all higher brain activity is lost. A patient in PVS does not need life support to remain physically alive, but shows no signs of consciousness and is not considered to have any hope of regaining consciousness in the future. He or she is incapable of any voluntary action and must therefore be artificially fed. In Britain, the case of Tony Bland gave the ethical and legal questions about PVS a high profile. He entered PVS as a result of injuries he sustained in the Hillsborough football stadium disaster in 1989, and after a long legal process, the House of Lords granted his parents' request that artificial feeding be withdrawn, allowing him to die (see Habgood 1998, 14–17 for an outline of this case). In the USA, the case of Karen Quinlan raised similar questions (see chapter 2, p. 42–44).

The answers we give to these and other questions about the end of life rest on our deepest convictions about life and death. It is often said that two opposite attitudes towards death can be discerned in contemporary Western societies such as Britain and the USA (cf. Guroian 1996, 3–18). On the one hand, death is regarded as the ultimate catastrophe, to be postponed, avoided or denied at all costs. On the other, euthanasia may be promoted as an easy alternative to terminal illness and intractable suffering.

Stanley Hauerwas, in the first reading, suggests that both of these opposite responses – regarding death as the ultimate catastrophe and welcoming it too easily and unambiguously as a friend – are inadequate from a Christian point of view. Our attitude to death must be more nuanced than either: we should regard it as 'both a friend and an enemy'. It is a friend because it sets a limit on our present life, and by facing us with the prospect that our life will end, teaches us to value what is worthwhile in love; it is an enemy in that it takes from us those things that it has taught us to value. But in a Christian perspective, it is emphatically not the worst thing that can happen to a person. Hauerwas, furthermore, suggests that much of our perplexity over death and how to care appropriately for the dying arises because we have forgotten how to speak of the dying person's moral responsibility to die a 'good death'. To die well, he argues, is not to conform to a general pattern or notion of what a good death looks like, but to die 'in a manner that is morally commensurate with the kind of trust that has sustained him or her in life' (p. 136). For the Christian, a good death should witness both to the human relationships that have sustained us and to our ultimate trust in God, the ultimate giver of life who has freed us from the curse of death through Jesus Christ.

The second reading, by Vigen Guroian, is part of the Christian vision of death which he articulates from an Orthodox perspective. He discusses the connection between sin and death, and argues that the complete meaning of death, while it includes biological demise, is much more than a merely biological phenomenon: it is above all a spiritual reality. With reference to Orthodox burial rites, he explores the journey through death. He points to the importance of repentance, not indeed in reversing the process of physical death, but in opening the way to a psychological and spiritual healing and hope made possible by the death and resurrection of Christ.

## References and Further Reading

Robin Gill (ed.), *Euthanasia and the Churches*. London: Cassell, 1998.

Vigen Guroian, *Life's Living Towards Dying*. Grand Rapids: Eerdmans, 1996.

John Habgood, *Being a Person: Where Faith and Science Meet*. London: Hodder & Stoughton, 1998.

Gregory Rutecki, 'Christian Care for the Dying', in John F. Kilner et al (eds.), *Bioethics and the Future of Medicine: A Christian Appraisal*, 279–290. Carlisle: Paternoster/Grand Rapids: Eerdmans, 1995.

D. W. Vere, 'Brain Death', in David J. Atkinson and David H. Field (eds.), *New Dictionary of Christian Ethics and Pastoral Theology*, 199–200. Leicester: IVP, 1995.

# Religious Concepts of Brain Death and Associated Problems

STANLEY HAUERWAS

## The Limits of Theological Determination of the Moment of Death

Theologians are considered an odd lot today. We sense the public's bemusement as soon as we try to explain what we do, because we are immediately subject to suspicious questioning. If you are fortunate, your listener misunderstands theology for geology and assumes you are engaged in an honest endeavor. However, if you go on to explain that you are not a geologist, but a theologian, you are confronted with a quizzical stare that makes you feel that an explanation, if not an apology, is in order. Generally, I assume that this means that people do not think it is odd for someone to spend his or her life thinking about rocks, but that it is an aberration to spend your life thinking about God.

There is, of course, good reason for this judgment – thinking about rocks seems to have some payoff in a way that thinking about God does not. Rocks are connected to oil in an immediate and direct way, and even the best prayer will not make a car run without gas. Therefore, when theologians are invited to speak at conferences on such matters as the determination of brain death, they are extremely anxious to please. Such conferences represent an opportunity to show that theology has concrete relevance.

Therefore you will understand how disappointed I am to have to tell you that there is nothing in Christian convictions that would entail preference for one definition of death over another. That is not to say that there have not been a lot of perceptive and incisive things said by theologians about the determination of the moment of death. However, it remains unclear what connection there is between their theological views and their judgments about death.

The claim that a connection must be demonstrated between Christian conviction and determination of the moment of death may seem odd. After all, physicians often deal with people who tell them that their Christian

From *Suffering Presence: Theological Reflections on Medicine, the Mentally Handicapped and the Church*, pp. 87–99. Edinburgh: T & T Clark, 1988.

convictions have something to do with their death. There seems to be good reason for this claim, since basic biblical texts deal with death. Thus in Paul's letter to the Romans we are told

> If we have died with Christ, we believe that we shall also live with him. For we know that Christ being raised from the dead will never die again; death no longer has dominion over him. The death he died to sin, once for all, but the life he lives he lives to God. So you also must consider yourselves dead to sin and alive to God in Christ. (Rom. 6:8–11)

In even more ringing terms Paul says

> Who shall separate us from the love of Christ? Shall tribulation or distress or persecution or famine, or nakedness, or peril, or sword? As it is written, 'For thy sake we are being killed all the day long; we are regarded as sheep to be slaughtered.' No, in all these things we are more than conquerors through him who loved us. For I am sure that neither death, nor life, nor angels, nor principalities, nor things present, nor things to come, nor powers, nor height, nor depth, nor anything else in all creation, will be able to separate us from the love of God in Christ Jesus our Lord. (Rom. 8:35–39)

These are powerful and substantive claims. Yet Paul Ramsey, a theologian who has dealt extensively with death and dying, stated with regard to a theological definition of the moment of death that 'a theologian or moralist as such knows nothing about such questions; the determination of death is a medical matter; and a theologian or moralist can offer only his reflections upon the meaning of respect for life and care of the dying, and issue some warnings of the moral complexities surrounding such matters' ([8], p.104).

In this essay I will explain why Ramsey is right to deny that there is a theological definition of the moment of death. Christians hold some very substantive beliefs about death itself, however, and I want to suggest how in general those beliefs help to provide a framework for the moral and practical considerations connected with definitions of the moment of death. In the foregoing passages from Paul death is described theologically and morally. I will try to show how those perspectives on death help to set the kind of questions that should be asked about the meaning and status of any proposed definition of the moment of death.

## The Meaning and Status of Brain Death

In order to understand the reluctance of theologians to provide a 'religious concept of brain death,' it is necessary to be clear about what brain death means. There is no reason for me to go over the work that Veatch [9] has done so well, but I will center my concerns about the very helpful distinction he provides. Veatch's central point is that the concept of death should not be confused with the criteria that determine when death has occurred. He rightly argues that the concept of death involves a philosophical judgment of a significant change that has happened in a person. Thus the concept of death is a correlative of what one takes to be the necessary condition of life, e.g., the capacity for bodily integration or the potential for consciousness.

Correlative to different concepts of death are certain loci and criteria of death. Loci are places where we look to determine whether or not the person is dead, i.e. heart, brain, neocortex. The criteria of death are those empirical measurements that can be made to determine whether a person is dead, such as cessation of respiration or a flat EEG. The subtle point of Veatch's analysis is that there is no necessary connection between certain concepts of death and the determination of the locus and criteria of death ([9], p. 51). Rather, the claim is made that certain associations of the loci and criteria of death with certain concepts of death seem more appropriate than others, but these associations are pragmatic and contingent, not conceptual and necessary. Thus it seems reasonable to identify the locus of death with the brain if one understands the concept of death to involve the irreversible loss of capacity for bodily integration. It also seems appropriate to use the criteria of the Harvard report as an indication of when death has occurred. 'Brain death' is an empirical standard for verifying a death, but it does not involve one and only one concept of death. So Veatch is right to suggest that 'terms such as brain death or heart death should be avoided because they tend to obscure the fact that we are searching for the meaning of death of the person as a whole' ([9], p.37).

For those dealing with dying patients this kind of analysis may seem to be question-begging. However such an analysis is but a reminder that genuinely practical matters often raise deep theoretical issues. These issues are absolutely crucial if we are to consider questions such as how to determine the moment of death without confusing them with questions concerning the worth of prolonging life under certain circumstances. For nothing could be more dangerous than the attempt to substitute a definition of the moment of death for a moral question concerning our obligation to keep ourselves and others alive under conditions of distress. A definition of death should not preclude the question of the worth of a life. The question regarding the worth of Karen Quinlan's life should not be precluded by defining her as dead.

This distinction helps to clarify why the issue of defining the criteria of death should not be determined in terms of the need for transplant organs. Whatever the concept of death we think appropriate, the criteria of death should take into account the dying person's needs. If the phrase 'right to die' makes any sense at all, it should at least mean that we should be allowed to die without the meaning of our death being determined by someone else's needs.

More important for the purpose of this paper, however, is the distinction between the concept of death and the loci and criteria of death to help make clear the role of Christian convictions about death. As I suggested, there may not be a religious concept of brain death. That does not mean, though, that Christian beliefs may not contribute to an understanding of the concept of death. This issue has been confused in the past by assuming that the use of a metaphor like the 'heart' in religious discourse implied a position about the locus or criteria of death. But 'heart' so used is not an empirical description of a part of the body, but rather an indication of the whole person's engagements with life. Thus the question arises of how Christian beliefs about the nature of death might make a difference in how the concept of death is understood.

## Sacredness of Life and the Concept of Death

The claim that Christian convictions make a difference in how the concept of death is understood remains ambiguous. Note how abstract such phrases as 'irreversible loss of the soul from the body,' or 'irreversible loss of capacity for bodily integration,' or 'loss of consciousness' are when compared with the life plans of people. For example, I have known some 'good old boys' who felt strongly that when you became too old to ride a horse you might as well be dead. If you told them that they were thereby committed to assuming death to consist of 'loss of consciousness,' thereby making the neocortex the locus of death and the criterion a flat EEG, they would probably tell you that they don't give a damn.

Christian beliefs about death work like 'riding a horse,' i.e. the beliefs shape the Christian's conception of death. The Christian is concerned not with life as an end in itself, but rather as the medium for service in God's kingdom. Put differently, no one lives just to live. We each live for some purpose or purposes. These purposes set certain boundaries that determine the meaning and significance of death. Christians believe that their lives have been determined by the purposes of God as manifest in the history of Israel and Jesus' cross and resurrection. Thus for Paul the 'death' that concerns him the most is the death that reigns in this life through the power of sin. The problem is that there is no clear inference that can be drawn from this sense of the purpose of life concerning which concept of death is most appropriate for the Christian.

With respect to life, however, it has recently been claimed that the basic stance of Christians toward life is that it is sacred. This obviously has been claimed in questions concerning death and dying and abortions. There is surely much about the phrase 'sanctity of life' in which Christians have a stake. We believe that God has sanctified every living thing and that each of his creatures, even the most wayward, cannot escape his care – in both life and death.

This claim regarding the sacredness of life often indicates the refusal of the Christian to separate the spirit from the body. Although there is much talk about the soul in Christian discourse, Christians always maintain the Jewish sense of the body's significance. Thus Ramsey maintains that

> Just as man is sacredness in the social and political order, so he is a sacredness in the natural, biological order. He is a sacredness in bodily life. He is a person who within the ambience of the flesh claims our care. He is an embodied soul or ensouled body. He is therefore a sacredness in illness and in his dying . . . The sanctity of human life prevents ultimate trespass upon him even for the sake of treating his bodily life, or for the sake of others who are also only a sacredness in their bodily lives. ([8], p. xiii)

This at least means that Christians will be suspicious of any concept of death that associates the death only with so-called 'higher forms of our life.' Of course that does not mean that the neocortex is ruled out as the locus of death, since it may well be the best indication that the bodily conditions necessary for our consciousness can no longer be sustained.

It is a mistake to assume that 'sanctity of life' is a sufficient criterion for an appropriate concept of death. Appeals to the sanctity of life beg exactly the question at issue, namely that you know what kind of life it is that should be treated as sacred. More troubling for me, however, is how the phrase 'sanctity of life,' when separated from its theological context, became an ideological slogan for a narrow individualism antithetical to the Christian way of life. Put starkly, Christians are not fundamentally concerned about living. Rather, their concern is to die for the right thing. Appeals to the sanctity of life as an ideology make it appear that Christians are committed to the proposition that there is nothing in life worth dying for.

When this happens Christians unwittingly embody the modern view that death is the one thing we can be sure about in life and that it is to be avoided as long as possible. As my former colleague, Rev. John Dunne, C.S.C., has pointed out, Descartes said 'I think, therefore I am,' while modern man says 'I am going to die, therefore I am.' Our identity is no longer anchored in life, but in death. As a result, death becomes the overriding enemy. But such an attitude is antithetical to the Christian belief that our identity is anchored in God's love as revealed in the cross. Even death itself cannot separate us from that.

Thus the phrase 'sanctity of life,' when used as an ideology, dangerously suggests that for a Christian life is an end in itself. Our sacredness rests on something such as rationality. But as Ramsey has suggested

One grasps the religious outlook upon the sanctity of human life only if he sees that this life is asserted to be surrounded by sanctity that need not be in man; that the most dignity a man ever possesses is a dignity that is alien to him . . . The value of a human life is ultimately grounded in the value God is placing on it. Anyone who can himself stand imaginatively even for a moment with an outlook where everything is referred finally to God – who, from things that are not, brings into being things that are – should be able to see that God's deliberation about the man need have only begun. ([7], pp. 11–12)

Therefore life for Christians is not sacred in the strict sense. Christians view life as a gift, but a gift for which they must care [2]. Thus the claim that life is sacred is not really so much a statement about ourselves as it is an indication of the kind of respect that we owe our neighbor. Our life and the lives of our neighbors are to be protected, since they are not ours to dispose of. For our dying as much as our living should be determined by our conviction that we are not our own.

But what do these homiletical flourishes have to do with the concept of death? They at least make clear why Christians have an aversion to the connotation of hastened death associated with the unhappy word *euthanasia* [2]. However, these considerations also help us to understand why Christians, in spite of their condemnation of euthanasia, have assumed that death need not be prolonged in all cases. This distinction between ordinary and extra-ordinary means of prolonging life, a distinction that is more trouble than it is worth, was the result of Christians' attempt to balance the sense that their lives were not at their disposal with their sense that death is not to be opposed unconditionally. Veatch is right to suggest that reflection on the right to refuse treatment is a much better means to consider such questions ([9], pp. 116–163).

Moreover, Ramsey has argued that the question of 'updating the criteria' of death in the context of Christian convictions is better described as an attempt to develop a criterion for when to use a respirator ([8], p. 81). I think it is useful to note why Ramsey thinks he has a theological stake in describing the issue in this manner. He fears that 'brain death' might be taken to indicate that a person's primary value is determined by intelligence rather than by his or her existence as one of God's children. Thus he can argue that the criteria of 'brain death' are not essentially different from 'heart death' criteria, but rather denote a procedural difference that has come about because of the extensive use of life-supporting techniques ([8], p. 87). Ramsey therefore has no objection to the criteria of death suggested by the Harvard report, since he assumes that the heart and lungs can only function artificially when there is total brain death. Thus there is no moral or theological commitment to continue using a respirator in such a case.

However, it would seem that Ramsey would have difficulty approving the definition of brain death as a 'dead' cortex accompanied by a brain stem still capable of maintaining heart and lung function. I mention this because Veatch has argued that, all other things being equal, the death of the neocortex should be sufficient to indicate that death should be declared. There are, of course, empirical issues involved in this proposal (i.e., whether an EEG unfailingly predicts the irreversible loss of consciousness associated with the death of the neocortex). My concern, however, is whether or not there is any theological issue at stake in this difference between Ramsey and Veatch.

Ramsey might well argue that Veatch assumes that the value of human life is only related to our consciousness and capacity for social interaction, and thus fails to see that the value of life should primarily be determined by God. However, this kind of argument assumes that there is a strong logical connection between the criteria of death and the concept of correlative worth of life. Veatch is not saying that the value of life is associated only with consciousness, but rather that consciousness is the necessary condition for any values. Moreover, Veatch's concern is primarily practical. His question is whether there are any indications that might help us to know when not to subject those who are dying to a mercy grown cruel through the power of our technology. While it is cruel not to try to sustain life, it may be just as cruel to extend care unconditionally. Interestingly, it is in terms of these practical issues that Christian convictions may be the most relevant.

## The Christian Way of Death

With respect to the practical issues surrounding the care of the dying I now want to provide a slightly different perspective. Briefly, I want to suggest that we have had trouble considering how we should care for the dying because we have not thought enough about what kind of responsibilities the one who is dying should have. In other words, the moral street here is not one way – the dying person has obligations to the living that are important for us to understand in the care of the dying. The attempt to determine the moment of death may be an attempt to avoid determining when it is time to die.

Today there is much talk about learning to care for the dying. Generally this means that the patient ought to be regarded as primary, that he or she is someone to whom something terrible is happening, and that we ought to help if we can. The assumption is that death, like a serious illness, robs persons of almost all claims to moral agency. The primary issue, then, is embodied in the question of the kind of care we ought to give someone so struck.

Also, the admonition that we must learn to care for the dying is an attempt to recover the personal side of medicine. What the dying often need is not further medical care, especially if that care is used only to prolong the dying process; but it is claimed that the patient needs personal care. Care is not synonymous with cure and it is argued that the doctor and nurses should help the patient in a psychological and moral way. These admonitions to learn how to care for the dying are salutary, but they assume that the care of the dying is primarily concerned with the attitudes of the living toward what is essentially a passive object.

However, as Milton Mayeroff has reminded us, care must be extended in such a manner that the one cared for is given the freedom to care also:

> To care for another person, in the most significant sense, is to help him grow and actualize himself. Consider, for example, a father caring for his child. He respects the child as existing in his own right and striving to grow. Caring is the antithesis of simply using the other person to satisfy one's own needs. Caring, as helping another grow and actualize himself, is a process, a way of relating to someone that involves development, in the same way that friendship can only emerge in time through mutual trust and a deepening and qualitative transformation of the relationship. ([6], p. 1)

This sense of caring cannot help but strike us as a little odd when it comes to caring for the dying, because the dying seem to be ending their growing. Interestingly, we have recently come up with an answer to this problem. We can help the one who is dying to accept his or her death in the manner suggested by Kübler-Ross [5]. We are thus engaged in the extremely odd enterprise of encouraging people to die better than they have lived. No one can die angry or apathetically because it becomes imperative that we all die with a quiet, brave acceptance.

There are some deep problems associated with this kind of proposal. By transforming her descriptive stages into normative recommendations, Dr Ross runs the risk of developing an extraordinarily manipulative strategy to deal with dying. More importantly, there is nothing associated with Christian beliefs that should require us to want our death. However, these beliefs do make a great deal of difference with respect to our learning how to die.

It is clear from the passages from Paul cited at the beginning of this paper that death is not the worst thing that could happen to a Christian. But neither is it a good thing. According to Paul, a Christian may desire death in a manner that denotes lack of trust in God's triumph over death. Death is both a friend and enemy. It is a friend in that without it we would not be forced to value one thing in life over another. Ironically, death creates the economy that makes life worthwhile. But because death is a friend it also becomes our enemy, for what we come to value and love we want to continue to value and love [3].

Moreover, the language associated with the acceptance of death must be carefully used. If the one who is dying accepts death too well, it plays a cruel trick on the living. One who is too willing to die can make us feel that our own lack of care caused the one who died to leave life without wishing to retain anything. (Of course, we are talking here about a gradual rather than sudden or accidental death.)

It is important, then, that the one who is dying exercise the responsibility to die well. That is, the person should die in a manner that is morally commensurate with the kind of trust that has sustained him or her in life. In terms of the language that I used earlier, it means that we should die in such a manner that others see that they are sustaining us and that correlatively due credit is given to God as the ultimate giver of life.

The very idea that we should take responsibility for how we die may strike many as odd. That such is the case is but an indication of our society's general attitude toward death. For example most people when asked how they want to die say in their sleep or suddenly – i.e., in a manner that they do not have to prepare for their dying. In contrast medieval people most feared sudden death since such a death would prevent them from preparing for their death both in terms of their social responsibilities and their eternal destiny. Thus they preferred death in battle, since they had time beforehand to prepare, and cancer was not for them the dreaded disease it is for us. The necessity to define the 'moment of death' is partly the result of our attempt to avoid preparing for death and thus making the moment of our death unexpected.

Thus the concern to recapture the meaning of 'natural death' is salutary. Daniel Callahan has recently tried to define natural death as when (1) one's life work has been accomplished; (2) one's moral obligations to those for whom one has responsibilities have been discharged; (3) one's death will not seem to others an offense to sense or sensibility, or will not tempt others to despair and rage at human existence; and (4) one's process of dying is not marked by unbearable and degrading pain [1].

Callahan notes that all four points are filled with ambiguity (e.g., it makes a lot of difference how you conceive your life's work and whom you think you have responsibilities to) and that it is hard to die without offending someone. However, there is much to commend Callahan's suggestion. As Eberhard Jungel has argued, the Christian conviction that we have been freed from the curse of death by Jesus Christ implies that

> Human life has a natural end which comes when the time allotted to life has expired. Man has a right to die this death and no other. One of the duties of Christian faith is to see that this right is recognized. There is therefore an immediate connection between the proclamation of the death of Jesus Christ and the concern that man should have the right to die a natural death. ([4], p.132)

There are a couple of qualifications that need to be made with respect to Jungel's and Callahan's defense of the idea of 'natural death.' First, we should avoid the phrase 'right to die.' The term is unclear and Callahan observes that no society can guarantee that there will be no 'deaths of the kind that lead people to fear their own death, or wonder about the rationality and benignness of the universe' [1]. Secondly, I suspect that the phrase 'natural death' is too misleading to be of much help. In a sense no death is natural, but is, as Veatch suggests, the result of some human choices. To perpetuate the fiction of 'natural death' may give us the feeling that we are relieved of responsibility, but it does so at the 'expense of continuing the suffering of death striking out in random and unregulated viciousness . . . [Natural death] is the death of the animal species, but in being so it is subhuman. If man is a responsible agent charged with the task of creating and sustaining life and his environment, then such fictions are escapist. Such fiction may give freedom, but the result is tyranny. To escape from responsibility to the imagined comforts of natural death cannot be a sustainable defense' ([9], p.302).

It seems to me, however, that Callahan's proposal does not hinge on a notion of natural death, but is really an attempt to indicate what an acceptable or perhaps even a good death would entail. A good death is a death that we can prepare for through living because we are able to see that death is but a necessary correlative of a good life. Thus a good death is not natural in the sense that it may well occur before our natural machinery runs down, but it is good if it is commensurate with those commitments that sustained our life. For Christians this means that while we do not wish to die, we do not oppose death as if life were an end in itself. For as Augustine said, 'Death is [to not] love God, and that is when we prefer anything to Him in affection and pursuit.'

Finally, what do these kinds of concerns have to do with the issue of brain death? They remind us that 'brain death' does not function just as a locus of death, but as a symbol of when it is time to die. But I am suggesting that if we are to die a good death, we must not allow the symbol of brain death to tyrannize us by requiring that we delay death so long that we can no longer die a good death. 'Brain death' may well serve as an indication of when the dying are released from certain claims having to do with the care of the dying, but it should not be used as a substitute for the responsibility each of us has to die our own death. 'Brain death' or 'heart death' should not remove the responsibility and risk that are the necessary concomitants of our willingness to die a good death.

## Bibliography

1. Callahan, Daniel. 1977. 'On Defining "Natural Death." ' *Hastings Center Report* 7, no. 3: 32–37.
2. Hauerwas, Stanley. 1977. *Truthfulness and Tragedy: Further Investigation in Christian Ethics*. Notre Dame, Ind.: University of Notre Dame Press. See especially pp. 101–115.
3. Hauerwas, Stanley. 1974. *Vision and Virtue: Essays in Christian Ethical Reflection*. Notre Dame, Ind.: Fides Press; rpt. University of Notre Dame Press, 1981. See especially pp. 166–186.
4. Jungel, Eberhard. 1974. *Death: The Riddle and the Mystery*. Philadelphia: Westminster.
5. Kübler-Ross, E. 1969. *On Death and Dying*. New York: Macmillan.
6. Mayeroff, Milton. 1971. *On Caring*. New York: Harper and Row.
7. Ramsey, Paul. 1971. 'The Morality of Abortion.' In James Rachels, ed., *Moral Problems*. New York: Harper and Row.
8. Ramsey, Paul. 1970. *The Patient as Person*. New Haven: Yale University Press. See especially pp. 59–164.
9. Veatch, Robert. 1976. *Death, Dying and the Biological Revolution: Our Last Quest for Responsibility*. New Haven: Yale University Press.

# The Vision of Death

VIGEN GUROIAN

## The Vision of Death

Death is as much of a mystery as life itself – a mystery that neither natural nor divine science is able to explain. As the Anglican theologian Austin Farrer so rightly said, 'God does not give us explanations; he gives up a Son.'[1] The Christian faith is not a theodicy; it provides no final rationale or explanation for death. At the core of the Christian vision of death lies Scripture's proclamation of salvation in Jesus Christ. Death is an evil that is defeated once and for all by the willing sacrifice of the Son of God on the cross and by his glorious resurrection and ascension to the right hand of the Father.

The twentieth-century Russian Orthodox theologian Georges Florovsky summed up the Christian realism about death when he wrote that 'death is a catastrophe for man' and asserted that this is the foundational principle of Christian anthropology.[2] He held fast to the belief that death signifies the need for salvation – this in contrast to both the standard demythologized secular view of death as the inevitable and ordinary end of personal existence and the reigning therapeutic view that we should accept death as perfectly natural and reconcile ourselves to our place in nature's cycle of birth, death, and new birth.

Alexander Schmemann, another contemporary Orthodox theologian, has pointed out the incompatibility of these secular views of death with the Christian faith. 'It falsifies the Christian message to present and to preach Christianity as essentially life-affirming without referring this affirmation to the death of Christ and therefore to the very fact of death,' Schmemann explained; it will not do 'to pass over in silence the fact that for Christianity death is not only the end, but indeed the very reality of *this world*.'[3]

The Christian vision of death affirmed and defended by Schmemann and Florovsky is rooted in Jesus' life and ministry, death and resurrection. Throughout his earthly ministry, wherever Jesus confronted sickness, he cured it, even to the point of bringing his friend Lazarus back from death. Through his crucifixion and resurrection, Jesus overcame death and made

From *Life's Living Towards Dying*, pp. 41–61. Grand Rapids: Eerdmans, 1996.

our lives immortal. These are the basic facts supporting the Christian vision of death.


## Sin and Death

The classical Christian teaching is that death originated in the sin of Adam and Eve and spread to all of humankind, since all sinned (Rom. 5:12). St. Paul said that 'the wages of sin is death' (Rom. 6:23) and 'the sting of death is sin' (1 Cor. 15:56). This mystery is deeply and profoundly embedded in human personal and social reality and is not subject to scientific or empirical verification. Yet both experience and modern medical science tell us something about it. We have established statistical correlations between overeating (gluttony) and heart disease, sexual promiscuity and dangerous sexually transmitted diseases, and excessive drinking and liver disease, to name just a few. We are only beginning to realize how the stresses generated by various kinds of deception, vengefulness, and manipulation in the workplace and the home can lead to a whole range of life-threatening illnesses. Where the vices rule, death draws near.

All of the great Christian writers since St. Paul have made essentially the same argument: sin and death are profoundly and mysteriously mixed together. The Orthodox Christian tradition grounds its theology of death in two core beliefs that expand on this Pauline teaching: (1) that the first couple was created with the potential for immortality and (2) that death as we know it in a fallen world is not the same thing as the natural cessation of life that Adam and Eve might have experienced had they not sinned.

The fifth-century Armenian catechismal text *The Teaching of Saint Gregory* comments on the creation story in Genesis 2 as follows: 'Only the will of man ... [is] independent to do whatever he wills. And he has been constrained in nothing more than what was warned: not to eat of the tree [Gen. 2:17], that thereby He [God] might make him worthy to receive greater things in return for lesser, and that by virtue of his having grace for his task, he might receive from the Creator, as recompense for lesser deeds, greater grace.'[4] This early Christian catechism clearly identifies this 'greater grace' with immortality. Had the first couple respected 'the enviable God-given wisdom, through the observance of the command,' they would have gone on to enjoy 'the inalienable glory of the existent one [God].'[5] The catechism distinguishes between creaturely temporality and the eternity of God: even before the fall, personal human life was destined to have a beginning and an end. But, had Adam and Eve not sinned, the 'natural' cessation of their earthly lives would have been different from the death that results from sin, which is the only form of death that we are acquainted with. Had the first couple not succumbed to the temptation of the serpent in the garden, the cessation of their earthly existence would have marked a satisfactory completion and fulfillment of life and seen them through an uninterrupted passage into immortality with God.

The fall rendered the dying and death of human beings emblematic of failed and doomed existence. Contrary to God's desire, the first couple chose to live *out from themselves* and *back to themselves* rather than toward God, and human beings have behaved the same ever since. This is how humanity became subject to the natural law of death that, apart from divine intervention, permanently dissolves the individual organism into its elemental constituent parts. The Greek church fathers used the term 'corruptible death' to describe the evil and abnormality of such a death for creatures whom God created in his own image and likeness. The early patristic writers generally agreed that death according to the natural law of the cessation and dissolution of an organism is a profoundly 'unnatural' thing for human beings. Georges Florovsky summarized the patristic consensus about corruptible death as follows: 'Strictly speaking, it is only man that dies. Death indeed is a law of nature, a law of organic life. But man's death means just this fall or entanglement into this cyclical motion of nature, just what ought not to have happened . . . Only for man is death contrary to [human] nature and mortality is evil.'[6] The anthem of St. John of Damascus in the Byzantine rite of burial describes vividly the ugly and humanly unnatural visage of corruptible death: 'I weep and wail when I think upon death and behold our beauty, fashioned after the image of God, lying in the tomb disfigured, dishonored, bereft of form.'[7]

Precisely because the human person is created in the image and likeness of divine personhood, human death amounts to more than mere animal death, even if it has a similar appearance. Human life – even sinful human life – amounts to more than the mere unfolding of a determinate nature. It is the enactment of a history marked by freedom of will. As we make the choices to determine our history, sin misdirects our will in ways that steer both our personal biography and our collective history toward dissolution and nothingness rather than into fullness of being in communion with God. That is the sense in which Florovsky speaks of human death becoming entangled in the entropy of natural existence. 'In the generic life of dumb animals, death is . . . a natural movement in the development of the species; it is the expression rather of the generating power of life than infirmity. However, with the fall of man, mortality, even in nature, assumes an evil and tragic significance . . . Death strikes at personality.'[8] . . .

St. Athanasius and the Armenian *Teaching of Saint Gregory* both maintain that the disobedience of Adam and Eve brought into existence a kind of death that would lead to extinction were it not for God's overriding intent for human beings to be immortal. The disobedience of the first human couple not only put immortality into jeopardy – one might say suspended it – but introduced what St. Paul called 'the sting of death' (1 Cor. 15:56). Human experience is suffused with the typically vague but sometimes acute sense that everything of value and joy in life is disintegrating and being despoiled. We all experience moments when the harmony of the body-and-soul union is assaulted or severely weakened, moments when our body or mind seems out of control and our identity and relationship with the world seem to be at risk. These descents into sickness are what dying in sin is ultimately about.[9]

As in the prayer of St. John of Damascus, death, as the dissolution of the union of body and soul, is described and lamented in the liturgies of the Orthodox churches. The Armenian burial service describes this corruptible death as having been summoned by God and 'poured . . . out upon creatures, in order that the wickedness that had befallen might not remain immortal.'[10] Note that the prayer does not say that God created death but rather that God allowed the sinful creature to lapse into the elements out of which it was made. The Byzantine Orthodox tradition even includes a prayer that beseeches God to mercifully hasten this process of dissolution so that 'the destructible bond' of body and soul might be dissolved – the body to 'be dissolved from the elements out of which it was fashioned,' and the soul to be 'translated to that place where it shall take its abode until the final Resurrection.'[11] Orthodox Christians pray for this dissolution not because they believe that death is good or out of despair but because they set their sights past death to the hope and promise of resurrection.

## Spiritual Death

Corruptible death lies beyond the scope of physical, biological, or psychological science because in origin and end it transcends space and temporality, that which is physical and that which is psychological. Human sickness and death are also spiritual and eschatological. The medical notion of a precise moment of death measured in terms of cessation of brain function or the 'closing down' of the body's system of vital organs is clinically useful, but it scarcely captures the complete reality or meaning of death. The demise of the biological individual is only a portion of death. Alexander Schmemann explained: 'In the Christian vision, death is above all a *spiritual reality* of which one can partake while being alive, from which one can be free while lying in the grave. Death here is man's *separation from life*, and this means from God who is the only Giver of life.'[12] Such a death may be a part of living: it does not belong exclusively to the biological demise of a person. The Christian vision of death encompasses scientific definitions of death as the terminus of biological life, but it also embraces spiritual and eschatological dimensions of human personhood. God, not nothingness, is the beginning, ground, and 'end point' of all persons. Thus, contrary to modern perceptions and secular beliefs, human death is not the opposite of immortality. We come from God and are bound to return to God. But even if unrepentance obstructs our way back to God, our fate is not nothingness. God is Lord of both life and death, and death leads either to an unceasing separation from God and from the company of saints (Luke 16:19–31) or to a union in the company of the Holy Trinity of Father, Son and Spirit. Sadly, many modern Christians seem to have lost hold of this vision of death and its place in God's salvation plan.

## The Journey through Death

The great prayer attributed to St. Basil in the Armenian rite of burial reveals its vision of death in a sweeping narrative that explores the spiritual and eschatological dimensions of death I have just touched on and asks God to grant to the deceased person 'a goodly journey' back to the Garden and the Tree of Life.

> We thank thee, Father of our Lord Jesus Christ, who because of thy love of mankind has visited us, and saved [us] from the machinations of the traducer [of] the race of men that were driven out and banished afar. For Satan was jealous of us, and drove us out of eternal life by his deceits and wiles, proscribing and banishing us unto our destruction and ruin. But thou, O God, who art benevolent and lovest mankind, didst not permit the bitterness of his poisoned fangs to remain in us. Wherefore thou didst summon death, and poured it out upon creatures, in order that the wickedness that had befallen might not remain immortal: but by removing us from this life, and cutting us from our sins, the punishment of the beneficent One became salvation.
>
> But in the last days thou didst send thy only-begotten Son, beloved in the image of the death of sin; and he condemned sin in his own body, and by his voluntary crucifixion shattered the hosts of the enemy. He became the firstfruits of them that slept, and by his divinely marvelous resurrection he invited us to share in his own immortality.
>
> Now this thy servant believing in him has been baptized into the death of thy Christ . . . Remit to this man his debts incurred either willingly or unwillingly, and heal all the wounds which the disincarnate enemy hath inflicted . . .
>
> And . . . heal his wounds, and convey him peacefully past the principalities of darkness . . . And efface the handwriting of their influences and inworkings, which they have sown in him and vouchsafe to him a goodly journey. Let there be held far away from him and stayed the flaming sword, with which they guard the path of the Tree of life . . . Let him through the same [so that he may] arrive at the place of safety where all thy saints are massed and wait for the great wedding, when

the great God and Saviour shall appear, Jesus Christ, at the sound of the great trumpet ... Then ... at the glance of the judge the earth shall be shaken, and sealed sepulchres be opened. The bodies that were turned to dust are built up afresh, and the spirits swooping down like eagles reach them and array themselves in the incorruptible body ... [13]

In this tradition, death in Jesus Christ is a spiral that breaks free from the natural cycle of birth, death and rebirth.[14] The lowest point of the spiral is death. But then the line curves upward beyond earthly life into eternal life. Christ gave death this upward curve by recapitulating our living and dying and then adding something else – a new creation. St. Paul describes it as the fruit of planting:

But someone will ask, 'How are the dead raised? With what kind of body do they come?' Fool! What you sow does not come to life unless it dies. And as for what you sow, you do not sow the body that is to be, but a bare seed ... God gives it a body as he has chosen ... So it is with the resurrection of the dead. What is sown is perishable, what is raised is imperishable. It is sown in dishonor, it is raised in glory. It is sown in weakness, it is raised in power. It is sown a physical body, it is raised a spiritual body. (1 Cor. 15:35–38, 42–44)

This sheds important light on the meaning of the Easter proclamation that death has been overcome once and for all in Christ Jesus. Christ abolished the corruptible form of death of which physical death is but a portion and a visible sign. The physical death that medicine knows, studies, and endeavours to delay is not the first issue here. God in Christ has taken the sting, the spiritual poison of sin, out of death through his own death so that our physical death becomes a sign of our destiny of communion with God.

## Penance and the Reversal of Corruptible Death

The wounded surgeon plies the steel
That questions the distempered part;
Beneath the bleeding hands we feel
The sharp compassion of the healer's art
Resolving the enigma of the fever chart.
                                    T.S. Eliot, 'East Coker'

No description of the Christian vision of the origin, nature, and course of death is complete without the element of the doctrine and practice of penance. The first words of Jesus' teaching are: 'Repent, for the kingdom of heaven has come near' (Matt. 4:17). Some have suggested that Jesus' command echoes God the Father's desire for repentance following Adam and Eve's decision to eat of the fruit of the Tree of Life. The Armenian *Teaching of Saint Gregory* speculates that immediately after they ate the forbidden fruit, God gave Adam and Eve one last opportunity to repent and to reverse the course of corruptible death. A key biblical passage is Genesis 3:9–10: 'But the Lord God called to man, and said to him, "Where are you?" He said, "I heard the sound of you in the garden, and I was afraid, because I was naked; and I hid myself." ' The *Teaching* interprets this passage to mean that '[God] wished by being somewhat indulgent to capture him [Adam], that the gentleness of God might lead them to penitence.' Instead, the couple made excuses for themselves. 'Then he [God] set judgment, passed sentence, which they paid and returned to dust [Gen. 3:19]; for the judgment of God is true over those who work evil.'[15] One can see how the author of this catechism might have arrived at this speculation, for the Genesis story indicates that God expels the first couple from the Garden and from proximity to the Tree of Life only after he speaks to them this last time. And only then does Adam blame Eve for what he has done and Eve blame the serpent for what she has done (Gen. 3:12–13) – excuses and deceptions that seal God's judgment and invite corruptible death.

Since that point, say our sources, repentance alone has not been sufficient to reverse the process of corruptible death. St. Athanasius reasoned as follows: 'Had it been a case of trespass only, and not of subsequent corruption, repentance would have been well enough; but when once transgression had begun men came under the power of corruption proper to their nature and were bereft of the grace which belonged to them as creatures in the Image of God.'[16] The *Teaching of Saint Gregory* concludes, 'For which reason, the God-seeing, holy prophets took care, like wise doctors [of faith], to prepare the medicine of cure for the pain of the illness, to remove and extirpate the scandal [of death] and destroy it completely.'[17] As Eliot's poetry notes so profoundly, the last prophet and true doctor is Christ, who cured our sickness unto death, defeating death itself by his own righteous sacrifice on the cross.

## Repentance and Healing

Death remains the outworking of sin in the human being, but it has also been transformed by Christ into the revelation of true life. In the Old Testament, the Hebrew word for 'salvation' derives from *yasha*, which means 'to save from a danger.' God delivers us not only from our enemies and from persecution but also from sickness and from death itself. In the New Testament, the Greek *sozo* comes from *saos*, meaning 'healthy.' Penance is for the sin that attaches to all 'flesh' and makes this flesh subject to corruptible death; penance issues from the belief that God desires to heal our infirmities and make us whole.

The Orthodox sacraments of holy unction and burial amplify and deepen

the meaning of this etymology of salvation. The Byzantine Rite of Holy
Unction opens with a recitation of Psalm 143 and 51, which set the tone and
direction of the entire rite.

> Hear my prayer, O Lord;
> give ear to my supplications in your faithfulness;
> answer me in your righteousness.
> Do not enter into judgment with your servant,
> for no one living is righteous before you . . .
>
> Answer me quickly, O Lord;
> my spirit fails.
> Do not hide your face from me,
> or I shall be like those who go down to the Pit.
> Let me hear of your steadfast love in the morning,
> for in you I put my trust.
>                         (Ps. 143:1–2, 7–8)
>
> Have mercy on me, O God,
> according to your steadfast love;
> according to your abundant mercy
> blot out my transgressions.
> Wash me thoroughly from my iniquity,
> and cleanse me from my sin.
>
> For I know my transgression,
> and my sin is ever before me.
> Against you, you alone, have I sinned,
> and done what is evil in your sight,
> so that you are justified in your sentence . . .
> Indeed, I was born guilty,
> a sinner when my mother conceived me.
>
> You desire truth in the inward being;
> therefore teach me wisdom in my secret heart.
> Purge me with hyssop, and I shall be clean; . . .
> Let me hear joy and gladness;
> let the bones that you have crushed rejoice.
> Hide your face from my sins,
> and blot out all my iniquities.
>
> Create in me a clean heart, O God,
> and put a new and right spirit within me . . .

> Restore to me the joy of your salvation,
> and sustain in me a willing spirit.
> (Ps. 51:1–10, 12)

The acts of repenting and asking God for forgiveness and healing are related to a profound understanding not only of death but of healing that encompasses the whole human being – spiritual and psychological as well as physical. In the Byzantine rite, a reading from the Epistle of James introduces this holistic interpretation of healing and sets the stage for anointing with oil:

> Be patient, therefore, beloved, until the coming of the Lord ... As an example of suffering and patience, beloved, take the prophets who spoke in the name of the Lord. Indeed we call blessed those who showed endurance. You have heard of the endurance of Job, and you have seen the purpose of the Lord, how the Lord is compassionate and merciful ...
>
> Are any among you suffering? They should pray. Are any cheerful? They should sing songs of praise. Are any among you sick? They should call the elders of the church and have them pray over them, anointing them with oil in the name of the Lord. The prayer of faith will save the sick, and the Lord will raise them up; and anyone who has committed sins will be forgiven. Therefore confess your sins to one another, and pray for one another, so that you may be healed. The prayer of the righteous is powerful and effective. (5:7, 10–11, 13–16)

Anointing with oil symbolizes the prayer, penance, forgiveness of sin, healing and salvation that this passage mentions. Anointment indicates the deep connection between sickness and the mystery of God's redemptive purpose. It is not a substitute for medical care, but it reveals the telos of medicine nonetheless. The story of the Good Samaritan from the Gospel of Luke (10: 25–38) introduces anointing, offering the assurance that even in the face of sickness and death God does not forget or abandon us, because his love is like that of the Samaritan, only stronger. Then a prefatory prayer reminds everyone present that God has made a lasting covenant with the Christian through baptism and chrismation and that God continues to honor this covenant as healer and redeemer in life and through death:

> For thou art a great and marvelous God, who keepest thy covenant and thy mercy towards them that love thee; who givest remission of sins through thy Holy Child, Jesus; who regenerates us from sin by Holy Baptism, and sanctifiest us with the Holy Spirit; who givest light to the blind, who raisest up them that are cast down, who lovest the righteous, and showest mercy unto sinners; who leadest us forth again out of darkness and the shadow of death.[18]

## A Tolstoyan Image of Penance

Tolstoy explores this deep signification of holy unction in his great short novel *The Death of Ivan Ilych*. Many Christian scholars have criticized Tolstoy for his advocacy of heterodox views in this novel and elsewhere in his fiction. Rather than stopping to assess this criticism, I want simply to propose an interpretation of this story that commends it as a forceful artistic exploration of the meanings of sin and death and penance and healing.

Most of the story consists of a retrospective description of the life that Ivan Ilych led until he was stricken by a mortal illness. This background shows us why Ivan's death is not merely physically painful but also spiritually and mentally agonizing. In the midst of dying, he discovers the court of his own conscience and comes to see himself guilty in the eyes of God. His understanding of his life is stripped of illusion and excuse. He is convicted of his pride and arrogance and the hollowness and superficiality of his relations with colleagues and family, and in the end he is led to repent.

Tolstoy masterfully draws his reader into the innermost thoughts and emotions of the dying man.

> His mental sufferings were due to the fact that at night, as he looked at [his servant] Gerasim's sleepy, good-natured face with its prominent cheek-bones, the question suddenly occurred to him: 'What if my whole life has been wrong?' . . . And his professional duties, and the whole arrangement of his life and of his family, and all his social and official interest might all have been false. He tried to defend all those things to himself and suddenly felt the weakness of what he was defending. There was nothing to defend.[19]

Ivan Ilych is moved by these shattering thoughts to take holy communion. Holy unction is not mentioned in the text, but Tolstoy's Russian readers would have assumed it as a matter of course, because in Orthodox practice communion is given in such circumstances only in conjunction with holy unction.[20] This unwritten subtext of the story is important, because it establishes the context of Ivan's subsequent thought and behaviour. It clarifies the sequence of emotions that Ivan experiences: short-lived hope, crushing remorse and despair, and, finally, penance.

After the priest comes to hear his confession, Ivan feels 'a relief from his doubts and consequently from his suffering, and for a moment there came a ray of hope. He again began to think of the vermiform appendix and the possibility of correcting it. He received the sacrament with tears in his eyes.'[21]

At the outset Ivan naively expects that he will be miraculously cured. His disappointment when this does not happen and when, in fact, his condition further deteriorates is especially meaningful in the context of the sacrament of holy unction. The healing that God works in the penitent person transcends mere physical healing. God may or may not heal our physical infirmities, depending on the requirements of his unwavering purpose to redeem us for eternal life. The evil of corruptible death may be overcome even as a person's biological life draws to an end.

During the last three days of his life – three symbolic days of death and resurrection – Ivan Ilych perfects his last act, the act of dying, and his death is transformed into a redemptive event. Tolstoy's description is haunting:

> For three whole days, during which time did not exist for him, he struggled in that black sack into which he was being thrust by an invisible, restless force ... And every moment he felt despite all his efforts he was drawing nearer and nearer to what terrified him. He felt that his agony was due to his being thrust into that black hole, and still more his not being able to get into it. He was hindered from getting into it by his conviction that his life had been a good one. That very justification of his life held him fast and prevented his moving forward, and it caused him torment.[22]

This passage defines the crux of Ivan's penance and conversion.

Ivan's 'conversion' follows the pattern of the dark night of the soul described by the Christian mystics and incorporated into Christian hagiography. This is the final surrender to death of the sinful self as a repentance opens onto the ineffable divine light. The crucial moment of grace and forgiveness in the story is marked by the loving kiss and holy tears of Ivan's young son, which dissolve the last obstacle of pride that has prevented him from surrendering himself to God and his eternity.

> 'Yes it [his life] was all not the right thing ... but that's no matter. It can be done. But what is the right thing?' he asked himself, and suddenly grew quiet. This occurred at the end of the third day, two hours before his death. Just then his schoolboy son had crept softly in ... The dying man was still screaming desperately and waving his arms. His hand fell on the boy's head, and the boy caught it, pressed it to his lips and began to cry. At that very moment Ivan Ilych fell through and caught sight of the light, and it was revealed to him that though his life had not been what it should have been, this could still be rectified.[23]

## Conclusion

> We must all die; we are like water spilled on the ground, which cannot be gathered up. But God will not take away a life. (2 Sam. 14:14)

In this discussion of *The Death of Ivan Ilych*, I have underlined and commended its redemptive vision. Yet there may be an even greater lesson to be learned, not from what the story says but from what it leaves unsaid. For I do not think that the pathos or tragedy of Ivan's life is wholly resolved by the ending that Tolstoy has supplied. What Ivan Ilych only begins to understand about living and dying at the end should ideally have been learned throughout the whole of his life ... [Remembrance] of death is a virtue commended to Christians at their baptism and in all the sacraments. God calls every Christian to live toward dying by way of this mimesis and remembrance. Practicing this virtuous habit throughout life will prepare us for dying in a manner that preserves hope.

This wisdom is the core of Christian ethics of caring for the dying. It amounts to much more than the formal presentation of rules and principles of moral decision making that often count for what is called medical ethics and pastoral training in many professional schools and seminaries. A habit of affirming life in all circumstances without averting one's eyes from the awful reality of death belongs to a whole way of life, a faithful way of living toward dying that all the Christian churches need to teach and cultivate. This fundamental instruction in Christian living toward dying is the necessary precondition for the ethic of caring for the dying ...

## Notes

1. Farrer, 'The Country Doctor,' in *Austin Farrer: The Essential Sermons*, ed. Leslie Houlden (Cambridge, Mass.: Cowley Publications, 1991), p. 204.
2. Florovsky, *Creation and Redemption*, vol. 3 of *The Collected Works of Georges Florovsky* (Belmont, Mass.: Nordland Publishing, 1976), p. 111.
3. Schmemann, *For the Life of the World* (Crestwood, N.Y.: St. Vladimir's Seminary Press, 1973), p. 96.
4. *The Teaching of Saint Gregory: An Early Armenian Catechism*, trans. Robert W. Thomson (Cambridge: Harvard University Press, 1970), pp. 45–46; italics mine. The catechism is included in *The History of the Armenians*, purported to be written by Agathangelos. The text of the catechism is attributed to Agathangelos by St. Gregory the Illuminatory, who converted Tiridates, king of the Armenians, to Christianity in the early fourth century.
5. *The Teaching of Saint Gregory*, p. 48.
6. Florovsky, *Creation and Redemption*, p. 106.
7. Cited by Florovsky in *Creation and Redemption*, p. 386.
8. Florovsky, *Creation and Redemption*, p. 106.
9. For this point, I owe a debt of gratitude to William F. May's essay 'The Sacral Power of Death in Contemporary Experience,' in *On Moral Medicine: Theological Perspectives in Medical Ethics*, ed. Stephen E. Lammers and Allen Verhey (Grand Rapids: William B. Eerdmans, 1987), especially pp. 181–82.
10. *Rituale Armenorum: The Administration of the Sacraments and Breviary Rites of the Armenian Church*, ed. F. C. Conybeare (Oxford: Clarendon Press, 1905), p. 130. Gregory of Nyssa says the same: 'Divine providence introduced death into human nature with a specific design so that by the dissolution of body and soul, vice may be drawn off and man may be refashioned again through the resurrection' (Quoted by Florovsky in *Creation and Redemption*, p. 108).

11. *Service Book of the Holy Orthodox-Catholic Apostolic Church*, ed. and trans. Isabel Florence Hapgood (Englewood, N.J.: Antiochian Orthodox Christian Archdiocese, 1975), p. 366.

12. Schmemann, *Of Water and the Spirit* (Crestwood, N.Y.: St. Vladimir's Seminary Press, 1974), p. 62.

13. *Rituale Armenorum*, pp. 130–31.

14. I have drawn in this analysis from Jaroslav Pelikan's extraordinary little book *The Shape of Death* (Nashville: Abingdon Press, 1961), esp. chap. 5.

15. *The Teaching of Saint Gregory*, pp. 51–52.

16. *St. Athanasius on the Incarnation* (Crestwood, N.Y.: St. Vladimir's Seminary Press, 1982), p. 33.

17. *The Teaching of Saint Gregory*, p. 51.

18. *Service Book of the Holy Orthodox-Catholic Apostolic Church*, p. 344.

19. Tolstoy, *The Death of Ivan Ilych*, in *Great Short Works of Leo Tolstoy*, trans. Louis Maude and Aylmer Maude (New York: Harper & Row, 1967), p. 299.

20. The association of holy unction with communion in this sort of context is evident in Tolstoy's account of the death of Nicholas Levin in *Anna Karenina*: 'Next day the patient received Communion and Extreme Unction. During the ceremony he prayed fervently. In his large eyes, fixed upon an icon with a coloured cloth, was a look of such passionate entreaty and hope that Levin was frightened at seeing it. He knew that his passionate entreaty and hope would only make the parting from the life he loved more difficult' (*Anna Karenina*, ed. George Gibian, trans. Louis Maude and Aylmer Maude [New York: W. W. Norton, 1970], p. 453).

21. Tolstoy, *The Death of Ivan Ilych*, p. 300.

22. Tolstoy, *The Death of Ivan Ilych*, p. 301.

23. Tolstoy, *The Death of Ivan Ilych*, p. 301.

# CASE STUDY:
## The Right to Die?

Diane Pretty was diagnosed as having motor neurone disease (MND) in 1999. By the time her case came to public attention, Mrs Pretty was paralysed from the neck down and wanted to be able to end her own life when she chose, but because of her disease she was physically unable to commit suicide. Therefore, she wanted her husband to be able to help her take her life without fear of being prosecuted under the Suicide Act (1961), which outlaws assisting another person to commit suicide. The Director of Public Prosecutions refused to guarantee that Mr Pretty would not be prosecuted, so Mrs Pretty took her case to the High Court, to the House of Lords and finally to the European Court of Human Rights in Strasbourg. Her lawyers argued that the Suicide Act breached her human rights by denying her the right that able bodied people have to take their own life. However, all three courts ruled that her human rights were not breached by the Act. The Law Lords recognised the harrowing situation she was in, but said that they were not a legislative body, and that the law as it stood did not allow her plea to be granted. The Strasbourg judges warned of the risk of abuse if an exemption for cases like Mrs Pretty's were built into the Act. After the Strasbourg case, Mrs Pretty said, 'The law has taken all my rights away.' She died in a hospice in May 2002.

## Questions
- Is there such a thing as 'a good death', and what should we understand by it?
- What light might a Christian understanding of 'a good death' shed on the morality of euthanasia and suicide?
- How, if at all, might a Christian vision of life and death help someone face a painful and undignified death?

**Sources**
Anon, 'In Brief', *British Medical Journal* 324, 1174 (2002).
Clare Dyer, 'Dying Woman's Demand for Right to Assisted Suicide is Rejected', *British Medical Journal* 323, 1326 (2001).
——, 'Dying Woman Loses her Battle for Assisted Suicide', *British Medical Journal* 324, 1055 (2002).

# 6

# PROFESSIONAL–PATIENT RELATIONSHIPS

## Introduction

At the heart of the healing and caring work done by doctors, nurses and other health professionals are relationships between those professionals, on the one hand, and patients and those close to them, on the other. When these relationships are good, their contribution to the care and healing of patients is immense. Imagine, for example, the story of a patient who has suffered for many years from a rare and serious condition, and has been treated for much of that time by the same specialist. Over the years, they have developed a relationship of mutual respect in which they have learned much together about her condition and its management. In a phrase of Paul Ramsey's, they have become 'joint adventurers in a common cause' (Ramsey 1970, 5–6).

The importance of these relationships is also illustrated, negatively, by the serious consequences when they go wrong. Extreme cases like the Alder Hey affair described in the case study are, thankfully, relatively rare. But such cases show in an extreme way the trauma that can be caused when good communication is neglected and trust abused in such relationships, as well as highlighting the need for systems and structures that support good communication and restrain abuses (cf. Bauchner and Vinci 2001). And quite apart from such scandals, there are everyday pressures that can make good relationships difficult to sustain in a clinical setting: a heavy workload and scarce resources, for example, may make it difficult for professionals to find adequate time to talk with patients; or the inevitable imbalance in knowledge, authority and status between a doctor and his or her patient may leave the patient feeling helpless and disempowered.

There has been much discussion by Christians and others of appropriate models for clinical encounters which may help to minimise these dangers and promote good relationships between professionals, patients and their relatives. Some writers have suggested that the relationship between professional and patient should be viewed as a contract, which would seem to offer some scope for correcting the imbalance of power and enabling patients to play a more active part in their care (cf. Portmann 2000).

Others, however, have been critical of contractual models, fearing that they might reduce the relationship to a legalistic transaction in which the professional makes no more commitment to the patient's well-being than is specified by the written or unwritten 'contract' between them. The alternative model of *covenant* has commended itself to many Christian writers, seeming to allow for a richer and deeper commitment (Ramsey 1970, May 1983, Messer 1996). In recent years, however, the covenant model has itself come under attack for failing to deliver the resources it seemed to promise for addressing the problems and pressures noted above (McKenny 1994).

Although much of the emphasis in this discussion is on the way that health professionals should behave, some authors also draw attention to the moral responsibilities of *patients* and the virtues that they should cultivate (cf. Hauerwas and Pinches 1997). A further factor which may significantly affect these relationships is the enormous increase in information about health care available through the media and the Internet. This may significantly shift the balance of power between patient and professional, requiring the professional to become more guide than gatekeeper of knowledge.[1]

The two readings in this chapter, drawn from the same collection of essays, approach these questions in very different ways. William F. May, a long-standing advocate of the covenant model, here combines that model with an inquiry into the particular virtues that can be expected of a professional – in this case, of a physician. He identifies prudence (in the Aristotelian sense of 'practical wisdom'), fidelity and public-spiritedness as the virtues that should characterise the practice of medicine.

Karen Lebacqz, by contrast, examines the clinical encounter from the perspective of the patient rather than the doctor, and focuses on moral principles rather than virtues. Drawing on an autobiographical account by the well-known neurologist Oliver Sacks, she shows how even someone with Sacks' intelligence, experience and status can be profoundly disempowered if he finds himself a patient. Sacks found that his healing required not only a physical cure, but also a social and spiritual restoration that would address his sense of diminished status, value and worth.

Lebacqz goes on to show that disempowerment in the clinical setting can be immeasurably more serious for those who are multiply disadvantaged to begin with. For example, she describes the experience of a group of poor Hispanic women in the United States who were sterilised without their consent. For people who experience this degree of multiple disempowerment, writes Lebacqz, 'nothing short of a change in the system' of health care provision will be required to restore their status and well-being (p. 180). This insight may have considerable importance for health care in other countries, too: in Britain, scandals like the Alder Hey affair are often found to expose not only failures in the conduct of individuals, but also systemic weaknesses in the delivery, regulation and supervision of health care. And the day-to-day pressures experienced by professionals in their dealings with patients and relatives are likely to have a great deal to do with the economic and organisational constraints of the systems in which those professionals work.

## References and Further Reading

Howard Bauchner and Robert Vinci, 'What Have We Learned from the Alder Hey Affair?' *British Medical Journal* 322, 309–310 (2001).

Tom L. Beauchamp and James F. Childress, *Principles of Biomedical Ethics*. 5th ed., Oxford and New York: Oxford University Press, 2001.

Stanley Hauerwas and Charles Pinches, 'Practicing Patience: How Christians Should be Sick', in *Christians Among the Virtues: Theological Conversations with Ancient and Modern Ethics*. Notre Dame: University of Notre Dame Press, 1997.

Gerald P. McKenny, 'Introduction', in Gerald P. McKenny and Jonathan R. Sande (eds.), *Theological Analyses of the Clinical Encounter*, vii–xx. Dordrecht: Kluwer Academic Publishers, 1994.

William F. May, *The Physician's Covenant: Images of the Healer in Medical Ethics*. Philadelphia: Westminster, 1983.

Neil G. Messer, *The Therapeutic Covenant: Christian Ethics, Doctor-Patient Relationships and Informed Consent*. Cambridge: Grove, 1996.

John Portmann, 'Like Marriage, Without the Romance', *Journal of Medical Ethics* 26, 194–197 (2000).

Paul Ramsey, *The Patient as Person: Explorations in Medical Ethics*. New Haven and London: Yale University Press, 1970.

## Notes

1. I am grateful to Dr Caroline Berry for pointing this out to me.

# The Medical Covenant:
# An Ethics of Obligation or Virtue?

WILLIAM F. MAY

A covenantal ethic, above all else, defines the moral life responsively. Moral action (such as selling, refraining, respecting, or giving) ultimately derives from and responds to a primordial receiving.

In its ancient and most influential form – the biblical covenant – covenantal obligation arises from specific exchanges between partners that lead to a fundamental promise which, in turn, defines the identity and therefore shapes the future of both parties to the agreement. The biblical covenant included the following four elements:

1. an original exchange of gifts, labor or services;
2. a promise based on this original or anticipated gift;
3. the acceptance of an inclusive set of moral obligations that will shape the future life of both partners; and
4. the provision of ritual and other means for the renewal of life between partners in the course of their subsequent alienation from one another.

The scriptures of ancient Israel are littered with such covenants between men and women and between nations, but they are controlled throughout by that *singular covenant* which embraces all others: the covenant between God and Israel. The latter includes the aforementioned elements: first, a gift (the deliverance of the people from Egypt); second, an exchange of promises (at Mt. Sinai); and third, the shaping of all subsequent life in response to the original gift and the promissory event. God 'marks the forehead' of the Jews forever, as they accept an inclusive set of moral commandments by which they will live. These commands are both specific enough to make the future duties of Israel concrete (e.g. laws governing protection of the weak) yet summary enough (e.g., 'Love the Lord thy God with all thy heart ... ') to require a fidelity that exceeds a legalistic specification. Fourth and finally, the biblical narrative marks out those ritual means whereby Israel returns regularly to those foundational events that shape her life (the dietary laws, the Sabbath

From Gerald P. McKenny and Jonathan R. Sande (eds.), *Theological Analyses of the Clinical Encounter*, pp. 29–44. Dordrecht: Kluwer Academic Publishers, 1994.

and the holidays). These elements variously reappear in the horizontal covenants between sovereigns and subjects, treaties between nations, and the all important covenant of marriage. For Christians, God's covenant with Israel structurally prefigures the inclusive covenant that will spread across the whole of humankind in God's Son [3, 4, 5].

The subsequent meaning of the word has not always carried forward the biblical sense of a covenant. The word, indeed, has often referred to a variety of unsavoury practices – real estate covenants that keep blacks or Jews out of particular neighborhoods; loyalty to the professional guild which sometimes takes precedence over professional duties to patients and clients; country club agreements that build invisible walls around the playing fields of the well-favored; hiring practices and referral systems that toss jobs and businesses to those with an 'in'. Further, the religiously disposed have often confused the divine covenant with an utterly parochial loyalty, reducing God to their gender, race, nation, class, neighborhood, or kinship group. The ancient prophets condemned the resulting amalgam and confusion as the worst sort of idolatry, the worship not of the idol that frankly tempts at a perceptible moral distance from the holy of holies, but of the counterfeit that slyly mounts the altar in the sanctuary itself and wraps itself in a stolen glory.

In its biblical form, the concept of a covenant offers resources for criticizing the narrowness and exclusivity of these various types of idolatry. God, the creative, nurturant, and donative source of all beings, establishes the primary covenant that measures all others. Loyalty to God, whatever its particular implications, requires loyalty to all God's creatures. Thus the covenant that distinguishes Jews and Christians from others requires them at the same time to deal open handedly with others – not only with familiars but also with strangers. The prophets, Amos and Isaiah, and the gospel writer, Luke, the physician, make abundantly clear that the biblical covenant must open outwardly towards others in servant love. The primary covenant with God serves as a critical standard for all those lesser covenants that people enter into and that tempt them to turn away from the stranger and the needy.

In this essay, I reflect on the bearing of this four-part, covenantal, story line on the medical covenant and, even more particularly, reflect on whether covenantal thinking leads to an emphasis in moral theory on obligations or virtues. That particular assignment invites me to jump one way or another into the current debates on the subject of theoretical ethics. The field of ethics conventionally requires coverage of at least three topics: the moral agent, the agent's action and the results of that action. Virtue theorists usually concentrate on the agent and his or her character; obligation theorists focus either on the agent's action (duty theorists) and/or on the results of that action (utilitarians or pragmatists).

While I will explore the implications of a covenantal ethic for the virtues,

I am not prepared to claim that such an ethic can do without the obligation theorists such as Paul Ramsey and James F. Childress who have developed principles and rules to shape medical practice. Covenantal fidelity defines the ruling principle in Ramsey's pioneering work, *The Patient As Person*, which he has rigorously applied to such issues as experimentation on human subjects, high risk therapy, organ transplants, care for the dying, genetic engineering, abortion and in vitro fertilization. Childress, also a religious obligation theorist, has co-authored *The Principles of Biomedical Ethics*, the most influential book in the field, that appeals to the principles of non-maleficence, beneficence, respect for autonomy, and justice as the comprehensive ground for all subsidiary moral rules in biomedical research and practice.

The influence of these obligation theorists derives largely from their excellence, but from other factors as well, religious, philosophical, societal and organizational . . .

[Therefore] I cannot dismiss the agenda of obligation theorists for medical ethics. Principle-oriented theory has some validity, philosophically and religiously; and it serves variously a religiously pluralist and secular society dominated by large organizations. But I also believe that a covenantal ethic must attend to the question of the moral agent and his or her virtues. Covenanted men and women do not simply accept a set of rules and principles guiding their actions, they also bind themselves over in the course of an event which alters and continuingly defines their identity. At Mt. Sinai, God marked the forehead of the Jews forever; through baptism, Christians acquire their very name and identity. As a covenanted people take up the particulars of their several vocations, their identity will display itself in the virtues that ought to characterize their practice. No ethic that adequately explores the medical covenant can focus simply upon the quandaries that emerge in medical practice and the bearing of moral principles upon those quandaries; it must also explore the identity of those agents who profess medicine. Virtue theory is the name we give to ethics as it focuses on such questions of identity and character.

Principle-oriented moralists concentrate on the question, 'what should we do?' Virtue theorists pose a second question behind the first, 'whom shall we be?' Practitioners' answer to the latter question of identity may more fatefully affect, for good or ill, their actual practice than the articulation of those principles which obligation theorists associate with applied ethics. What does it mean to be a physician? Is the physician simply a hybrid, an aggressive mix of technician and entrepreneur, or something more, a professional? If the practitioner is simply a careerist who puts his skills up for grabs to the highest bidder, then answers to the questions of truth-telling, price-charging, guild-policing, and resource allocation will simply reflect at best the driving force of enlightened self-interest. The practitioner simply sells time and services, throwing in an occasional act of charity to air blow the image and salve the conscience. Only in acknowledging his or her identity as a professional does the practitioner assume the full burden of those moral principles which obligation theorists emphasize.

## Professional Identity

'To profess' means 'to testify on behalf of,' 'to stand for,' or 'to avow' something that defines one's fundamental commitment. A profession opens out toward an as yet unspecified transcendent good that defines the professor. In contrast, a career is self-referential; a career reminds us of the word 'car,' a self-driven vehicle. We all breathe easier if we have a career that supplies us with a kind of self-driven vehicle through life whereby we enter into public thoroughfares but for our own private reasons and with our own private destination in mind. The Hippocratic Oath acknowledged a transcendent element in the profession of healing when the young physician avowed, 'I swear by Apollo Physician, and Asclepius and Hygieia, and Panaceia and all the gods and goddesses, that I will fulfil according to my ability and judgment this oath and covenant' ([2], p. 6) . . .

What does it take to make good on that [commitment]? Abraham Flexner, the mother of all reformers in medical education, identified six distinguishing marks of a professional which, in my judgment, reduce to three: intellectual, moral, and organizational. Each of these marks, in turn, calls for a primary virtue. The three marks and their correlative virtues set the agenda for the rest of this essay.

## The Intellectual Mark and Prudence

A professional draws on a complex and esoteric body of knowledge not available to everyone but to which he or she has direct access. This direct access to first principles distinguishes professional education from mere training. Trained people can perform specific routines but, argued Flexner, they don't know *why* they perform them. They quickly lapse into undeviating patterns; they don't adapt or grow. A knowledge of first principles, however, lays the foundation for the profession's future growth.

The need for direct acquaintance with basic principles led Flexner to insist on locating professional education in universities and on closing the so-called proprietary schools which smacked of mere training. He further insisted on the university site for medical education since a profession must, in some range of its work, engage in scientific research which expands the profession's knowledge base and thus serves its advancement and progress. Not any and all professionals must be researchers, but somewhere within the profession – usually at the university – the research enterprise must be supported.

If the physician's intellectual mark consists of scientific knowledge, no more, the student might need little more than the virtue of perseverance to acquire it. While a lowly virtue, perseverance is indispensable to the acquisition of scientific knowledge under the trying conditions of a lengthy professional education today. But healing is an art, not simply a science, requiring something more than the virtue of perseverance. Additionally, the physician needs the virtue of prudence.

Contemporary medical literature, however, offers little help on the meaning of the phrase, 'the healer's art' that would help us connect the art with prudence. When practitioners plump for medicine as an art rather than a science, they sound rather apologetic, as though they want to defend a place for themselves and their slender store of experience in turf largely occupied by scientists and the huge warehouses of knowledge and equipment over which they preside in tertiary care centers. Alternatively (and sometimes patronizingly), scientists accept healing as an art only in the provisional sense that they cannot yet reduce any and all cases to investigative techniques. Had we fuller knowledge, then the instinctive surmise would disappear. Only because of gaps in our scientific knowledge do we need to venture into the intuitive and the imaginative. Thus the art of healing provides but a temporary station on the way to a more perfect science of healing.

Healing, as an art, like other arts, displays a cognitive and a creative aspect; it is both a knowing and a doing. The cognitive component in the healing process – both diagnostic and prognostic – acts partly as science but partly as art. As science, it requires specialized and abstract investigatory work. Each medical specialty rests on its peculiar knowledge base; it relies on a series of indicators that signal the presence of diseases that its technical interventions can affect. This specialized knowledge and activity systematically abstracts from the patient as a whole, by ignoring the technically irrelevant.

But the cognitive component of healing includes a further element. The healer must attempt not only to cure the disease but address the illness of which the disease forms a part. As Dr. Eric Cassell has put it, 'Disease is something an organ has; illness is something a man has' ([1], p. 48). The host may be incidental to the disease (sometimes, not always), but the host is rarely incidental to the state of illness. The healer who would 'make whole' stricken patients cannot rest content with a specialized and abstract knowledge, as much as that may contribute to the enterprise. The healer must look at the whole patient, the full range of somatic and psychic structures disrupted by disease. Such a knowledge must ultimately unite and specify, situating the disease in a particular person and in his or her idiosyncratic social history. The knowledge resembles more the coordinations of an experienced fisherman scanning the sea or a hunter wary in the woods or a cook fully experienced in the kitchen than it resembles the reductions of a particular case to a general law.

Finally, the healer's knowing aims at doing. The healer's art creates as well as knows, and the constructive activity in which the healer engages includes more than curing disease. The fully rounded work of healing reconnects the patient with the world and recovers his or her self-control and self-confidence. The treatment plan at its best offers a coherent total program for as much recovery as a particular patient can achieve under the circumstances. Preventive medicine and chronic care, just as much as acute and rehabilitative medicine, require artistic intervention. Admittedly, such care has its routines, techniques, and tricks. No art form lacks its conventions. But these activities ultimately aim to reorder comprehensively a human life. That work, in the nature of the case, must unite and specify.

The fully developed physician needs the virtue of prudence since the physician's art of knowing is artful as well as scientific. Ethical theorists who orient to principles sometimes tend to downgrade the importance of prudence as they rely on general principles rather than the concrete insight of the moral agent. Some theorists trivialize prudence into a merely adroit selection of means in the pursuit of ends, into a crafty packaging of policies. The virtue of prudence, to be sure, deals with fitting means to ends. But, as a virtue, it consists of much more than the 'tactical cunning' to which Machiavelli and many in the modern word diminish virtue. Thomas Aquinas noted,

> . . . in order that a choice be good, two things are required. First, that the intention be directed to a due end . . . Secondly, that man take rightly those things which have reference to the end: and this he cannot do unless his reason counsel, judge and command aright, which is the function of prudence and the virtues annexed to it . . . (*Summa Theologica*, Pt. 1–11, Q. 58, Art. 5, Trans. Dominican Fathers).

The ancients gave a primary place to prudence as the 'eye of the soul.' The medievalists ranked prudence as the first of the cardinal virtues on the grounds that 'Being precedes Truth and . . . Truth precedes Goodness'([6] p. 4). Diagnosis and prognosis precedes apt therapy. One must discern what is there in order to be there for it. An openness to being underlies both being good and producing the good in and for others. The art of prudent discerning includes three elements, especially if one hopes to discern fully a human being:

a) *memoria* – being truly open to the past (rather than retouching, coloring, or falsifying the past);

b) *docilitas* – defined, not as a bovine docility, but as an openness to the present, the ability to be still, to be silent, to listen and take in what makes itself present; and

c) *solertia* – a readiness for the unexpected, the novel, an openness to the future, a disposition sometimes in short supply in those who only too quickly subsume the new case under old routines.

This disciplined openness to the past, present, and future fairly summarizes what the distressed patient needs from the healer and the moral tradition that argued for it long precedes Freudian wisdom on the subject of the therapeutic relationship.

Such prudence demands much more than a facile packaging of what one has to say or do. *Discretio* presupposes metaphysical perception, a sense for what the Stoics called the fitting, a sensibility that goes deeper than tact, a feel for the other and one's own behavior that is congruent with reality. Without discernment, the professional does not deal with the whole truth in diagnosis and prognosis, that is, with the truths of illness, as well as disease; and without discernment, the professional does not mobilize the full power of healing, which exceeds that of laser, knife, and drug.

## The Moral Mark and Fidelity

Professionals who stand for, or avow something, do so on behalf of someone. They profess not simply any and all knowledge, but a particular body of learning that applies tonically to a specific range of human problems. Unlike earlier knowledge merchants, such as wizards and magicians, who may use their knowledge simply to display their virtuosity, professionals must orient altruistically to serve human need, and not simply their own needs or those of their friends and relatives, but those of the stranger. 'Hanging out one's shingle' symbolized from the seventeenth century forward the professional's readiness to direct knowledge to the needs of the stranger.

The symbol of the shingle is ambiguous. It invites the stranger, but it does so, at least partly, in the setting of the marketplace. The professional differs from the amateur in that the amateur does it for love and the professional for money. Only a species of angelism would argue otherwise. Professionals are not disembodied spirits. They earn their bread and pay their bills in the course of serving others. The professional exchange with patients and with the institutions for which they work partly conforms to a marketplace exchange of buying and selling. It therefore requires the traditional marketplace virtues of industry, honesty, and integrity.

But the professional exchange also transcends or ought to transcend, the case nexus. It requires the further virtue of fidelity. A sustaining commitment to the being and well-being of the patient presumably distinguishes it from the marketplace assumptions about an exchange between two relatively knowledgeable, frankly self-interested parties. Ultimately, the interest and well-being of the patient must trump the physician's own self-interest. The patient's own perceptions of self-interest will not adequately protect the patient. Usually, patients cannot obey the marketplace warning, 'buyer beware,' because an asymmetry exists between the professional's knowledge and power and the patient's relative ignorance, powerlessness, and oftentimes urgent distress which does not permit comparative shopping. This imbalance requires that the professional exchange takes place in a fiduciary setting of trust that transcends the marketplace assumptions about two wary bargainers. Only the physician's fidelity to the patient in the disposition of his or her knowledge and power justifies that trust.

Fidelity to the patient should constrain the physician's notion of what he or she has to sell. If I walk into a Volvo showroom, I do not expect the salesperson to question whether I actually need a Volvo. No one in a Volvo showroom has ever suggested to me that, as an academic, I ought to trot across the street and buy at half the price a Toyota Tercel. The salesperson takes it as a challenge to sell me a car and thereby meet his quota for the month. I am a pork chop for the eating. But if I visit a surgeon, I must be able to assume that he or she sells two items, not one. The surgeon is not simply interested in the business of selling hernia jobs, but also the further, detached, disinterested, unclouded judgment that I need that wretched procedure. Otherwise, the physician abuses disproportionate knowledge and power and poisons a fiduciary relationship with distrust. Instead of sheltering, the surgeon takes advantage of the distressed.

Herein lies the ground for professional strictures against conflicts of interest. The professional must be sufficiently distanced from his or her own interests and that of other patients to serve the patient's well-being. However, serving the patient's welfare faces subtler pitfalls than gross conflicts of financial interest. Physicians must take care that their eagerness to recruit their patients into high risk research protocols does not obscure their primary duty to their patients' welfare. Otherwise, they act as double agents, pretending concern for their patients while serving, in fact, the drug companies or the advancement of their own careers as researchers.

The professional exchange differs in a second way from a marketplace transaction. In addition to its disinterestedness, it is, for want of a better word, transformational, and not merely transactional. The healer must respond not simply to the patient's self-perceived wants but to his or her deeper needs. The patient suffering from insomnia often wants simply the quick fix of a pill. But if the physician goes after the root of the problem, then she may have to help the patient transform the habits that led to the symptom of sleeplessness. The physician is slothful if she dutifully offers acute care but neglects preventive medicine.

The term 'transformational,' however, awakens legitimate fears of paternalism. The prospect of the physician, the lawyer, the manager, and the political leader engaged in transforming habits provokes memories of overbearing authority figures who haunt the American past.

Transformational leadership slips into parentalism unless teaching becomes its chief instrument. Teaching becomes one of the few ways in which one can engage in transformation while respecting the patient's intelligence and power of self-determination. No one can engage properly in preventative, rehabilitative, chronic, and even terminal care without properly teaching his or her patients and their families.

This fidelity to the patient in his or her deeper needs brings the discussion back to the virtue of prudence. Prudence is sensitive not only to ends but to fitting means to those ends. The end of medicine is healing, but the art of healing must pass through rational self-determining creatures. In securing patient compliance, in acute care and patient partnership in the tasks of preventative, rehabilitative, and chronic care, the physician must honor fully the person who hosts the disease. The physician does not succeed in these tasks unless she lets herself be taught by the patient in the course of the interview and teaches the patient aright in turn. Teaching aright poses the question: how does one teach the sick and stricken? If teaching is the means, what are the means to the means? How does one teach? Pedantically? Naggingly? Vindictively? Scoldingly? Scripture answers that question concisely: speak the truth in love. Therewith prudence and fidelity fully knit together.

## The Organizational Mark and Public-spiritedness

This mark traces back to the medieval guild and, still further back, to the Hippocratic covenant of the young physician with his teacher who helped initiate him into his professional identity. Continuing with this tradition, Abraham Flexner believed that physicians should organize in order to maintain and improve professional standards. A professional guild ought to differ from a trade association in that it aims at self-improvement, not self-promotion. So goes the ideal.

Until recently in the United States, it appeared that the organizational mark had all but faded, except for purely defensive and self-promotional activities upon the part of the guilds. In addition to the general American myth of the self-made man, the medical profession subscribed to the myth of the free-lance physician who ran his own office, made the rounds of his patients in their homes, and managed a practice partly by cash and partly by charity. But since the 1930s medicine has increasingly organized to produce medical goods in the setting of large hospitals and to expect compensation for the distribution of these goods and services through huge third-party payers. (The professional guild has been much less disposed to accept responsibility for controlling the quality of medical goods through the mechanism of self-regulation and discipline.)

This organizational mark calls for the professional virtue of 'public-spiritedness,' which I would define as the art of acting in concert with others for the common good, in the production, distribution, and quality control of health care.

Why do professionals owe something to the common good? Physicians, along with other professionals, are rulers in a society such as ours. We do not transmit power today on the basis of blood. We largely wield and transmit a knowledge-based power acquired in the university. This derivation of power from a university inescapably generates an indebtedness to the society. A huge company of people contribute to the making of practitioners as they zigzag their way through college and professional schools: the janitors who clean the johns, the help in the kitchen, the secretaries who make the operation hum, the administrators who wrestle with the institution's problems, the faculty who share with students what they know, the vast research traditions of each of the disciplines that set the table for that sharing, and the patients who lay their bodies and sometimes souls on the line, letting young physicians and surgeons practice on them in the course of perfecting their art. And behind all this, the public moneys and gifts that support the enterprise, so much so that tuition money usually pays for only a small fraction of the education. When professionals treat education as providing them with a private stockpile of knowledge to be sold on the market to the highest bidder, they systematically distort and obscure the social origins of knowledge, and therefore the power which that knowledge places within their grasp.

Further, the power which modern professionals wield vastly exceeds that of their predecessors. What physicians do fatefully affects the society at large. They have even less reason than their predecessors to bend their power to serve purely private, entrepreneurial goals. When they do so, they conform to Aristotle's definition of tyranny, that is, the channeling of public power to private purposes. Somehow we have managed to normalize power directed to private purposes alone under the conditions of a marketplace democracy without recognizing the despotic element in its exercise. It ill behooves professionals to sever their calling from all questions of the common good and to instrumentalize it to private goods alone. The social source of power's derivation and the public consequences of its exercise should elicit from professionals the virtue of public-spiritedness, the art of acting in concert with others for the common good.

## Public-spiritedness and the Production of Medical Goods

In professing a body of knowledge which they place at the service of human need, physicians do not do so as purely private performers. Medicine today is increasingly a social art practiced by a health care team in the setting of a very large institution. Until recently, the hospital has served as the physician's workshop, where he or she performed services and made money under the third party payment system with few controls over either those services or the money to be made. However, hospitals now operate under the restriction of a federal payment system, which controls the amount of money that the hospital (and indirectly the doctor) can make off a given disease, and under growing pressures from insurance companies and from corporations negotiating health care contracts. Physicians must increasingly accept some responsibility for not only their personal professional values but also the values shaping the institution in which they work. In effect, physicians need to recognize the hospital as a *polis*, a political entity, in which they must help set policies on the relative weight of ends served and the resources deployed to reach those ends. The ill require for their healing not only covenanted individuals but covenanted institutions that profess, testify on behalf of, or stand for something. Such institutions, in turn, need physicians skilled not simply in the art of medicine, but in the art of acting in concert with others for the common good.

Physicians need the virtue of public-spiritedness for the further reason that, whether in the hospital, clinic, or in group practice, they rarely work today as solitary gunslingers, but as members of a health care team. Medical education and residency training programs have only partly recognized the importance of cultivating the professional as a member and leader of the health care team. They concentrate exhaustively and almost exclusively on educating students in the sciences and developing their technical skills, while paying much less attention to their maturing as team members.

Further, the very conditions of residency training often distract and disrupt effective teamwork. The constantly changing caste of specialists, attending physicians, residents and nurses often leaves patients and their families wondering just who is their physician. The system also can signal to the impressionable resident that team membership is incidental and subordinate to technical performance. The ever shifting composition of the team with rotation shifts makes it difficult to deliver continuous, coherent service to a particular patient, however conscientious team members may be. The accidental intersection of a variety of needed technical services does not spontaneously mesh into a coherent program of care. Clearly, the effective team requires not only self-conscious efforts to prepare young members for participation and leadership but also the rethinking of schedules and agendas so as to honor the team's unitary responsibilities.

## Public-spiritedness and the Distribution of Medical Goods

The notion of the just and public-spirited professional calls for more than a minimalist commitment to what the moral tradition has called *commutative* justice, that is, the fulfillment of duties between two private parties based on contracts. Public-spiritedness suggests a more spacious obligation to *distribu-*

*tive* justice which seeks to meet the health care needs of all members of society, a goal which has not been, and cannot be, met solely through the mechanism of the marketplace and supplements of charity. Physicians and other professionals have a duty to distribute goods and services targeted on basic needs without limiting those services simply to those who have the capacity to pay for them. Some would deny this obligation to distributive justice altogether. Others would argue that the services of the helping professionals should be distributed to meet such basic human needs, but that this obligation rests on the society at large and not on the profession itself. This approach, which argues for a tax-supported third party payment system, would eliminate *pro bono publico* work as a professional obligation.

Still others, myself included, perceive the obligation to distribute professional services to be both a public and professional responsibility. Professionals exercise power through public authority. The power they wield and the goods they control are of a public magnitude and scale. Although the state has a primary responsibility for *ministering* justice (an old term for distributive justice), professional groups, too, have a ministry, if you will, to perform. When the state alone accepts responsibility for distributive justice, a general sense of obligation tends to diminish in the culture at large, and the social virtue upon which the impetus to distribute depends loses the grounds for its renewal. Professionals particularly need to accept some responsibility for ministering justice to sustain that moral sensibility in the society at large. Otherwise, the idealistic motives that originally prompted the founding of institutions (such as mental hospitals) will peter out, and the institutions deteriorate into custodial bins.

Further, such *pro bono publico* work does not merely serve the private happiness of those individuals who receive services; it eventually redounds to the *common* good and fosters public happiness. Those who receive help are not merely individuals but *parts* of a whole. Thus the whole, in so serving in its parts, serves its own public flourishing; it rescues its citizens mired in their private distress for a more public life. In the absence of *pro bono publico* work, we signal, in effect, that only those people who can pay their way into the marketplace have a public identity. To this degree, our public life shrinks; it reduces to those with the money to enter it. Public-spirited professionals not only receive private distress, they help preserve our common life, in a monetary culture, from a constant source of its own perishing.

## Public-spiritedness and Professional Self-regulation and Discipline

Physicians need the virtue of public-spiritedness not only to perform satisfactorily on health care teams in hospitals and to distribute the good of health care widely, but also to control the quality of the good produced and distributed. Professional self-regulation and discipline is the name for that quality control.

For many reasons, physicians duck responsibility for professional self-monitoring. Like any professional group, they find themselves in complex, interlocking relations with fellow professionals which make actions against a colleague awkward, the defense of abused patients inconvenient. Unlike lapses on the part of other professionals, the physician's therapeutic misadventure can be fatal or irreparable in its effects. Since the stakes are so high in the case of a physician's malpractice, professionals are tempted to draw their wagons into a circle to protect a challenged member. Unlike lapses on the part of other professionals, the physician's misadventure can irreparably harm or kill. Further, Americans, in general, press charges against their neighbors or colleagues only reluctantly; they are morally averse to officiousness. Unlike some of their European counterparts, Americans show little stomach for playing amateur policeman, prosecutor, judge, when they themselves are not directly or officially involved in an incident. In many respects, this *laissez faire* attitude is an admirable trait in the American character.

Yet this morally attractive nonchalance cannot justify permissiveness in professional life, for professionals are power wielders, *de facto* rulers in modern society. They reserve the right to pass judgment (in professional matters) on colleagues or would be colleagues; and the society supports this right in establishing educational requirements and licensing procedures. To be sure, patients profit from this through higher standards, but the profession also profits – handsomely – in money and power. Professionals have not justified this state created monopoly if they merely practice competently themselves. The individual's license to practice depends upon the prior license to license which the state has to all intents and purposes bestowed upon the guild. If the license to practice carries with it the obligation to practice well, then the prior license to license carries with it the obligation to judge and monitor well. Not only individuals but a guild must be accountable. Am I my colleague's keeper? The brief answer is, yes. And that responsibility may sometimes require not simply disciplining the troubled colleague, but finding positive ways to help him. Public-spiritedness in this always disturbing activity of professional discipline calls for the attendant virtues of courage, fairness, and compassion.

In my opening comments on the biblical covenant, I mentioned the elements of gift, promise, and moral and ritual action. The discussion of prudence and fidelity highlighted only the element of promise. The physician professes his or her art (prudence) on behalf of someone (fidelity). The discussion barely adumbrated the moral advisories and the ritual/habitual routines that flow from this double profession and promise. But, in closing, I need to make explicit the element of gift that precedes and generates the power of this double promise to something on behalf of someone. Otherwise, we interpret the professional either contractually as the seller of services or contractually/philanthropically as a combined seller/giver of services but not covenantally as a person whose actions rest upon a comprehensive receiving. We interpret the physician as benefactor but overlook his or her deepest identity as a beneficiary. Thereby we fail to trace the three covenantal virtues to their original source and their final resource to which the virtues of gratitude and hope testify.

Before specifying the antecedent gifts implicit in the foregoing account of the three professional virtues, I must concede that one cannot fully appreciate the indebtedness of a human being by totting up the varying sacrifices and investments made by others to his or her benefit. The sense that one inexhaustibly receives presupposes a more transcendent source of donative activity than the sum of gifts received from others. The formula borrowed from Josef Pieper – 'Being precedes Truth and . . . Truth precedes Goodness' [6] – neatly captures the element of transcendent gift upon which the virtues depend. Knowing depends upon the taking in of Being; and goodness (or doing aright) depends upon that receptive knowing. In the biblical tradition, this transcendent source is a Being which is a Being-true, which, in covenant fidelity secretly gives root to every gift between human beings. The secondary gifts in the human order of giving and receiving can only (and imperfectly) signify this primary gift.

But giving at the human level also contributes to the physician's knowing and doing. The discussion of public-spiritedness has already made that clear. No one can graduate from a modern university and professional school and think of himself or herself as a self-made man or woman. Practicing physicians cannot survive a single day without drawing upon the massive research traditions of their profession that support whatever prowess is theirs in diagnosis, prognosis, and therapy. Not only past generations of researchers, but countless patients, many of them poor, have submitted to the experiments that now make the physician seem so smart in the office, the clinic, or the hospital. Further, that research tradition does not effectively connect with the individual patients unless the patient himself presents, complains, lays bare his vulnerability and distress. The successful interview with the patient requires addressing, but also being addressed, giving, but also taking in, the tongue, but also the ear.

Thus professionals who, in fidelity, benefit their patients do not do so as pure benefactors. Idealistic members of the helping professions like to define themselves by their giving or serving alone – with others indebted to them. A reciprocity, however, of giving and receiving is at work in the professional relationship that needs to be acknowledged. The physician has received abundantly from her patients, not only in all the aforementioned ways but also by their petitions for help which confer upon the physician her identity.

Patients help give the professional her calling. In answering the call, the professional gets back nothing less than what she is – a remarkable gift indeed.

However, in trying to make good on their calling, professionals discover that they fall short. They promise a deep-going, core identity with their patients, but discover that drawing close to misery and deprivation threatens to suck them into a whirlpool. They risk getting mired down in the mess and confusion of their patients' lives. Some physicians respond to human affliction somewhat heroically and grimly, playing the role of savior, the anointed defender and guardian of the woe beset. Others, discouraged, recognize the very limited, partial, and temporary nature of the relief which they can offer; they burn out. Still others respond self-protectively, finding a way to shield themselves defensively from the stricken, radio-active patient. While differing, these varied responses have in common a metaphysical gloom; they raise the question of the place of the virtue of hope in the helping professions.

The virtue of hope does not enter into the picture if a covenantal ethic generates a moral principle of unconditional fidelity, but nothing more. Indeed, as a moral principle alone, it only intensifies professional burdens and increases the possibility of moral exhaustion and burnout. A covenantal ethic, however, depends upon the conviction that one's own promise-keeping rests, not simply on a moral principle of keeping one's promises, but upon an all-surrounding promissory event. God has made and will keep his promise to humankind. This promise defines men and women not only retrospectively in gratitude but prospectively in hope. It comforts them in the midst of their professional excesses, shortfall, and burnout with the knowledge that God will not abandon his creatures, either those who give or those who receive care. God's promise gives to human promise-keeping some buoyancy. To the degree that professionals persist in 'being-true' to their promises, even with some small measure of resiliency, they offer their troubled patients a tiny emblem of that ultimate hope.

## Bibliography

1. Cassell, E.: 1979, *The Healer's Art*, Penguin Books.
2. Edelstein, L.: 1967, *Ancient Medicine, Selected Papers of Ludwig Edelstein*, Owsei Temkin and C. Lillian Temkin (eds.), John Hopkins Press, Baltimore, MD.
3. May, W. F.: 1983, *The Physician's Covenant*, Westminster Press, Philadephia, PA, now in Louisville, KY.
4. May, W. F.: 1984, 'The Virtues in a Professional Setting', in *Soundings*, vol. LXVII, No. 3 (Fall), 245–266.
5. May, W. F.: 1991, 'The Beleagured Rulers: the Public Obligation of the Professional', the *Kennedy Institute of Ethics Journal*, vol. 2, No. 1, 25–41.

6. Pieper, J.: 1954, *The Four Cardinal Virtues*, University of Notre Dame Press, Notre Dame, Indiana.
7. Wolin, S.: 1960, *Politics and Vision*, Little, Brown and Company, Inc., Boston.

**Notes**

1. This essay draws on the three sources in my writings cited in the Bibliography, but it orders the thought in a way I have not heretofore proposed.

# Empowerment in the Clinical Setting

KAREN LEBACQZ

In *Professional Ethics: Power and Paradox* [17], I proposed that the power of the professional person is morally relevant to determining what should be done in the practice setting and that justice or empowerment of the client becomes a central norm for professional practice.[1] The time has now come to see what justice as empowerment means for the clinical setting. The task is particularly crucial in light of Kapp's recent definition of empowerment as advocating for oneself and participating maximally in one's own significant decisions ([14], p. 5). Under this definition, to choose dependence upon others is to 'forego' empowerment ([14], p. 6). I will explore below the adequacy of this definition.

Just as we learn about justice by exploring experiences of injustice [16], so we may learn about empowerment by exploring disempowerment. Disempowerment, and therefore empowerment, within the clinical setting will differ from setting to setting and from population to population. I will examine two populations: those who begin with power and become disempowered in the clinical setting, and those who begin from a position of relative powerlessness and experience the clinical setting from that perspective.

## The Disempowerment of the Powerful

Hans Jonas argued that the ideal research subject is a doctor: the doctor is best positioned to understand the risks and implications of the research and to give a truly voluntary and informed consent [13]. In short, the doctor as subject is most likely to be empowered in the research setting. Similarly, the doctor as patient is most likely to be empowered in the clinical setting. By looking at the disempowerment experienced by those most likely to retain power in the clinical setting, we begin to develop a sense of what constitutes disempowerment and therefore what would constitute empowerment. So we begin with those who experience no language, cultural, knowledge, or sexual barriers to empowerment.

From Gerald P. McKenny and Jonathan R. Sande (eds.), *Theological Analyses of the Clinical Encounter*, pp. 133–147. Dordrecht: Kluwer Academic Publishers, 1994.

Yet even white, male, well-educated doctors, when they become patients, experience disempowerment in the clinical setting. The film 'The Doctor,' based on *A Taste of My Own Medicine* by Ed Rosenbaum [22] and just released at the time of writing this essay, demonstrates precisely this disempowerment. Here is a physician, a surgeon, accustomed to ordering people around in the hospital who must now wait in line, fill out forms by the hour, be told 'sorry, the doctor is late today,' and undergo any number of forms of indignity experienced routinely by patients.

A similar story is told in Oliver Sacks' delightful treatise *A Leg to Stand On* [24]. Sacks broke his leg in a climbing accident. Not only was the leg broken; Sacks also lost all sense of feeling in the leg, and all ability to move or exercise control over it. He lost 'proprioception,' the sense of owning one's own limbs and having command over them. Ironically, proprioception is one of the foci of Sacks' work as a neurologist. Thus his story is the story of a man who moves not only from the status of physician to the status of patient, but indeed to the very kind of patient that he himself treats. He thus learned to see from the 'inside' what his patients had tried to communicate to him.

## Two Miseries, Two Empowerments

To be a patient – at least under critical circumstances – is to live in an altered world. It is almost as though one has entered the 'twilight zone.' Perceptions are distorted, time and space appear to be different, even everyday conversations can loom threateningly: ' "Execution tomorrow," said the clerk in Admissions. I knew it must have been, "Operation tomorrow," but the feeling of execution overwhelmed what he said' ([24], p. 46).

Illness takes place on two levels. Sacks calls it 'two miseries'. One is the physical disability, the 'organically determined erosion of being and space' ([24], p. 158). The other he calls the 'moral' dimension associated with 'the reduced stationless status of a patient, and, in particular, conflict with and surrender to "them" – "them" being the surgeon, the whole system, the institution . . .' ([24], p. 158).

Illness is not just a matter of physical disability. The clinical setting involves also, and even more importantly, a change in one's structural and sociological status. One becomes a 'patient.'

Even the most powerful of patients therefore feel disempowered in two ways. First, they have lost some ability previously possessed – in Sacks' case, the ability to walk and even to feel his own leg. Loss of ability is annoying at best, frightening at worst: 'I found myself . . . scared and confounded to the roots of my being' ([24], p. 79). This is the first 'misery' with which the patient deals, and it is often overwhelming in itself, undermining one's ability to deal normally with the world.

But other patients have also lost normal status in the world. For Sacks, and for many others, it is the role of patient as much as physical disability itself that inflicts misery and requires empowerment. 'I felt morally helpless, paralyzed, contracted, confined – and not just contracted, but contorted as well, into roles and postures of abjection' ([24], p. 158). For example, Sacks asked for spinal rather than general anesthesia, and his request was denied. He writes, 'I felt curiously helpless . . . and I thought, Is *this* what "being a patient" means?' Sociologists have described the 'sick role' or status of patient. From the inside, this status is often a feeling of diminishment. Sacks calls himself a 'man reduced, and dependent' ([24], p. 133).

The role of patient is reinforced by institutional structures and practices: 'we were set apart, we patients in white nightgowns, and avoided clearly, though unconsciously, like lepers' ([24], p. 163). As Alan Goldman puts it in his examination of professional ethics,

> Life in hospitals . . . continues to be filled with needless rituals suggestive of patient passivity, dependence, and impotence. The institutional setting is still structured in such a way as to block the exercise of rights at least partially accepted intellectually . . . Patients are rarely permitted to see their charts; pills are almost literally shoved into their mouths . . . Often newly admitted patients perfectly capable of walking are taken to their rooms in wheelchairs, an apt symbol of the helpless pose they are made to assume from the time of their entrance into this alien and authoritarian setting ([10], pp. 224–5).

Ultimately, suggests Sacks, he indeed became an 'invalid': in-valid ([24], p. 164). Sacks resisted the patient role at every step. Yet he recognized that both he and the surgeons were, in a sense, 'forced to play roles – he the role of the All-knowing Specialist, I the role of the Know-nothing Patient' ([24], p. 105).

If illness is composed of two miseries, then recovery will require two empowerments. 'Now we needed a double recovery – a physical recovery, and a spiritual movement *to* health' ([24], p. 164). The patient needs physical healing – in Sacks' case, surgery and physical therapy so that he could once again walk, run, jump, and do things that his body had 'forgotten' how to do. But as much as the physical healing, the patient needs recovery from the abject, reduced, dependent status of patient.

Both miseries are disempowering. But it is the 'contortion' into roles and postures of abjection that is the core of the power gap between physician and patient. Such contortion need not accompany physical deterioration. Different structures, a different approach in the clinical setting, might significantly reduce the second 'misery.'

Nor is such contortion necessarily diminished when physical healing takes place. Too often, we assume that once health is restored, the patient automatically becomes a non-patient and experiences restored moral status. In my experience, this is not true. Effects of dependent status can linger, making future contacts difficult and undermining patients' sense of their own worth and being. While the patient may literally move outside the hospital or clinic and cease being a patient in a technical sense, the psycho-sociological effects of dependent patienthood may remain. Moreover, during the time of clinical care, the dependent status of patient can adversely affect medical treatment.

What can be done to empower patients? The loss of function, the physical disability, is the initial presenting problem. The best the medical team can do in the face of it is to try to heal. But is the loss of status, the diminished sense of personhood that often accompanies being a patient, also necessary? Must there be two miseries? Is there a way to reduce the second misery, to hasten recovery from it, and to empower the patient who experiences it? Using Sacks' experience, we can examine the disempowerment of the powerful and suggest how different structures and responses might empower the patient.

## The Central Role of Communication

The clinical context begins with communication. Disempowerment begins with failures of communication. One of the most disempowering things that happens in the clinical context is shutting down the patient's words.

In Sacks' case, this began with his first attempts to share what had happened. 'They wanted to know the "salient facts" and I wanted to tell them everything – the entire story' ([24], p. 47). Something had *happened* to Sacks. It was his story. He wanted to tell it. And he wanted to be heard. So from the first 'intake' interview in which Sacks tried to tell the 'entire' story and the medical team asked for the 'salient facts,' things went awry.

Failure to communicate went far beyond this first incident. Sacks knew that something was wrong with his leg because he had lost all feeling in it. He waited (and waited and waited!) for the surgeon to come in order to raise his concerns. The surgeon finally appeared, only to state briskly, 'there's nothing to worry about' and disappear before Sacks could say more than 'but . . .' Sacks was given no *time* to communicate.

As the days went by and the leg failed to respond to physiotherapy, Sacks became desperate to communicate his concern: 'Desperately now, I wanted communication, and reassurance' ([24], p. 88). Above all, he recognized a need to communicate to the surgeon and have the surgeon understand. While he wanted reassurance, he was prepared to accept the truth if no reassurance could be given: 'I should respect whatever he said so long as it was frank and showed respect for me, for my dignity as a man' ([24], p. 93).

When the surgeon came, he neither looked at Sacks nor spoke to him, but turned to the nurse and said, 'Well, Sister, and how is the patient now?'

([24], p. 104). Rather than respect and frankness, Sacks was treated as a nonentity. He was not even addressed by the surgeon, but talked about as if he were not there. Sacks was given no *respect* for himself as a communicator; all the communication was with those around him. Using Kapp's definition of empowerment as advocating for oneself and participating 'maximally' in one's own significant decisions, Sacks was clearly disempowered.

Sacks persisted in raising his concern and tried, falteringly, to tell the physician what was wrong:

> It's ... it's ... I don't seem to be able to contract the quadriceps ... and, er ... the muscle doesn't seem to have any tone. And ... and ... I have difficulty locating the position of the leg ([24], p. 104).

I have quoted this speech as Sacks describes it. If it is an accurate representation of what he said, this fact alone is significant. Sacks is a literary man. He writes eloquently, powerfully.[2] It is difficult to imagine him at a loss for words, or stumbling over his words. Yet, confronted with the power of the physician, and in his own dependent state as patient, stumble is apparently what he did. He seems to have stammered, acted hesitant and evidenced confusion.

There may be an important lesson here for empowerment in the clinical context. Few medical people realize how dis-empowering the very context is. Patients generally feel inadequate in their descriptions of what is wrong. They hesitate, stumble, try to find the right words. Nothing seems to come out right. The patient who stumbles over her words is not necessarily stupid, but may simply be experiencing, as Sacks did, a diminishment of her capacity to verbalize.

I went to my physician complaining of pain in my hip joint. He asked me to stand and turn in certain ways, and then declared flatly that it could not be my *joint* that was hurting. It must be the *tendon*, not the joint. To him, this technicality and diagnostic accuracy is important. I do not care whether the pain originates in the joint, technically speaking, or in the tendon. I care only about what can be done to alleviate it, since I live in a house full of stairs. But his focus on the technicalities made it difficult for me to persist in my query. I had been told that I was *wrong*. I felt inadequate and unable to communicate. I gave up, and no treatment was forthcoming.

Sacks suggests that there is among doctors, 'in acute hospitals at least, a presumption of stupidity in their patients' ([24], p. 171). Whether all doctors do in fact consider their patients stupid, in acute or other contexts, failures to communicate often have the subtle effect of giving the patient a sense that she or he is not only stupid but also not worthy of the physician's time and effort.

Failure to hear the patient's story, impatience to get to salient facts, lack of time to listen, failure to address the patient at all, focussing on technicalities or calling the patient's understanding wrong – all these are disempowering in the clinical context. The patient who has been treated this way often gives up on the effort to communicate.

Many feel keenly their 'ex-communication' ([24], p. 110). Not only have they been shut down from the healthy world literally – stuck in the hospital, wrapped in white gowns, and avoided by healthy people – but they are now shut out symbolically by failure to communicate, to listen, to honor their perspective. 'As a patient in the hospital I felt both anguish and asphyxia – the anguish of being confronted with dissolution, and asphyxia because I would not be heard' ([24], p. 209). Thus does Sacks describe the life-killing effect of having communication shut off.

Lack of communication is not the only thing that is disempowering in the clinical context. Being denied a legitimate request (e.g. for spinal rather than general anesthesia), being forced to wear unattractive hospital gowns that strip one's individuality, being shunted from department to department like a sack of potatoes – all these and many other routine aspects of clinical care also take power away from patients. But many of these ills would be compensated by careful communication that leaves patients feeling as though they have been treated as persons, as though they can advocate for themselves and participate maximally in decisions. As Sacks puts it, he would have been content with whatever he was told, so long as it was told with respect.

## The Liberating Word

If failures of communication are the beginning of disempowerment, then communication can be the beginning of empowerment: 'The posture, the passivity of the patient, lasts as long as the doctor orders . . .' ([24], p. 133). Sacks points to the importance of the liberating word on several occasions. In order to heal, to regain use of his leg, he had to walk. Rehabilitation is based on action. Yet that action was birthed not just by himself, but by others: 'I had to *do* it, give birth to the New Act, but others were needed to deliver me, and *say*, "Do it!" ' ([24], p. 182). He calls this speaking the essential role of the teacher or therapist. It is a form of midwifery. Only as others granted permission could he find the way to do something new.

Once he missed a memorial service that he would have liked to attend, and lamented to the nurse that he was unable to go. 'Why not?' she queried. By challenging the limitations he had set for himself, she had removed them: 'The moment she spoke and said, "Why not?" a great barrier disappeared . . . Whatever it was, I was liberated by her words' ([24], p. 184).

Words of support ('do it') and words of challenge ('why can't you?') can both be liberating. Both can set the patient free to take a new step in the healing process and to claim skills and territory that the patient has not been able to claim by herself.

## Empathy

But communication goes far beyond words. When Sacks was first injured, a young surgeon danced into his room, and leaped on the bed-side table. This surgeon had once had a broken leg, and showed Sacks the scars from surgery. 'He didn't talk like a text-book. He scarcely talked at all – he acted. He leapt and danced and showed me his wounds, showing me at the same time his perfect recovery' ([24], p. 44). This visit made Sacks feel 'immeasurably better.' Here, he encountered someone who had been through it and could demonstrate that there is light at the end of the tunnel. Later, another surgeon came to see Sacks, and Sacks felt that he could communicate with this man. *'I've been through this myself,'* said the surgeon, *'I had a broken leg . . . I know what it's like'* ([24], p. 183). The empathy that comes from experience communicates and empowers.

Empathy gives authority to speak: 'So when Mr Amundsen said that the time had come to graduate, and give up one crutch, he spoke with authority – the only real authority, that of experience and understanding' ([24], p. 183). Sacks reflects on his own change as a physician because of what he went through as a patient, 'Now I *knew,* for I had experienced myself. And now I could truly begin to understand my patients' ([24], p. 202). At the end of the film 'The Doctor,' the protagonist puts all his physicians-in-training through the experience of being a patient in the hospital. Sacks suggests that there is an 'absolute and categorical difference' between a doctor who knows and one who does not, and that this difference is because of the personal experience of 'descending to the very depths of disease and dissolution' ([24], p. 203).

There is here, then, an important epistemological question that relates to empowerment. One who knows what the patient suffers and can truly hear the patient can empower the patient. But how does one 'know' what the patient suffers? Those who have been through a similar experience have readiest access to empathy. This suggests that, where possible, medical care teams should include at least one care-giver who has experienced what the patient suffers. Where this is not possible, groups of patients with similar problems might be assembled. Patients often feel more secure about their position and more enabled to question medical practice when they are with a group that shares their experience.

## Art and Religion

Sacks found several other things empowering as well. When he was rebuffed by the surgeon who told him that his concerns were 'nothing,' he felt as though he had entered a scotoma, 'a hole in reality itself' ([24], p. 109). 'In this limbo, this dark night,' he writes, 'I could not turn to science. Faced with a reality which reason could not solve, I turned to art and religion for comfort . . .' ([24], p. 114). Two additional sources of empowerment, then, are art and religion.

A friend loaned Sacks a tape recorder with only one tape: Mendelssohn's violin concerto. 'Something happened' to Sacks from the first playing of the music. The music appeared to reveal the creative and animating principle of the world, and thus began to give him hope for animation of his own portion of the world, his leg. 'The sense of hopelessness, of interminable darkness, lifted' ([24], p. 119). When he first tried to walk on crutches, he was unable to do so until suddenly the music began to play in his mind, and then he found that he could move to the rhythm.

In his own medical practice, Sacks finds that music can 'center' his patients. It appears to restore a sense of the inner self that has been lost through neurological injury or disease ([24], p. 219). Because healing and empowerment involve both physical rhythms of the body and also the 'center' of the self, music might be a powerful tool for empowerment. 'Music,' writes Sacks, 'was a divine message and messenger of life. It was quintessentially quick – the 'quickening art,' as Kant has called it . . .' ([24], p. 148). This makes me wonder what would happen if our hospitals provided not television sets but stereos equipped with the great masterpieces of music from the centuries!

Art is not the only response to realities which reason cannot solve. 'Science and reason could not talk of "nothingness," of "hell," of "limbo;" or of "spiritual night." They had no place for "absence, darkness, death." Yet these were the overwhelming realities of this time' ([24], p. 114). In order to find a language adequate to describe his experiences, Sacks turned to religion. The patient who faces dissolution of her world needs a language adequate to give voice to that dissolution and to provide a framework within which it can be understood, accepted, and overcome. The language of science and reason is often too sterile for this task. The language of religion, precisely because it is often poetic [5] and mysterious, is adequate to the task.

Sacks gives eloquent expression to the power of religious language when he writes, 'In a sense my experience had been a religious one – I had certainly thought of the leg as exiled, God-forsaken, when it was "lost" and, when it was restored, restored in a transcendental way' ([24], p. 190). While he admits that his experience was also a 'riveting scientific and cognitive' experience, it had transcended the limits of science and cognition. A language beyond science was needed.

Moreover, it is not only the *language* of religion that is empowering. Sacks went home for a night to see his family. While there, he attended synagogue. Here he experienced 'inexpressible joy': 'Behind my family I felt embraced by a community and, behind this, by the beauty of old traditions, and, behind this, by the ultimate, eternal joy of the law' ([24], p. 189). Religion is not just a language. It is a community, a set of laws and rituals, a sense of belonging to something larger and more grounding than one's own family or personal universe. All of these things have empowering possibility. They also suggest that Kapp's definition of empowerment is too individualistic and based too much on an autonomy model. Empowerment includes community and connection; it includes strengthening and honoring relationships.

## Summary

What Sacks needed was a 'leg to stand on.' He needed it in two senses: the literal, physical healing of his limb, and the symbolic, 'moral' healing of his status in the world. Because there were two miseries, two empowerments – two 'legs' – were needed. The second leg is social and spiritual. Although the empowering possibilities of physical healing should not be underestimated, neither should the need for the second leg be neglected. It has to do with the meaning system of the patient, with hope and fear, with anxiety and joy, with community and solidarity. It is a leg composed of the liberating word. The communication that comes from empathy, the centering power of music and art, the adequacy of religious language and the solidity of religious ritual and community.

## The Disempowerment of the Powerless

Oliver Sacks was one of the lucky ones. White, male, well-educated, a physician to boot, he was in a position to be as powerful as any patient can be. The mere fact that one so powerful experienced two 'miseries' and needed two empowerments gives us many clues as to what happens in the clinical setting. But it does not cover the situation of those who are not powerful at the outset. What about those who suffer language, educational, racial, or sexual barriers when confronting the medical establishment?[3] The experiences of patients who are female, non-white, poor, not well-educated, or in some other way less powerful than the white male physician suggest some additional dimensions of disempowerment and therefore of empowerment. Those who begin in a more powerless position have many more barriers to empowerment. For them, it will take not only a change in communication, a bit more thoughtfulness, or a little music to give them back their moral status and sense of wholeness. For them, it will take nothing short of a change in the system.

## Consent and Rationality

Consider, for example, the case of Maria Diaz, whose doctors recommended tubal ligation while she was in the last stages of a difficult labor. 'I told them I would not accept that. I kept saying no and the doctors kept telling me that this was for my own good' ([7], p. 108). Maria Diaz never agreed to be sterilized and signed no consent form for the procedure but she was sterilized during caesarian section. Later, she and other Hispanic women brought a suit against U.S.C.-L.A. medical center where the procedure was performed. In a subsequent study, Dreifus and her colleagues found that nine of 23 physicians interviewed had either witnessed coercion or worked under conditions that border on coercion: 'hard-selling, dispensing of misinformation, approaching women during labor, offering sterilization at a time of stress, on-the-job racism'([7], p. 116).

Maria Diaz was disempowered in two ways. First, she was treated not simply without her consent but against her explicit will. In spite of her constant advocacy for herself, she did not participate even minimally in a very significant decision. Using Kapp's definition, she was disempowered.

But she was disempowered in another way as well. Sterilization is a life-changing operation with earth-shattering ramifications for women from 'machismo' cultures. In 'machismo' culture, a man's stature may be measured by the number of children he sires. He may divorce or abandon a woman who cannot bear children. Indeed, this is what happened to Lupe Acosta, whose common-law husband of eight years left her after she was sterilized against her will ([17], p. 107). She ended up on welfare, experiencing not only medical disempowerment, but social and economic disempowerment as well. A decision to refuse sterilization that may not seem 'sensible' or 'rational' in one culture may be very sensible in another. Empowerment in this context would require sensitivity to such cross-cultural issues, and recognition of the devastating consequences of what might seem a 'sensible' decision in white North American culture.

Oliver Sacks may not have been told everything that he wanted to know, and may not have had the kind of communication that he desired. But at no time did he experience the kind of disempowerment that these poor, multi-parous women with language and cultural barriers experienced. He was not treated *against* his will, nor was a foreign rationality imposed on him.

## Medical Harm

Practices such as forced sterilization would be condemned as unjust by most observers. Harder to uncover are the injustices, the disempowerments, built into ordinary routine medical practice. Here, there are two levels on which we must look for disempowerment and therefore empowerment. In Sacks' case, the primary disempowerment came with the social *role* of patient – with losing control, being ignored, and not having social power.[4] But for many women, these social concomitants of the role of patient are only part of the picture. Medical practice historically has contributed not only to this second 'misery' for women, but also to the first 'misery,' the phenomenon of physical disintegration itself.

Feminists and concerned women over the years have exposed a range of obstetrical and gynecological practices that actually *endanger* women's health. Unnecessary hysterectomies [15], use of the Dalkon shield [6], clitoridectomies [4, 23] – any number of practices with serious deleterious impact on women's health have been 'routine' or common at one time in our history. For example, a number of studies have documented the movement from child-birth to the 'delivery' of children in obstetrical units [11, 29]. Historical evidence suggests that midwifery was safer than obstetrics at the time when the (largely male) medical profession pushed out the (largely female) mid-wives. Many women have objected to the health risks presented for both mother and child by routine obstetrical practices. Ethel, who bore 16 children, puts it plainly:

> I had all mine at home except the last six . . . [I]t was easier to have them at home than to have them at hospital . . . They'd take me to the hospital and they'd strap me down. I'd like to never have the baby! When I was home, you know, I'd walk till the pains got so bad that I had to lay down then I'd lay down and have the baby. Without any anesthetic and never no stitches or nothing, because they waited till time. Now they cut you, you know, and they don't give you time to have it . . . That's what ruins women's health ([3], p. 229).

That such practices actually are dangerous has been argued by several commentators [21, 25].

In this context, empowerment for women includes having control over one's own body and important medical decisions. The dimension of decision-making that Kapp lifts up remains important. But empowerment also includes better health care practices that do not endanger women or children.

In a study of court cases, Miles and August found that when the patient was a man, the court constructed his preferences for treatment in 75% of cases and allowed those preferences to be determining. But when the patient was a woman, the court constructed her preferences in only 14% of cases, and her preferences were not determinative of treatment decisions. Miles and August conclude that 'women are disadvantaged in having their moral agency taken less seriously than that of men' ([20], p. 92). If Sacks had difficulty being heard and treated as a moral agent, imagine what he might have faced had he been a woman instead of a man. Thus, on the level of the second 'misery,' which Sacks calls the moral level, women are not treated equally with men. Empowerment in such a case means not having a double standard: both male and female patients should be treated with attention to their own expressed preferences as well as to their familial connections.

But it is not only at the second level of 'misery' on which women are not treated equally. Ayanian and Epstein found that 'women who are hospitalized for coronary heart disease undergo fewer major diagnostic and therapeutic procedures than men' ([2], p. 221). Steingart et al. argue that it is 'disturbing' to find that women report more cardiac disability before infarction than do men, but are less likely to receive treatments known (in men) to lessen symptoms and improve functional capacity ([26], p. 230). Just as Miles and August found that women's statements of not wanting to be kept alive were dismissed as 'emotional' rather than 'rational' desires, so it is possible that women's complaints of chest pain may not be taken as seriously as men's. Empowerment for women in the clinical setting clearly begins with having our voices honored and appropriate interventions utilized.

## Empathy and the Non-treatment of Women's Issues

Another subtle form of disempowerment is the non-treatment of or non-focus on women's issues. Coronary artery disease is the leading cause of death in women ([26], p. 226). Yet our common image of 'heart attack' is an image of a middle-aged professional man, not an image of a woman. The studies just cited make clear that there is much we do not know about how to treat heart disease in women. We have focussed on men's needs, but not on women's.

Similarly, more women die *each year* of breast cancer than men died of AIDS in the first *ten years* of the epidemic [30]. It is estimated that one out of every three women will get cancer during her lifetime, and the breast cancer incidence rate has increased 32% in the last decade [27]. Yet, there is neither the commitment of funds for research and development of new treatments and interventions nor the commitment of public energies and attention to breast cancer that we currently experience for AIDS. Empowerment means *attending* to women's issues, and making them a priority for clinical research and treatment.

The reasons for the relative lack of attention to issues so central to women's lives are complex. Lack of women physicians and researchers may be an important contributing factor. A history of exclusion of women from top ranks of the medical profession leaves its legacy. Walsh concludes her historical study of the discrimination against women in the medical profession with these cautioning words: 'There is an interrelationship between discrimination against women as medical students and physicians and against women as patients – resulting in the present lack of research on breast cancer, excessive rates of hysterectomies and surgery on women . . . and generally deficient health care for women' ([28], pp. 281–282).

Lack of women physicians not only influences choices about research and clinical emphasis; it also influences the possibilities for empathy, so important in Sacks' experience of healing. What male physician can truly empathize with the birth pains of a woman patient, or with what it means to a woman to lose a breast to surgery? If empathy is important for empowerment, then women will experience less empowerment than men when they are treated in a system that does not encourage women physicians. Similarly, white care-givers have difficulty empathizing with women and men of color; the well-to-do will not even imagine some problems experienced by those who are economically disadvantaged; and so on. Empowerment in the clinical context will require a change in the system that encourages different care-providers.

## Problems of Access

While the focus of this essay is on empowerment *within* the clinical setting, some of the most important empowerment issues for those who are relatively powerless have to do with access *to* the clinical setting. Ectopic pregnancy is now the leading cause of maternal death among African-American women [19]. But in 1982 there were 44,000 women in New York state identified as at 'high risk' who became pregnant, had no health insurance, and were not eligible for Medicaid ([19], p. 58). Without health insurance or the means to pay, these women do not get *into* the clinical setting. Their empowerment must begin outside that setting, with changes in political, social, economic policies, Medicaid eligibility, and access to health care. Similarly, for older women, changes in Medicaid to allow access to needed health care are critical.

While some problems of access raise larger social and political issues, there are some things that can be done within the clinical setting to address these problems. For instance, would women who are eligible for Medicaid be able to find a physician who accepts Medicaid patients? 'The worst medical problems I've had really,' says Ethel, a poor mountain woman with 12 living children, 'has been since I been on welfare. Trying to see the kinds of doctors that's needed for the children and myself, and they don't take the card – needing to see specialists, and specialists don't take the card' ([3], p. 231). At the same time that we are experiencing the 'feminization of poverty,' with women increasingly among the poor who must depend on Medicaid, we are also experiencing a time in which ob-gyns, who specialize in women's dis-eases and reproductive processes, have the lowest rate of Medicaid participation of all primary care physicians ([19], p. 57). Women who cannot get into the health care system at all are doubly disempowered.

Empowerment in this context means the willingness of clinical care pro-viders to 'take the card' and deal with the government red tape, the bureaucratic form-filling, and the loss of income represented by accepting those patients. If more physicians 'took the card' and had to deal with these inconveniences, perhaps we would see a faster move toward a more equitable system of access for the poor, many of whom are women.

## Alternative Structures

Under these circumstances, it is no wonder that many women and other relatively powerless people have felt that empowerment cannot happen within the system. Empowerment means not only advocating for oneself and participating in significant decisions, but receiving care from a radically re-oriented system.

Some have moved to establishing alternative health care systems. One such organization was called 'Jane' [1, 12]. Run by women on a non-hierarchical basis, 'Jane' helped women get access to safe abortion during the time that abortions were largely illegal in the United Sates. 'Jane' was part of a larger movement that involved teaching women about their bodies, their sexuality, and their own medical care [8, 9]. Alternative clinics were set up where women were trained to do their own vaginal examinations and to monitor their gynecological health. These organizations were empowering for women because they gave women knowledge, allowed women to help each other in non-hierarchical structures, and kept control of important bodily processes largely in the hands of women themselves. They strengthened relationships among patients and providers, and tried to deal with issues that were central from the perspective and rationality of women of different cultures.

But alternative structures outside the system are not the only solution. Recognizing the rise of breast cancer and the crucial place of mammograms in diagnosis and early treatment, The Medical Center of Central Massachusetts set out to discover why women were so reluctant to come in for mammograms and whether something could be done about it. They asked women to talk about what keeps them from having mammograms. Among the factors that keep women away, they found these:

1. Lack of child-care;
2. Cold and unattractive hospital gowns;
3. Lack of privacy;
4. Inadequately trained technicians, with resulting pain and discomfort;
5. Lengthy waiting times between testing and results.

The mammography unit was redesigned to address these problems; it now provides child-care, privacy, specially trained technicians, attractive and warm clothing, immediate test results, and so on. Such structural changes provide empowerment not just for individual patients, but for the entire class of patients and ultimately society as a whole.

## Summary

The lesson to be learned from those who are relatively powerless is that we need changes in the system, not just changes of attitude in a few care-providers. More thoughtful listening, a willingness to hear the 'whole' story and not just the 'salient facts' will still be important. But it is the system that must be scrutinized for how it disempowers those who are already powerless, and how it could be made more empowering instead.

Empowerment in the clinical setting will require allowing patients to be their own advocates and to participate in significant decision-making. It will require not treating patients against their will, nor assuming that one culture's 'rationality' makes sense for all cultures. It will require honoring those forms of rationality, such as art and religion, that offer a language 'beyond' reason and science, a language that may be more appropriate to the patient's needs. It will require recognizing the network of community and relationships that affect patients' lives and decisions. But above all, it will require changing the system so that those who are relatively powerless have access to health care, for without that access, all talk of empowerment within the clinical setting is void.

## Bibliography

1. Addelson, K. P.: 1986, 'Moral Revolution', in M. Pearsall (ed.), *Women and Values: Readings in Recent Feminist Philosophy*, Wadsworth, Belmont, CA., pp. 291–309.
2. Ayanian, J. Z., and Epstein, A. M.: 1991, 'Differences in the Use of Procedures between Women and Men Hospitalized for Coronary Heart Disease', *New England Journal of Medicine* 325(4): 221–230 (July 25).
3. Baker, D.: 1977, 'The Class Factor: Mountain Women Speak Out on Women's Health', in C. Dreifus (ed.), *Seizing Our Bodies*, Random House, NY, pp. 223–232.
4. Barker-Benfield, G. J.: 1977, 'Sexual Surgery in Late Nineteenth Century America', in C. Dreifus (ed.), *Seizing Our Bodies*, Random House, NY, pp. 13–41.
5. Brueggemann, W.: 1989, *Finally Comes the Poet: Daring Speech for Proclamation*, Fortress Press, Minneapolis.
6. Dowie, M., and Johnston, T.: 1977, 'A Case of Corporate Malpractice and the Dalkon Shield', in C. Dreifus (ed.), *Seizing Our Bodies*, Random House, NY, pp. 86–104.
7. Dreifus, C.: 1977, 'Sterilizing the Poor', in C. Dreifus (ed.), *Seizing Our Bodies*, Random House, NY, pp. 105–120.
8. Frankfort, E.: 1977, 'Vaginal Politics', in C. Dreifus (ed.), *Seizing Our Bodies*, Random House, NY, pp. 263–270.
9. Fruchter, R. G., et al.: 1977, 'The Women's Health Movement: Where Are We Now?', in C. Dreifus (ed.), *Seizing Our Bodies*, Random House, NY, pp. 271–278.
10. Goldman, A. H.: 1980 *The Moral Foundations of Professional Ethics*, Rowman and Littlefield, Totowa, NJ.
11. Haire, D.: 1972, *The Cultural Warping of Childbirth*, International Childbirth Education Association, Seattle.
12. 'Jane': 1990, 'Just Call "Jane" ', in M. G. Fried (ed.), *From Abortion to Reproductive Freedom: Transforming a Movement*, South End Press, Boston.

13. Jonas, H.: 1970, 'Philosophical Reflections on Human Experimentation', in P. Freund (ed.), *Experimentation with Human Subjects*, George Braziller, NY, pp. 1–31.
14. Kapp, M. B.: 1989, 'Medical Empowerment of the Elderly', *Hastings Center Report* 19(4), (July–August).
15. Larned, D.: 1977, 'The Epidemic of Unnecessary Hysterectomy', in C. Dreifus (ed.), *Seizing Our Bodies*, Random House, NY, pp. 195–208.
16. Lebacqz, K.: 1987, *Justice in An Unjust World: Foundations for a Christian Approach to Justice*, Augsburg Publishing House, Minneapolis, MN.
17. Lebacqz, K.: 1985, *Professional Ethics: Power and Paradox*, Abingdon Press, Nashville, TN.
18. Lebacqz, K.: 1986, *Six Theories of Justice: Perspectives from Philosophical and Theological Ethics*, Augsburg Publishing House, Minneapolis, MN.
19. McBarnette, L.: 1988, 'Women and Poverty: The Effects on Reproductive Status', in C. A. Perales and L. S.Young (eds.), *Too Little, Too Late: Dealing with the Health Needs of Women in Poverty*, Harrington Park Press, New York.
20. Miles, S. H., and August, A.: 1990, 'Courts, Gender and "The Right to Die" ', *Law, Medicine, and Health Care* 18(1–2): 85–95 (Spring/Summer).
21. Rich, A.: 1986, *Of Woman Born: Motherhood as Experience and Institution*, W. W. Norton, NY.
22. Rosenbaum, E.: 1988, *A Taste of My Own Medicine*; now published as *The Doctor*, Ivy Books, NY.
23. Rothman, B. K.: 1979, 'Women, Health and Medicine', in J. Freeman (ed.), *Women: A Feminist Perspective*, 2nd ed., Mayfield Publishing Co., Palo Alto, CA.
24. Sacks, O.: 1984, *A Leg To Stand On*, Harper and Row, NY.
25. Sarah, R.: 1988, Power, Certainty, and the Fear of Death', in E. H. Baruch, A. F. D'Adamo, and J. Seager (eds.), *Embryos, Ethics, and Women's Rights: Exploring the New Reproductive Technologies*, Harrington Park Press, New York.
26. Steingart, R. M. et al.:1991, 'Sex Differences in the Management of Coronary Artery Disease', *New England Journal of Medicine* 325(4) (July 25), 226–230.
27. Steingraber, S.: 1991, 'Lifestyle Don't Kill. Carcinogens in Air, Food, and Water Do' in M. Stocker (ed.), *Cancer as a Women's Issue: Scratching the Surface*, Third Side Press, Chicago.
28. Walsh, M. R.: 1977, 'Doctors Wanted: No Women Need Apply': Sexual Barriers in the Medical Profession, 1835–1975, Yale University Press, New Haven.
29. Wertz, R. W., and Wertz, D. C.: 1977, *Lying-In: A History of Childbirth in America*, The Free Press, NY.
30. Winnow, J.: 1991, 'Lesbians Evolving Health Care: Our Lives Depend on It', in M. Stocker (ed.), *Cancer as a Women's Issue: Scratching the Surface*, Third Side Press, Chicago.

**Notes**
1. The definition of justice and dimensions of justice as empowerment are further explored in *Six Theories of Justice* [18] and *Justice in An Unjust World* [16].
2. I have also heard him speak and found his address strong.
3. Precisely because these patients are already relatively powerless in the system, they are less likely to write books about their experiences than are the more powerful who become patients.
4. Loss of control and autonomy is a typically male problem; feminist literature suggests loss of relationship might be more problematic for women.

# CASE STUDY:
## The Alder Hey Affair

In 1999 it emerged that many children who had died at the Alder Hey Hospital in Liverpool had had tissues and organs (including hearts and brains) removed during post mortem examinations without their parents' informed consent. In some cases consent had not been obtained, and in others the parents had not realised what they were consenting to. The result was that many parents had buried or cremated their children without knowing that some of their organs were missing. When they found out, many had felt the need for second, and even third and fourth, funerals as they found out about more retained body parts. The inquiry found that removal and retention of organs without fully informed consent was widespread throughout the UK – the report referred to 'paternalism' on the part of clinicians who believed that it was not in parents' best interests to be given detailed information about such a distressing subject. However, it found that the situation had been made worse at Alder Hey both because of the behaviour of individuals and because of inadequate supervision by hospital and university management. It made a wide range of recommendations, both about legal provisions and about the behaviour of hospitals and doctors.

## Questions
- Does the Alder Hey affair hold any wider lessons for the behaviour of health professionals towards patients and their families, or was it a tragic but extreme case that had little in common with more everyday clinical encounters?
- Might any of the theological perspectives included in this chapter help avoid similar scandals in the future?
- In the light of this chapter, what main obligations and responsibilities do you think health professionals have towards patients and their families?
- What obligations and responsibilities do patients and their families have towards health professionals?

## Sources

Howard Bauchner and Robert Vinci, 'What Have We Learned from the Alder Hey Affair?' *British Medical Journal* 322, 309–310 (2001).

Royal Liverpool Children's Inquiry, *Report*. London: HMSO, 2001.

# 7

# ECONOMICS AND BIOETHICS

## Introduction

Every health care system has to address the problem of scarcity: resources (whether money, equipment, personnel, materials or others) are always limited, while the demand is potentially unlimited. This means that choices about the allocation of resources are unavoidable. As Beauchamp and Childress point out, such choices operate both at the level of 'macroallocation' – for example, what proportion of a health care budget should be spent on different areas of care – and at the level of 'microallocation' – when individual patients are in 'competition' for a scarce resource, who should have higher priority. However, there is not a sharp dividing line between these two levels of allocation, and they often interact (Beauchamp and Childress 2001, 250).

Decisions about health care rationing or resource allocation are often hard, in the nature of the case: one patient's or one specialty's gain is likely to be another's loss. Sometimes they are tragic choices: if one donor organ becomes available, and there are two or more suitable recipients awaiting transplants, the allocation of the organ to one of them may be a decision who lives and who dies.

Rationing decisions, particularly at the macro-level, may be complex questions involving the management and co-ordination of many different resources. However, the ethical criteria on which they may be based are much easier to describe, though vigorously argued over. Resources may be allocated on the basis of *need*: those patients whose need is most urgent, or whose condition is most serious, should have the highest priority. They may be allocated on the basis of *merit*: patients who are judged to have the greatest social worth or potential to contribute to society might be given the highest priority for treatment. A famous example is the Seattle committee in the 1960s which selected patients for kidney dialysis (Ramsey 1970, 242–252).

Another version of allocation according to merit could occur if patients held to be responsible for their disease were given lower priority for treatment (cf. Beauchamp and Childress 2001, 248–249).

A third way of allocating resources is by likely *outcome*: resources should be used where they will bring about the greatest benefit. The best-known example of such a procedure uses the concept of the Quality Adjusted Life Year, or QALY (Beauchamp and Childress 2001, 209–212). A QALY is a year of life expectancy multiplied by a factor proportional to the quality of life, and it can be used as a measure of the cost-effectiveness of a medical treatment. Advocates of this approach argue that priority should be given to medical activity whose cost-per-QALY is low, so as to bring about the greatest possible benefit for a given cost. Such approaches clearly rely on the utilitarian principle that the right course of action is the one which will bring about the greatest happiness or benefit. As such, they are vulnerable to the criticisms often levelled at utilitarian theories. For example, they are unable to make sense of the notion that there may be actions which justice demands regardless of the consequences. (See Banner 1999, 136–162, for a Christian critique of the QALY concept.)

Fourth, we may decline to operate any criteria for prioritising some patients or areas of care over others, and instead distribute resources by a system of *random allocation*, such as a lottery or a first-come first-served rule.

In practice, rationing policies may contain elements of different criteria, and it may sometimes be difficult to differentiate between the various criteria that may be operating in a particular case. For example, suppose a centre refuses smokers non-urgent coronary bypass surgery unless they first give up smoking (cf. Persaud 1995). Whatever the reasons in any actual case of this sort, it is in principle possible to imagine several different justifications for such a policy: (1) smokers are held to be responsible for their own illness, and therefore less deserving of treatment than non-smokers; (2) withholding treatment may persuade them to give up smoking, which would be in their own medical interests; (3) the clinical outcome of surgery is likely to be poorer for smokers than non-smokers, so that treating smokers represents a less efficient use of resources in cost-per-QALY terms; (4) the outcome of surgery for a patient who smokes is less likely to be good enough to justify the risk and burden *for that individual*; or (5) a combination of some or all of these reasons.

The first reading in this chapter takes up this debate. It comes from a classic of the bioethical literature, Paul Ramsey's *The Patient as Person*. In the extract reproduced here, Ramsey considers the various possible criteria by which rationing decisions in health care could be made. Taking as a basic axiom the equal worth of each human life, he argues that this principle rules out any attempt to prioritise individuals or groups on merit. Rather, a system of random allocation is called for. The only exceptions to this general rule are in highly unusual situations such as disasters, when (for example) medical personnel who are among the injured might be given priority treatment because they are needed to help treat others. With these exceptions, writes Ramsey, a policy of random allocation is required because we are not to 'play God with human lives' by taking upon ourselves the authority to judge who shall live and who shall die. Rather, we are called to ' "play God" in the correct way: he makes his sun rise upon the good and the evil and sends rain upon the just and the unjust alike' (p. 198); if this is how God treats humans, we should not discriminate between people or groups in giving health care.

If sharing the fruits of biomedical science justly is a problem within one country and one health care system, it becomes almost immeasurably more complex and more serious when we consider the distribution of resources between countries. It is often pointed out that while there may be severe pressure on health care resources in a country such as the UK, in many developing countries a large proportion of the population lacks access even to basic health care. Some writers claim that such gross inequalities are not accidental, but are in some way built into the global economy, and can only be set right by a radical change to international economic systems and structures (cf. the reading by Boff in chapter 1).

In the second reading in this chapter, Márcio Fabri dos Anjos examines human genetic research – which requires an enormous investment of money, effort and expertise, but in which there are great profits to be made – from the perspective of the world's poor. He draws attention to the imbalance of power that results from inequalities of knowledge and wealth. People, communities and nations lacking the knowledge or the financial resources to initiate genetic research may be vulnerable to exploitation in a variety of ways by the corporations and research organisations that sponsor such research. For example, researchers may make use of local indigenous knowledge to discover and exploit genetically valuable plants, while denying the local community the opportunity to share in the profits from their discovery. Or again, poor patients with little access to health care may be easily induced to act as medical research subjects in ways that bring them little or no benefit.

However, dos Anjos also notes more hopeful signs. For example, the numerous internationally agreed codes of ethics for medical research indicate some level of 'ethical maturity on the part of global society' (p. 208), which could offer a basis for more just ways of proceeding in genetic research. Drawing on his Brazilian experience, he makes some general proposals for the safeguarding of the poor and vulnerable in this rapidly growing field.

## References and Further Reading

Michael Banner, *Christian Ethics and Contemporary Moral Problems*. Cambridge: Cambridge University Press, 1999.

Tom L. Beauchamp and James F. Childress, *Principles of Biomedical Ethics*. 5th ed., Oxford and New York: Oxford University Press, 2001.

Rajendra Persaud, 'Smokers' Rights to Health Care', *Journal of Medical Ethics* 21, 281–287 (1995).

Paul Ramsey, *The Patient as Person: Explorations in Medical Ethics*. New Haven: Yale University Press, 1970.

# A Human Lottery?

PAUL RAMSEY

In selecting the patients with fatal illness who are to be given treatment that is not available to everyone equally in need of it, the lawyer's norm of equal protection and due process and the moralist's norm of fairness, justice, or equal respect for human lives can be implemented only by one of three methods. Each of these methods is designed to exclude comparisons of the social worth of individuals, or of their extrinsic worth to others.

First, certain rules can be announced in advance which are not discriminatory but based on statistical medical probabilities. Thus we could state certain formal, if somewhat arbitrary, rules that put people in categories while excluding comparative judgments among them individually. If persons over 45 or 50 are to be excluded from hemodialysis, then no one need compare the worthiness of one 55–year-old man with another. If children should be excluded because they likely cannot endure the treatment and will not develop normal puberty, then no one need estimate the intelligence or family background of children, or take account of letters of reference. Even a policy of restricting the services of a given hospital to in-state residents is to be preferred to accepting 'notable' out-of-state applicants. These rules would be universalizable de facto standards of selection – a significant improvement over much current practice, but not yet a sufficient or a sufficiently moral principle of selection.

Second, random patient selection can be instituted, either by lottery or by a policy of 'first come, first served'. The Los Angeles County General Hospital Renal-Dialysis Center, for example, uses a lottery system to select among medically graded applicants on record, while the Detroit Receiving Hospital affords the same equality of opportunity by a policy of 'first come, first served'. These two procedures are in principle the same, and we will consider them as if they were one. 'First come, first served' amounts to an ongoing lottery. Moreover, in the use of sparse medical resources there will often in practice be medically suitable patients who have already come to the center among whom selection must be made when there is room for them on the program. We have then only two principles to choose between in choosing

From *The Patient as Person: Explorations in Medical Ethics*, pp. 252–259. New Haven: Yale University Press, 1970.

how to select patients: randomness among lives presumed to be equally valuable, and comparisons of social worthiness or extrinsic worth to others. I assume that physicians and only physicians are competent to make a prior medical selection; and, indeed, that their experience in an on-going lottery may be sufficient to uphold a judgment that a medically more suitable applicant will come next week for whom room on the program should be held open. This would be to allow maximum latitude to a doctor's distribution of sparse medical resources within the terms of the judgments he, and he alone, is competent to make. Still, randomness would ensure equality of opportunity to live, and not die, to every one of a class of patients, and it would forbid the physician from raising questions of comparative social merit as a means of determining who lives and who dies.

In the search for a more impersonal method of selecting who is to be saved from among the dying, the model is the casting of lots among passengers apparently doomed to die in an overloaded lifeboat, which is the rule in U.S. maritime law. The decision in *United States v. Holmes*[1] accepted lottery in such a desperate lifeboat situation as the procedure which alone would rule out arbitrariness and manifest equal respect for equal rights to life when not all can be saved. An English case, however, rejected a lottery as 'grotesque', expressing the same aversion to the idea of a 'human lottery' as did one member of the public committee at Seattle's Swedish Hospital. Instead, however, of endorsing judgments of comparative social worthiness to reach decisions concerning life or death, the English court ruled that all must wait and die or be rescued together.[2]

From this decision one might, abstractly, conclude yet another possibility for resolving conflicts of lives when not all can be saved. Overloaded dialysis centers, we might say, are to be compared with overloaded lifeboats. If neither social worthiness nor a 'human lottery' should be used in passenger or patient selection, the conclusion to be drawn would seem to be that there is no sound basis for choosing anyone to be saved, because not all can be saved and each one has a right to life equal to any other. This possibility will be discussed, obliquely at least, in the course of our examination of the justification for choosing randomness over social worthiness in patient selection. These remain the two realistic alternatives. Still, it is significant to note that random selection has as its model casting lots in the overloaded lifeboat situation; that from pondering such a procedure sensitive minds like Benjamin Cardoza and Edmond Cahn have been repelled by it; and that – far from going to selection in terms of social worth – they have felt impelled to say that when faced with choosing one life at another's expense no selection can ethically be made.

In analyzing the lifeboat cases in the applicability to the problem of patient selection, David Sanders and Jesse Dukeminier, Jr., seem to me to be mistaken in drawing a distinction between the law and the moral principle governing in cases of jettison and the law and moral principle governing in cases of rescue. These authors seem to believe there is a morally significant distinction between a decision to jettison some of the passengers from a lifeboat made by those who are also imperiled, and a decision to rescue some from the dying made by persons not doomed. 'Selection for hemodialysis,' they write, 'is analogous to a situation where there are thirty persons in a sinking boat and a second boat, with room for five persons, comes by. A committee on land is to decide and advise by radio which five persons will be transferred to the second boat.'[3]

Jettison initiated by doomed men and rescue initiated by men who are secure on shore with their well kidneys are, of course, different moral situations. But these situations do not differ in the principle of selection to be used if selection must be made. Sanders and Dukeminier need not have sought for another principle or a principle underlying the rule of equality in shipwreck cases. That rule of equality, and how alone to accord equality, applies to human rescue by third parties as well as to decisions to jettison by men who are themselves among the imperiled. In the Holmes case, the rescuers were aboard: the mate Holmes, who gave the order, and the rest of his crew were needed for rowing. Holmes made the decision to jettison in his official capacity, being the highest ranking officer aboard among the imperiled. The issue in human rescue or in jettison is how to exclude arbitrary decisions in determining who lives and who dies when not all can be saved.

Sanders and Dukeminier cite Professor Paul Freund in his Gay Lecture at Harvard Medical School: 'The governing principle is not the merit or need or value of the victim but equality of worth as a human being. The governing principle, it might be said, is that man shall not play God with human lives.'[4] I suggest that here Freund proposes two alternative statements of the same governing principle. Perhaps 'man shall not play God with human lives' is a principle that underlies or bases the rule of equality in shipwreck cases. If so, it is also a principle that underlies or bases the rule of equality in cases of human rescue. In the case of jettison or of rescue, 'the essence of playing God,' as Sanders and Dukeminier say, 'is to look at A and to look at B, assay them, declare B is worth more than A, and save B.'[5] True enough; but this is also the essence of a violation of the principle of equal rights to life in making forced selections either to jettison or to rescue. In both cases, it is 'equality of worth as a human being' that comes into competition with that of another human being. This equality of worth as a human being mandates the randomizing of selection if selection is the only way to avoid all perishing. Neither in jettison nor in rescue should worthy lives or lives having unequal worths to others be thrown into comparison. Granting that men are unequal to others in all sorts of respects, these are not relevant moral features to be reckoned in deciding who lives and who dies.

The moral difference between these two situations is only that, if I am among the doomed, I may be more in need of the constraints of a socially accepted governing principle of the equality of worth of every human being in order for me to be fully willing to place myself under a casting of lots and to see the justice of its outcome. Still, I allow that for someone safely on shore among the rescuers, 'the governing principle that man shall not play God with human lives' by making direct comparisons of the social worth of individuals in deciding questions of life and death may be a salutary expression of, and the ultimate ground and source of, 'the governing principle of the incomparable equality of worth which every man has as a human being.' How else am I going to be able to restrain my normal human propensity to do good by thinking more highly of some lives than I ought to think? How else am I going to be willing to have blood-washings fall upon the deserving and the undeserving alike, and good blood chemistry shine upon the needy no less than those who are needed?

When the ultimate of life is the value at stake, and when not all lives can be saved, it can reasonably be argued that men should stand aside as far as possible from the choice of who shall live and who shall die. Men should then 'play God' in the correct way: he makes his sun rise upon the good and the evil and sends rain upon the just and the unjust alike. This physicians do when in order to ensure equality of opportunity to live they devise a lottery scheme or adopt the practice of 'first come, first served' to determine who among medically equal patients shall be admitted to a kidney dialysis program or be given an implanted vital organ. The equal right of every human being to live, and not relative personal or social worth, should be the ruling principle. When not all can be saved and all need to die, this ruling principle can be applied only or best by a random choice among equals.

Random selection is preferable not simply because life is a value incommensurate with all others, and so not negotiable by bartering one man's worth against another's. It is sustained also because we have no way of knowing how really and truly to estimate a man's societal worth or his worth to others or to himself in unfocused social situations in the ordinary lives of men in their communities. The equal right of every human being to live ought generally to prevail since men and their communities are organized around a plurality of social goals and many sorts of manifestations of the uniqueness of personal beings. There can be a describable sort of 'exception' to this ruling principle (guaranteeing by random selection equal possibility of life when not all can be saved) if and only if a community and its members have (or have been reduced to) a single focus of purpose and goal under some quite extraordinary circumstance.

Professor Paul A. Freund of the Harvard Law School stated the ethical principle governing choice of who shall live and who shall die, and he also stated the sole qualification to be added to this ruling principle. 'My own submission,' Freund writes, 'was that in the matter of choosing life or death, not involving specific wrongdoing, no one should assume the responsibility of judging comparative worthiness to live on the basis of unfocused criteria of virtue or social usefulness, and that either priority in time, or a lottery, or a mechanical selection on the basis of age should be followed.'[6] Freund gave an illustration of a community of men reduced to 'focused criteria' in which comparative social usefulness can be and should be employed. This was the decision to allocate penicillin, in short supply in 1943 among the U.S. Armed Forces in North Africa,[7] to victims of venereal disease rather than to victims of battle wounds. What could possibly justify giving penicillin to men 'wounded in brothels' instead of to men wounded in battle?[8] The justification depended on the special requirement of the practice of medicine on men in battle. The restoration of a larger number of men more quickly to fitness for the limited purpose in which they were engaged was the only – and it was a sufficient – excuse. The particular decision of the Theatre Medical Commander in this case can be generalized into a universalizable stipulation designating the morally relevant features of situations which alone justify deciding questions of life and death in terms of comparative social worthiness. One may act in accord with a morality of social utility in a situation, such as this one, 'where objectives were closely defined – maximum fighting power as rapidly as possible.'

Two additional illustrations can be given. While in the lifeboat situation the ruling principle of equal right should be ensured to the passengers by random selection among them if not all can be saved, Freund's qualification of this rule applies to a choice between passengers and the crew if the latter are needed because of special knowledge and skill in rowing in order for any to be saved. Here again the objectives of all aboard are closely defined; they have one purpose: to endure the storm and reach shore or rescue.

The morality of triage in disaster medicine is the second illustration. In the case of natural or man-made disasters, victims most in need of help – on whom normally we would lavish resources – must simply be set aside, and nothing be done for them. First priority must be given to victims who can quickly be restored to functioning. They are needed to bury the dead to prevent epidemic. They can serve as amateur medics or nurses with a little instruction – as the triage officer directs the community's remaining medical resources to a middle group of the seriously but not-so-seriously injured majority. Even among these, I suppose a physician should first be treated. It is not enough to say that 'those casualties whose immediate therapy offers most hope for the conservation of the common good should receive first priority'.[9] We must go on to say that first priority should be given to those casualties whose immediate therapy offers most hope for the conservation of a quite specific, minimal common good, i.e., mere survival and the restoration of the conditions of there being any good or a good in common or a common good in any higher sense. When it comes to that, who can say who most matters? Or who should say who matters most when the consequence of doing so determines life and death? The good is not common that does not flow back upon all alike. How one participates and for what just rewards may vary or be debated in a society, but participation itself – life in the human community – cannot rightfully be made contingent upon quality of contribution. Triage decisions are all a function of the narrowly defined, exceptional purposes to which a community of men may have been reduced. In these terms, comparative social worthiness can be measured.

But as Freund says, 'life is rarely so circumscribed in its goals.' No one can tell the worth of an old man sitting on the porch watching a sunset, or ponder imponderables like the relative moral worth of comparative genetic inheritances, or say whether a disturbed or seemingly undisturbed child should be saved. When tragically not all can be saved the rule of practice must be the equality of one life with every other life, which in such a case can be implemented only by randomizing the choice that necessarily must be made among them. To begin to estimate comparative worthiness to live on the basis of unfocused criteria of virtue or social worthiness would be to presume to make a (nearly) total estimate of a man's life. 'The more nearly total is the estimate to be made of an individual, and the more nearly the consequence determines life and death, the more unfit the judgment becomes for human reckoning . . .' The more nearly total is the estimate made of an individual, the nearer we would be to presuming 'to act as gods on the Day of Judgment.'[10]

Here we see the important and informative distinction between a practice that 'plays God' and a practice that is fit for the reckoning of men who imitate rather God's care (before the Judgment Day!) alike for the good and the bad, the profitable and the unprofitable, the deserving and the un-deserving, and seeks to serve those who are only needy no less than those who are needed. In allocating sparse medical resources among equally needy persons, an extension of God's indiscriminate care into human affairs requires random selection and forbids god-like judgments that one man is worth more than another.

## Notes

1. 26 F. Cas. 360 (No. 15,383) (C.C.E.D. Pa.1842).
2. *Regina v. Dudley,* 14 Q.B.D. 273 (1884). Justice Benjamin Cardoza approved the English and rejected the American rule of law, saying, 'Who shall know when masts and sails of rescue may emerge out of the fog?' ('What Medicine Can Do for Law,' *in Selected Writings of Benjamin Nathan Cardoza,* Margaret E. Hale, ed. New York: Fallon, 1947, p. 390). One hears similar statements made in the medical ethical context in support of unending efforts to prolong life, because some new discovery or life-saving remedy may emerge like a sail of rescue out of the fog, but not in support of

the proposition that sparse life-sustaining remedies should be withheld while all wait and die until all can be rescued together.

3. David Sanders and Jesse Dukeminier, Jr., 'Medical Advance and Legal Lag: Hemodialysis and Kidney Transplantation,' in Reflections on the New Biology, U.C.L.A. Law Review 15, no. 2 (February 1868): 374–77.

4. Paul A. Freund, 'Ethical Problems in Human Experimentation,' New England Journal of Medicine 273 (1965): 687.

5. 'Medical Advance and Legal Lag,' p. 375.

6. Paul A. Freund, 'Introduction to the Issue Ethical Aspects of Experimentation with Human Subjects,' Daedalus, Spring 1969, p. xiii.

7. The same circumstance of the scarcity of antibiotics in England during the war morally permitted withholding them from a 'control group' of patients in order finally to prove their greater degree of effectiveness in contrast to established treatments.

8. The expression is Henry K. Beecher's, in agreement with Freund. Daedalus, Spring 1969, p. 280.

9. Thomas J. O'Donnell, S.J., 'The Morality of Triage,' Georgetown Medical Bulletin 14, no. 1 (August 1960): 70.

10. Paul A. Freund, in Daedalus, pp.xiii–xiv. The same point was made by David Sanders and Jesse Dukeminier, Jr., 'Medical Advance and Legal Lag', pp. 376–77: 'Opinions of social worth are infinitely more diverse than opinions concerning the design of a belfry ... Ad hockery is not the stuff from which constitutional guaranties of equal protection and due process are made.'

# Power, Ethics and the Poor in Human Genetic Research

MÁRCIO FABRI DOS ANJOS

Genetics today is recognized as a field in which the quest for knowledge and power has been concentrated. In the areas of crop cultivation and animal husbandry, its achievements have brought about a real revolution, not only in terms of food production, but also, thanks to recent advances, leading to new pharmaceutical products and even to organic elements that can be transplanted into humans. Researches in human genetics have formed part of this expansion of knowledge of biological processes, with a corresponding expansion in the power to control them. Here knowledge brings health and well-being, while at the same time increasingly promising to extend human power to programme life itself. This shows the truth of the axiom that 'knowledge is power', and knowledge and power, once joined, tend to empower each other, in a spiral of interaction.[1]

Among the many ethical questions raised by this subject, I should like to raise the place of the poor in human genetic research. What chances do countries, populations, groups and individuals lacking the resources to acquire genetic knowledge have of sharing in the research and benefiting from its results? Defining this question as an ethical concern, I propose to raise a few interrogatives from the perspective of the poor and also to sketch out proposals on proceedings in power relationships in this area.[2]

## Powers and Interests at Stake

In general, and without for the moment considering current tensions, the course of research into human genetics holds out most promise in the areas of health, longevity and quality of life. At the same time, these objectives are tied up with a chain of more pragmatic interests that result in the commercialization of the results obtained, whether services or products. It is worth noting that the mapping and sequencing of genes brings new resources for identifying and assessing human individuals, intervening in their

From Maureen Junker-Kenny and Lisa Sowle Cahill (eds.), *The Ethics of Genetic Engineering: Concilium* 1998/2, pp. 73–82. London: SCM/Maryknoll, NY: Orbis.

procreation, diagnosing hereditary diseases, preventing sicknesses, and bringing the possibility of genetic therapies.

These illustrations are enough to show the considerable political and economic potential wrapped up in human genetic research. We are generating a power to intervene in the very biological identity of persons, their prospects and chances of life. It is therefore easy to see why human genetics has become a field attracting huge financial investment, with strong prospects of large profits. The news media detail the vast sums involved in the economic aspects of this field: research with genetic materials is 'the latest frontier in science – and a market that promises to generate billions of dollars. The first vast contract has already been signed. The US corporation Sequana Therapeutics claims to have found the cure for asthma in an African coastal tribe. It has sold the DNA samples from this group to Boehringer, a German pharmaceutical laboratory, for US$70 million. None of the blacks involved has earned a cent from this operation.'[3] This little example shows that genetics has become a field of economic and political endeavour that national and international policies cannot ignore. It is no longer just a case of applying the results of research to individuals, but of rapidly accumulating options that can affect the whole of humanity.

Two interrelated forces constitute the requisite for entering this area of knowledge and power. In effect, the way to achieving results in genetic research has a long history of high monetary cost and highly developed scientific resources. Researchers have to be trained, research centres established, and projects financed. Those with the economic and scientific potential to do this can produce in genetics and enter into the developing competition, seeking to lead the race and capture the market. Those who lack this potential may be in a position of satisfying the requirements to become consumers of the results if and when these become available.

Those who have the economic and scientific potential to develop research and furnish its results fall into two main groups: on the one hand, the public authorities of various countries, concerned with the development of health programmes for their own populations, as well as with the economic exploitation of the services and products resulting from research; on the other, private initiatives, composed mainly of pharmaceutical industries and medical and health bodies, which seek to make human genetics a profitable enterprise for themselves on a national and a multinational level.

Beyond these, there are those dispossessed of the necessary potential to produce in genetics. On the present map of geo-power in genetics, the North is significantly stronger than the South. Economically poor countries (with a few exceptions, such as Cuba, which has made a special investment in public health), most of the black populations, and indigenous peoples in a general sense have no chance of leading in any initiatives taken in these fields.

## Vulnerability and Autonomy

As can be seen, the question of ethics in power relationships in human genetics is posed within a context of great economic inequality and of corresponding differentials in capacity for scientific production. I am not going to go over the ethical interrogatives hanging over the free-market economics dominant in the West, though these form an important underlying context to this study. Here I am less concerned with analyzing the competition, the play of forces and pressures among the 'strong'. I prefer to concentrate on the situation of the dispossessed in the midst of these power relationships.

Vulnerability is an interesting concept in bioethics insofar as it expresses the situation of those with limited capacity for autonomy and for defending their won rights in questions of research and of profiting from its results. Vulnerability is generally assessed by the limits to the capacity people have for taking decisions freely. It is well established that this capacity can be diminished or even annulled by the absence of conditions of understanding, culture and feeling (where the vulnerable include children, comatose patients, and those with no access to even a minimum knowledge of scientific procedures). The vulnerable would also include individuals subject to certain pressures, especially when subordinated to a hierarchy, such as the military and members of any institution that can exercise pressure. Perhaps less recognized are those whose vulnerability stems from economic pressures and from exploitation of situations that leaves them with few alternatives. Understanding these levels of vulnerability becomes easier when illustrated with some specific examples.

## Lack and the Attraction of Promise

The Brazilian newspaper report on 'sale of indigenous DNA'[4] is instructive for understanding some aspects of vulnerability. The paper related that the Corriell Cell Repositories Corporation, in the United States, was in 1996 offering for sale samples of DNA from two Brazilian indigenous groups, the Karitiana and the Surui, both from the State of Rondônia in Amazonia. On its internet page (www.arginine.umdnj.edu), Corriell mentioned that the samples came from the collections of two prestigious US universities, Stanford and Yale, and that the Yale doctor Ken Kidd had handed over the samples. Among the economic data provided was the statement that 'Corriell Cell calls itself a scientific concern, with no profit aims. It charges $500 for each DNA sample', but this amount barely covers the cost of collecting and processing.

The declaration by the village headman on the manner of collecting the samples is also revealing on the subject of vulnerability. According to the same report, in August 1996 researchers from the United States obtained authorization from FUNAI (the National Foundation for Indians) for research into the giant sloth in Karatiana territory. In the words of the headman Cizino Dantas Morais, the collection of samples took place like this: 'When we went into the jungle to show them the lair of the mapinguari (the legendary 'sloth-beast'), doctor asked Karitiana for blood. They said: we are going to see if you have anaemia, meningitis, AIDS, disease that kills quickly. Indian let them take blood.' The reporter concluded by saying that the Karitiana have not the least idea of what DNA is, but have now discovered that their blood is worth money: 'After finding out that their blood is on sale in the United States, they want money from any researcher who comes to collect blood on their territory.'

## Patients Who Have Never Had Treatment

The relationship between lack and promises of benefit shows that vulnerability is also defined by exploitation of those who find themselves in situations where they have few alternatives. In poor regions, there are innumerable 'patients who have never had treatment', who are quite beyond the reach of public health networks. For these, becoming subjects in a research project seems like a guarantee of salvation. Recently a many-centred research project on the efficacy of a drug to combat AIDS, 'the largest research into medicaments to combat AIDS undertaken outside the USA and Europe, involving 996 Brazilian volunteers', applied a monotherapic treatment to HIV-positive patients who had never had any treatment, to evaluate the efficacy of the drug (Indinavir). Now, as far as one can tell, the scientific community maintains the inefficacy of monotherapy in such cases. The American laboratory Merck Sharp & Dohme, which financed the project, confronted by a commission for ethics in research which raised ethical questions, suspended this branch of research.[5]

I am not passing ethical judgment here on the actions of this laboratory. But I mention the incident to show how understandable it is that an HIV-carrier's need for treatment can become a weak point that is easily exploited. In truth, this personal vulnerability is not isolated and simply the outcome of the patient's psychological state. It is connected with a broader weakness affecting society, which is supposed to protect individuals. Note that those 'who had never had any treatment' were sought out. This means that, to the extent that societies are incapable of defending those who suffer, or simply uncaring, they increase their vulnerability. So countries with precarious health systems and few rules governing research are always oases, not always ethical, open to those who have the economic and scientific potential to carry out research.

## The Vulnerability of Nations

I have already mentioned the vulnerability of indigenous peoples. Let us now look closer at the question of national sovereignty of countries with poor populations. A first aspect of weakness appears when a nation lacks a minimum of directives and resources to control research proceedings. The condition of many poor countries can be called calamitous in this regard, which in itself makes it difficult to name the countries with such limitations. In recent discussions on biomedical ethics with a view to signing treaties within Mercosul ('south trade'), it was found that some South American countries had (in 1996) no such thing as a Code of Medical Ethics. How, in such a situation, can one propose an ethics of research? It is easy to see how, in such a context, individuals are defenceless against those who have power without ethics.

The question of national sovereignty surfaced in acute fashion in researches into the Amazon rainforest.[6] The US laboratory Sharman Pharmaceuticals alone has investigated around 7,000 plant species from the Amazonian region. This major research project necessarily involves national sovereignty, both when the research is carried out and at the time when its results are patented and start earning royalties. The Royal Botanical Gardens of the United Kingdom, considering the question of rights on eventual discoveries a delicate matter, suspended its researches into the production of remedies based on Brazilian plants.[7] At the Rio ECO-92 Conference, a Convention of Biodiversity was signed, providing for the payment of royalties to the community or country of origin on products that utilize indigenous community knowledge or native raw materials.[8]

However, regulating research in poor countries is still not everything. Another aspect of national vulnerability is shown directly in international political and economic relationships, in which rights recognized can be subjected to various pressures and have to be negotiated. One example of this emerges from the laws governing patents. Regulation in this sphere is absolutely necessary, beginning with the need to defend not only nations but also businesses from bio-piracy. But this does not save regulation from being subject to a powerful play of interests. In Brazil, policy negotiations began in 1991 and took five years, ending by recognizing patents on genetically modified micro-organisms and conceding a validity of twenty years for patents on products manufactured from them. Now, given the increasing rate of change in all aspects of life today, twenty years can correspond to a hundred in earlier times. A concession as generous as this is inexplicable without political and economic pressures, a context of free-market ideology, and the need to attract foreign capital into the country.

## Deconstruction and Construction of Ethics in Research

What can be concretely postulated in terms of ethics, especially in societies or countries lacking in the relevant social regulation? Does one begin with norms or with laws? I am convinced there is an earlier step. Laws and norms will become necessary, but they depend on establishing a more solid ethical and cultural base if they are not to fall into legalism.

The first concern, therefore, has to be to dismantle a colonist mentality, and replace it with an ethical culture, informed by humanitarian convictions and invested with citizenship. I speak on the basis of the Latin American colonial experience: in other contexts the experience may be more imperialist or dictatorial, but the experiences are relatively analogous. The remnants of colonial culture have the effect of making territories and peoples 'no man's land', open ground for the first explorer to arrive to operate in with no rules other than those he makes himself. The force of inertia in this culture still persists today, imbuing many researchers with the omnipotence of not having to give satisfaction to their patients or subjects for research. A dictatorial context would treat territory and people as 'one man's land', with the same practical results.

We can point to two reciprocal dimensions of this process that need to be reversed. One shows in the interpersonal relations between researchers and the subjects of their research. In these, both researchers and their subjects need to learn ethical attitudes, to discover and respect the dignity of those involved in the relationship. The other concerns the socio-political sphere, affecting public state relationships. Here it is not just a question of respecting individual rights but of claiming and defending the rights of the collectivity. An interesting example of this dimension is provided by the projected Law of Biodiversity approved in the state of Acre, one of the states that makes up Brazilian Amazonia. By this law, researchers or foreign entities that propose to work in the region have to be associated with a Brazilian group; besides this, they have to leave part of the material they collect behind, in the hands of the state. The deputy responsible for this project commented emphatically: 'The time has come to put a stop once and for all to the neo-colonialism attacking Acre and the whole region of Amazonia.'[9]

Are these harsh judgments? Or do they just appear harsh simply because we have always counted on the compliance of colonialism? Once knowledge becomes power, overcoming colonialism and dependency means sharing knowledge itself, not just handing on its products. In other words, ethics in research is not upheld simply by interpersonal relations of respect between researcher and subject of research. We need to have the courage to confront also the tacit laws of the political, economic and cultural colonialism to which most poor countries are still subject.

The cultural construction of an ethics in research refers us, as we have seen, to the foundations of our human inter-connectedness. On the one hand, it requires us to strengthen our consciousness of the humanitarian commitments that unite us as like beings. On the other, it demands a sort of cosmic vision, a 'galaxy view', forcing us to accept that as planet Earth we are a tiny boatload navigating the expanse of the universe. The spirit of solidarity with and sharing of the planet, and therefore among nations, would be a basic rule of common sense.

As we well know, on the other hand, society is hardly governed by ethical ideals. So, laws and directives are needed. In building an ethical construct, norms and directives are often more appropriate than laws. Laws suppose sanctions and punishment; they involve enforcement officers; they lead to more directly juridical proceedings – which are obviously needed in certain cases. But directives and norms seem more effective in developing ethical formation and consolidating attitudes. The growth of the ethical conscious- ness of humanity on this subject has been marked by significant occasions, on which important international declarations were signed, setting out directives for ethics in research.

While, therefore, there are still motives for deploring the lack of ethics in many research proceedings, there are also, on the other hand, reasons to rejoice at these expressions of ethical maturity on the part of global society.

## Ethics in Day-to-day Research

In day-to-day research practices, ethics is well regulated by norms proposed or upheld by local and national committees of research ethics. There is an accessible bibliography on the functioning of such committees.[10] There are two distinct, though related, undertakings: working out national norms or directives governing ethics in research, and forming commissions or commit- tees to implement them. In Brazil, the first of these appeared in the 1960s, but took definite shape in the 1970s as 'Committees for Hospital Ethics'.[11] After this, local committees and national commissions with a broader remit began to be formed. Ethical concern is undoubtedly growing throughout the world, and it is to be hoped that all countries will soon organize the institution of these valuable bodies for promoting ethics.

What steps are needed to regulate the ethics of research, and what must such regulation comprise? In the Brazilian experience, in 1996, of reworking a National Resolution on *Ethics in Research involving Human Beings*,[12] we found that it was vital to begin with a democratic process for formulating directives, involving society in the actual elaboration of suitable norms. In such cases, participation is a potent factor in ethical education. So it is useful to organize a collection of suggestions, proposals and observations in which various sectors of society can take part. It is essential for research centres themselves to contribute, and interdisciplinary contributions are also very enriching.

The next stage is to plumb the ethical heritage of humankind. At first sight, the search for consensus would seem to be the next logical step after collecting contributions. But consensus can sometimes, to a greater or lesser extent, express the simple agreement of the strongest, and this is no guarantee of an ethical procedure. To counterbalance this disadvantage, one needs to be able to incorporate the experiences and ethical expressions of international agreements and the experiences of other countries. Contexts in which more humanitarian and egalitarian models of relationship in research have already been established can serve not only as an inspiration in drawing up norms but also as a policy instrument in overcoming imbalances and inequalities in the situation in one's own country.

The content of regulations for ethics in research will necessarily be complex in detail, and they can therefore be more conveniently adopted from regulations worked out in the various countries that already have them. Their principal tasks have to be: to include ethics in the scientific process itself; to require that the maximum of respect be shown for the subjects of research, paying particular attention to their 'free and informed consent';[13] to establish guarantees on risks and benefits; to ensure a structure of openness in research, in its installation, development and conclusion;[14] to establish a national commission and local committees for ethics, which can put the necessary directives into practice.

Finally, it needs to be said that day-to-day ethics in human genetics inevitably refers us to the broader socio-political conditions under which research takes place and under which the results it obtains are distributed and applied. Here, I must just note the need for regulations and laws that deal with more than the research process, protecting the ethical application of the results obtained. So poor countries, too, need good laws on biodiversity, bioprotection, patents, applications of therapies and especially of diagnosis. Defence of the poor and upholding the dignity of the vulnerable depend very largely on these legal dispositions.

## Conclusion

In conclusion, I should like to return to the question of the place of the poor in human genetic research. It is obvious that the course of research in this field involves colossal economic and political interest and therefore sets a complex interplay of forces in motion. Scientific progress depends on effort and the investment of energy and also relies on the attraction of the benefits and profits it can bring. The poor, as individuals, groups, or nations, are, in this interplay, an ethical challenge remaining present from the installation of research projects and throughout the whole process of their development, in both their methods of procedure and the use they make of their results. At each of these stages there are vulnerable and dispossessed persons requiring respect and needing signs of solidarity.

How effective can such a challenge be in the face of power play? First, it is right to recognize humankind's capacity for producing ethics, however profound the ambiguities we experience. Human power is not corrupt for being power, but through the lack of commitment with which it is invoked in relationships with our fellows.

Second, the poor have considerable allies in those who are using their power in research in an ethical manner, and also in those who are working for human rights in all sectors affected by human genetic research. In the end, however, the effectiveness of the ethical challenge posed by the poor depends on the poor themselves growing in consciousness of their dignity and of their social rights and responsibilities. It is also fundamental to add that the poor come into ethics as agents and co-workers, not needing to remain in their customary condition of recipients of compassion. In the research field, there are signs that social organizations are moving in this direction in the so-called Third World. And once the poor and vulnerable are no longer trampled on in this power play, humanity will have become more human. And would this not be one of the most important criteria for measuring real progress in human genetics?

## Notes

1. A. Toffler, *Powershift: The Overthrow of the Elites*, 1990.
2. I should like to express special thanks to L. Pessini, vice director of the S. Camilo Integrated Faculties, São Paulo, for his valuable help in this study.
3. M. C. Carvalho, 'Firm sells indigenous DNA', in *Folha S. Paulo*, 1 June 1997.
4. Ibid.
5. Pivetta, 'Ethical committee suspends AIDS research', in *Folha S. Paulo*, 22 March 1997.
6. 'The world market in remedies derived from plants is now approaching $32 billion, according to UN estimates', *Folha S. Paulo*, 6 July 1997.
7. J. C. Assumpçao, 'Forest becomes pharmacy', in *Folha S. Paulo*, 1 June 1997.
8. It is not in the least surprising that the United States refused to take part in this Convention.
9. *Folha S. Paulo*, 6 July 1997.
10. In view of the difficulty of compiling a bibliography accessible to all language areas in which this article is published, I note merely: W. T. Reich (ed.), 'Research Ethics Committee', in *Encyclopedia of Bioethics*, New York, 1995; D. P. Salas, 'Estructura y función de los Comités de Etica de la Investigación Clínica', in *Cuadernos del Programa Regional de Bioética*, Chile, OPAS/OMS, 1996, 3, 92–105.
11. C. A. Mühlen, 'Comitês de Etica em Pesquisa em Seres Humanos nos Estados Unidos da América', in *Bioetica*, Brasilia-DF 1993, 3, 45.
12. Ministry of Health, National Health Council, doc. 01960/96.
13. The *vulnerable* subjects, mentioned above, deserve special consideration here.
14. The Brazilian Resolution establishes a protocol containing the following elements in its description of research: 'detailed financial budget for research'; guarantee that 'the

results of the research will be made public'; 'declaration of the use and destination of material and/or data collected'; description of the procedure to be followed in obtaining 'free and informed consent'.

# CASE STUDY:
# Anti-AIDS Drugs in Developing Countries

The global AIDS pandemic is having a devastating effect in many parts of the world, particularly Africa. South Africa is one of the worst hit countries: at the beginning of 2002, about 4.7 million South Africans were infected with HIV, and it has been estimated that if present trends continue, five to seven million people in South Africa will have died of AIDS by 2010.

At the time of writing, the South African government has attracted serious criticism over its response to AIDS, particularly because anti-retroviral drugs (ARVs) have not been made widely available for a variety of reasons. The charity Médecins Sans Frontières (MSF) has been campaigning to have ARVs made widely available in South Africa. MSF reports a great contrast between South Africa and Brazil, where more than 100,000 people have received ARV treatment. This has been made possible by a variety of government actions, including the allocation of increased resources to health care and a variety of actions designed to force down the price of the drugs. According to MSF, Brazil is able to use 'generic' versions of some ARVs, which are around half the cost of brand-name versions even at the discounted prices which some brand-name manufacturers offer to developing countries.

MSF also report that the UN Global Fund on AIDS, tuberculosis and malaria requires US$8 billion per year to meet its global health care targets, but that by January 2002 only US$1.7 billion had been promised to the fund for a three-year period.

## Questions
- When there are urgent health care needs in a developing country, what parties share responsibility for meeting those needs, and what are the responsibilities of the different parties?
- What would be needed to ensure that all countries' citizens have access to basic health care?
- What if anything is the relationship between small scale rationing decisions in any one health care system and the disparities in health care between nations?

**Source**

Médecins Sans Frontières, 'Generic AIDS Drugs Offer New Lease of Life to South Africans, Importation of generics cuts price in half' (press release, 29 January 2002) and 'Brazilian generic drugs in South Africa – the background' (29 January 2002). Both available at www.accessmed-msf.org.

# 8

# HUMANS AND OTHER ANIMALS

## Introduction

In chapter 3, we saw that the question 'Who counts as a person?' is frequently asked in the context of bioethical debates, and often means something like, 'What individuals have rights?' or, 'What individuals have a moral status that requires us to treat them with respect and care?' Some approaches answer this question in terms of the capacities or potential that different individuals possess, which either do or do not qualify them to be counted as persons. On this basis some ethicists argue that not all human individuals count as persons or the bearers of rights (e.g. Singer 1993, 135–174); conversely, some non-human animals *do* qualify (Regan 1983; Singer 1993, 110–117). If they are right, radical changes are needed in our treatment of non-human animals: if some animals are to be considered as persons with rights, it is almost certainly unjustified to kill and eat them, and may be wrong to farm them for their milk, eggs and other products. Hunting, fishing and other sports that cause harm to such animals are likely to be ruled out. And their use in biomedical research which causes their suffering and death is seriously called into question, even if that research is necessary for the treatment of serious human diseases or the production and testing of vital medicines. After all, most of us do not think it right to use humans in seriously harmful or lethal medical research, even if the knowledge gained thereby would save many more human lives. If other animal species are the bearers of comparable rights, their use in this way will be similarly unjustifiable.

The first reading in this chapter is a robust exchange on the subject of animal rights between two very different Christian thinkers. Oliver Barclay, a zoologist, is highly critical of the notion of animal rights. He argues that it is unclear, that it involves the 'naturalistic fallacy' (that is, an illegitimate move in moral argument from an 'is' to an 'ought') and that it does not offer a secure basis for the humane treatment of animals. In the first part of the article from which this extract is taken, he has given a critique of Regan and other philosophers. In the extract reproduced here, he extends his critique to the theologian Andrew Linzey, who has written extensively on animals and theology, and has defended a theologically based understanding of animal rights.

The next reading is Linzey's reply to Barclay's critique. In response to Barclay, he stresses that his theory of rights is different from Regan's and others. Linzey's is a theory of 'theos rights': rights that are not grounded in any intrinsic properties or abilities of animals, but in the right of God their creator 'to have what is created treated with respect' (p. 224). The reading concludes with a brief response by Barclay to Linzey's comments.

Elsewhere, Linzey has argued for change in our treatment of animals on many other grounds, quite apart from arguments about rights. In particular, he has argued on the basis of biblical and other Christian sources that humans have moral obligations to other animals, not because they are equal to us, but precisely because they are *not*. The great power of humans and the weakness and vulnerability of other animals gives the latter a 'moral priority'; and the uniqueness of humans is best described as a distinctive calling from God to be the 'servant species', charged with the care of other animals and of the creation (Linzey 1994, 28–61). Some of these themes are taken up by Scott Bader-Saye in the third reading in this chapter. He explores the relevance of the Christian doctrine that human beings are made in the image of God (Gen. 1:26–28). This is closely related to the discussions of personhood in chapter 3. Bader-Saye is highly critical of the use of this doctrine as 'a category that released us from concern for certain of God's creatures, put a limit on our moral vision, and placed other animals in the category of those not "worthy of our compassion" ' (p. 231). Rather, he argues, it should be seen as a special calling of God, to live at peace with other animals and to be a blessing to them.

**References and Further Reading**

Donald Bruce and Ann Bruce (eds.), *Engineering Genesis: The Ethics of Genetic Engineering in Non-Human Species*. 2nd ed., London: Earthscan, 2002.
Stephen R. L. Clark, *Biology and Christian Ethics*. Cambridge: Cambridge University Press, 2000.
Andrew Linzey, *Animal Theology*. London: SCM, 1994.
Mary Midgley, *Animals and Why they Matter*. Harmondsworth: Penguin, 1983.
Tom Regan, *The Case for Animal Rights*. London: Routledge, 1983.
Peter Singer, *Practical Ethics*. 2nd ed., Cambridge: Cambridge University Press, 1993.

# From 'Animal Rights: A Critique'

OLIVER R. BARCLAY

## Christian Approaches in Terms of Rights

Although the concept of animal rights does not attract many Christian writers, there are two explicitly Christian writers who are especially important. Stephen R. Clark, another professor of philosophy, in his book, 'The Moral Status of Animals'[1] develops a vigorous case for the welfare of animals. He starts with 'a moral and philosophical sense' and emphasises our *moral* sense that it is 'not proper to be the cause of avoidable ill'. He goes on, 'if this minimal principle be accepted there is no other course than the immediate rejection of all flesh-foods and most biomedical research'.[2] Nevertheless he is hesitant about the use of the language of rights. He states: 'on absolute terms it is plausible to say that nothing has any positive rights: all is gift, whether to us or to jackdaws, or to the young lions that seek their prey from God',[3] or again he acknowledges, 'animals perhaps have no positive rights: it is difficult to see on what basis *we* have any either'.[4] He develops the view that *we* have no 'rights to their (i.e. animals') flesh or their service, or are in the right if we torment them'. Therefore, throughout his wide ranging argument he almost entirely avoids the use of the word 'rights'. He depends on our 'moral sense' of outrage at the treatment of creatures who have so much in common with us in physiology and in a lesser degree psychology. He also, like many non-Christian writers, holds that 'we have no extra standing in the world . . . the land is the mayfly's, the thrush's and the fox's as much as it is ours'.[5] The point is that he finds ample reasons for defending animals without resorting to rights. Few people could be stronger for the defence of animals, but the rights questions he finds too controversial to be useful.

The other important Christian writer who has achieved considerable influence is Andrew Linzey, who constantly uses the word 'rights' in relation to animals. In his book, 'Christianity and the rights of animals'[6] he says that in his earlier writings[7] he drew a line between those who must be protected, and those who need not, at 'the capacity to experience pain and pleasure'. He now believes that he must find another criterion because: 'What this

From *Science and Christian Belief*, vol. 4.1, pp. 57–61 (1992). The complete article comprises pp. 49–61.

criterion was searching for was some way in which the theological sense of community with animals could be assessed. To put it bluntly, I wanted to find some way in which the spiritual capacities of animals could be recognised as giving them a status beyond that of cabbages and greenfly'.[8] He starts with 'a theological sense of community with animals' and then looks around for arguments to defend it. One can debate the arguments, but it is very hard to argue with 'a sense of community'. When he calls it a theological sense one has serious doubts about its theological nature.

His first main point is entirely valid. This is that God is the Lord of all Creation and cares for it all. God has a claim on it all because he made it and maintains it in being. This is not open to dispute among Christians. He goes on, however, to develop a thesis which has two fatal weaknesses. Once more he is trying to claim too much for too few creatures. Because his case does not hold water it is in danger of ending up achieving too little for all animals.

Linzey writes about what he calls the 'theos rights of animals'. This depends on his agreed starting point that God values the whole of his creation. When he talks about the 'theos rights' of higher animals, however, he is introducing a confusion, because what he means is *God's* rights in his creation and this is an entirely different thing from animals having rights. He has in a sense turned the concept of rights around, but cannot resist the temptation to use the word rights of animals.

Linzey accepts Regan's position as approximately the same as his own in practice and quotes Regan that 'rights are possessed by humans and animals who are mentally normal mammals of a year or more' (why not birds?). But Linzey differs from Regan in that Regan 'makes no use of the concept of God as the upholder and sustainer of value'.[9] Linzey's whole position depends on the view that the value of the psychological and other features that Regan uses as a criterion 'can only be ultimately justified by reference to God's own right as sovereign Creator'.[10]

Secondly, Linzey adopts a description of those animals which come under the category of theos rights as 'Spirit-filled, breathing beings composed of flesh and blood'. Without dogmatism he is inclined to the view that only animals which come clearly within that definition are the subject of rights. The phrase 'Spirit-filled creatures' occurs frequently in his treatment. He leans to the view that this means that only warm-blooded animals fall *clearly* into the category of creatures possessing rights. Linzey as a Christian does make a distinction between man and animals, though its nature is not very clear. Regan, as we have noted, has virtually no distinction to make.

Linzey sometimes tilts at extremes, or positions that not many people would defend today – such as, that animals do not feel pain and they are not intelligent, or that man's 'dominion' described in Genesis 1:28 is equivalent to despotism or tyranny. This device often back-fires somewhat because those who do not agree with him feel that they have been misrepresented and are less sympathetic to the discussion. Linzey has some good things to say about man's dominion as a mandate to rule God's world in God's way and not in a selfish tyranny or exploitation, but he is a little frightened of the whole concept of dominion even though it is clearly biblical. He does not discuss some of the key biblical passages that others would use.[11] This is unfortunate and, like others, he over-reacts to its abuses and adds to non-Christian caricatures of it in White.[12]

Linzey's concept of 'Spirit-filled creatures' is crucial to his whole approach and it must be said that his biblical and other evidence for this is very weak indeed and in fact is quite seriously misleading. His position depends on a very loose use of biblical passages. When, for instance, he quotes Psalm 104:24–30 he forgets firstly, that it is about *all* God's creatures 'both small and great' that swarm on the land and in the sea (surely that includes crabs, sea urchins, worms and the aphids that he excludes). Secondly, it is not stated that they are Spirit-filled, but that God's spirit *creates* a new generation to renew the face of the earth, in the same way that God's Spirit in Genesis 1:1 was active in the creation of all things, including the inanimate world. Again he concludes from Romans 8:18–23 that animals can be redeemed, but what the passage says is that 'the *whole of creation* will be delivered from bondage to decay when the redemption of *mankind* is completed'. He always uses a capital S for 'Spirit-filled' thereby implying that they are in the same category as people. Like Skinner and Regan he is claiming too much for too few animals and so weakens his whole case. One might agree that some animals may be thought as possessing 'spirit' (small s), though the nature of this 'spirit' is very hard to define and describe. This, however, if it was carefully defined could be used as a distinguishing mark of the higher animals which makes them worthy of special respect. Such a difference of degree amongst animals is probably more clearly described in terms of 'consciousness'.

## Outlines of a Christian Response

The outlines of a Christian response could be put under the following headings, but cannot be elaborated here. Many of these points would be included in any discussion on the environment.[13]

1. *The worth of all creation.* The Christian ought to hold that the whole of God's creation is of value to him just because it is his. 'The sea is his and he made it and his hands prepared the dry land'.
2. People are throughout the Bible assumed to be in a special position in relation to God. At creation they are described as '*in the image of God*'. This does not apply to any other aspect of the creation and is repeated in the New Testament as a distinguishing mark of humans and a distinguishing

reason why they must be treated with special respect.[14] People have spiritual dimensions that no other created thing possesses.

3. *Dominion and greater value.* One of the classical passages here is Psalm 8 where it is explicitly said that whereas the whole of creation shows God's glory, his name is majestic in *all* the earth, his glory is chanted above the heavens, yet man is put in a special position of responsibility over the whole animal creation. Genesis 1, of course, announces man's position of responsibility and Jesus himself stresses that we are of more value than sparrows. But, as we have said, it is a matter of *more* value, which does not allow the rest to be treated as of no value.

4. *Stewardship of creation.* Man is therefore put in a position not of despotic rule, but of duty of stewardship over the whole creation for God. We are at best the tenant farmers. Sadly we have often abused our powers and must acknowledge that. Sometimes people have tried to give a religious sanction for cruel exploitation. The concept of stewardship and, because of our responsibility to future generations, of sustainable development, must be major themes in the whole environment discussion and apply especially to animals. Nevertheless, this and the responsibility of dominion mean that every time we dig our garden or plant a field we are interfering with the natural world, and we should do so not with apologies, but with confidence that this is what we are meant to do.

5. *Higher animals.* Leaving humankind aside, higher animals are in a special position because they suffer more and may suffer nearly as we do. Therefore there is obviously a greater responsibility for how we treat higher animals. Nevertheless, Jesus must have eaten meat at the Passover and certainly, even after his resurrection when free from all human limitations, ate fish.[15] The special position of animals does not mean that they may not be farmed or used for food. It requires special care in their treatment. But there is no line to be drawn above which we should not act and below which we may be more care-less.

6. *Cruelty to animals.* The Bible treats cruelty or thoughtlessness in the treatment of animals as a serious fault which is shown, for example, by our Lord's words where he confirms that even the most crucial of socio-religious commands, the keeping of the Sabbath, was to be over-ruled to avoid animal suffering.[16]

7. One of the problems with writers such as Linzey is that they manage constantly to create a situation of doubt, or possibly ill-conscience, about a responsible stewardship of the world and the use of animals. Thus he asks, 'is pet keeping immoral in itself?', or, 'are wild animals best left alone?' In the last case he thinks that 'it *could be* our responsibility to respect what God has given and let it be' (my italics). But we have to decide, is it or is it not our responsibility to let rats be? If the answer is no, then we must control the population with a good conscience. Simply

to question can give a guilty conscience about everything, and we need a certain toughness to stand up to this kind of approach and to say that it is our duty and that we may, and should act and also enjoy animal food, etc. 1 Timothy seems to have been addressed in part to attack asceticism in relation to food and marriage. Both can be abused, but in 1 Timothy 4:1–4 it seems that the Apostle is authorising the use of 'everything created by God' for food. We are to eat what God has given us with thankfulness and not with an uneasy sense that it is a grudging permission, or a concession to sin. It is God's provision for us in the world as we have it. It is sometimes argued that meat eating is a concession to sin,[17] but whatever its origin it is something which is God-given to us in our world, which is not utopia. 1 Timothy makes it plain that we should do so with a good conscience and indeed with positive thankfulness to God, *'everything is to be received with thanksgiving'*.

## Conclusion

I conclude that the term 'animal rights' should not be used. However it is developed it is a misleading application of what is a controversial concept even in relation to humanity. But although I believe that we should avoid the term, we should not simply leave a vacuum. We should be committed, as Christians have been for a long time, to the welfare of animals and their proper treatment in the context of our responsibilities for the whole of the natural world. The case for animal welfare will be spoilt if claims are made which cannot really be substantiated. One or two bad arguments can discredit the whole. Our approach should not be in terms of animal rights, but rather in terms of the positive mandate given to humankind to look after the earth and to use everything in it constructively and in respect for the marvellous and complex beauty of what God has created. This does not mean that we should say that: 'Animals have no rights'. That is a strong negative statement that implies far more than its strict logical sense. We should say that the term is inappropriate as applied to animals.[18] They will be better protected by developing the concept of animal welfare and our duties to and responsibilities for animals, in the context of our overall responsibilities for the whole environment.

## Notes

1. Clark, Stephen R. L. *The Moral Status of Animals*, Oxford and New York, OUP 1977, references to 1984 paperback edition.
2. *ibid*, preface to first edition, page 1.
3. *ibid*, page 27.
4. *ibid*, page 28.
5. *ibid*, page 113.

6. Linzey, Andrew, *Christianity and the Rights of Animals*, London, SPCK, 1987, page 80.
7. Linzey, Andrew, *Animal Rights: A Christian Assessment*, London, SCM Press, 1976.
8. Linzey (6) page 81.
9. *ibid*, page 82.
10. *ibid*, page 83.
11. Such as Genesis 1:26–28; Genesis 9:3; 1 Timothy 4:1–4 and Psalm 8.
12. White, Lynn Jr. 'The Historical Roots of our Ecological Crisis', *Science* (10 March 1967), page 1203–7.
13. See Berry, R. J. 'Christianity and the Environment' and 'A Bibliography on Environmental Issues' in *Science and Christian Belief* (1991) 3 (1) page 3–18.
14. e.g. James 3:9.
15. Luke 24:42, 43 and John 21:9–14.
16. Matthew 12:11; Luke 14:5. See also Exodus 23:4–5; Deut. 22:1–4, 25:4; Pro. 12:10.
17. It is argued that because the right to take animals for food is only explicitly mentioned after the Flood in Genesis 9 it cannot have been the original idea. It is, however, a gift of the covenant made with mankind at that point and from then on.
18. I owe this point to Mary Midgley, *Animals and Why they Matter*, Harmondsworth, Penguin, 1983, page 61. She follows it with a useful discussion of the problems of the legal and moral uses of rights terminology.

# Animal Rights: A Reply to Barclay

ANDREW LINZEY

1. *Human uniqueness.* Barclay prefaces his criticisms of my work by a discussion of the views of two philosophers, Peter Singer and Tom Regan. Inevitably my own contribution is seen as continuous with these philosophers and understood through the same critical lens. This is fair to some extent – since there are some continuities between us – but there are also discontinuities which Barclay fails to grasp. Singer and Regan must speak for themselves as to whether they have been misrepresented as at least in one instance Singer has been,[1] but Barclay's judgement that 'The (sic) animal rights literature rightly points out that their whole position depends upon refusing to draw any sharp distinction between animals and people' [not reproduced here – Ed.] is not relevant to myself. As Barclay acknowledges 'Linzey as a Christian does make a distinction between man and animals, though its nature is not very clear' (p. 218). In fact, one of the reasons I give for adopting the concept of 'theos rights' is precisely because the 'unique significance of man in this respect consists in his capacity to perceive God's will and to actualise it within his own life'.[2] Far from underrating the spiritual and moral significance of humankind, my thesis depends upon it.[3]

Barclay makes much of how animal rightists seek to deduce an 'ought' from an 'is' – in the matter of sentiency ... But he fails to see that he is open to entirely the same charge when it comes to human uniqueness. He emphasises human difference without explaining how and why it is morally relevant (see 2 below).

2. *Human dominion.* Barclay maintains that I am 'frightened of the whole concept of dominion even though it is clearly biblical' (p. 219). Untrue. In my book to which he refers, I go out of my way to explain how, while some Christian commentators have sometimes interpreted dominion as despotism, the idea as expressed within the Genesis text suggests otherwise. I summarise my position as follows: 'Jews and Christians have been right to point to man's God-given power over the non-human. Where they have been wrong in the past is in interpreting what this power means. If full weight is given to Christ as our moral exemplar, our power cannot be understood as legitimate except in service, which is necessarily costly and sacrificial'.[4] Barclay

From *Science and Christian Belief*, vol. 5.1, pp. 47–51 (1993).

fails to grasp this Christological argument completely. Human difference and power over the non-human are not by themselves sufficient moral justifications for our exploitation of animals. A further question has to be posed, namely, How are we to exercise our superiority? I argue that Jesus provides us with the essential model here, namely lordship exercised through service.

3. *Theos rights.* Barclay argues that: 'When (Linzey) talks about the "theos rights" of higher animals . . . he is introducing a confusion, because what he means is *God's* rights in his creation and this is an entirely different thing from animals having rights. He has in a sense turned the concept of rights around, but cannot resist the temptation to use the word (sic) rights of animals' (p. 218). Again, Barclay fails to understand that what I am doing is significantly different from Regan or Singer. Right at the start of my discussion of rights, I make it clear in what sense I use this term[5] and subsequently explain how this differs from other secular attempts.[6] This is not 'confusion', it is a *different* theory of rights. Barclay argues that God's rights are 'an entirely different thing from animals having rights' but the whole point of my discussion is to show how it is possible to ground the rights of the creature in the rights of the Creator to have what is created treated with respect. Barclay may legitimately disagree with my view, but he has no right to call it a 'confusion', or dismiss it *a priori* without argument.

Barclay maintains that '*The* Christian approach starts with duties or responsibilities and acknowledges rights only if they arise out of duties or responsibilities' [not reproduced here – Ed.]. This is breathtakingly dismissive of the long tradition of rights theory within Christendom. Roman Catholic rights theory has grown out of a long tradition of natural law, and in particular, the 'dignity and rights of the human person' was regarded by John XXIII as the dominating theme of modern catholic teaching.[7] Again, Dietrich Bonhoeffer – to take only one protestant example – strongly defends – on biblical grounds – the primacy of rights from which duties flow and not vice versa.[8] Barclay is free to challenge the tradition which holds to notions of rights; he has no right to claim his view as '*The Christian* approach'.

4. *Spirit and animal life.* Barclay does not like the way in which I draw the line between what I call 'Spirit filled, breathing creatures composed of flesh and blood' – whose rights we should respect – and other creatures. Indeed he appears to deny that it is the special operation of the Spirit which gives life to animal beings. He writes that 'Like Skinner (here he presumably means Singer) and Regan, (Linzey) is claiming too much for too few animals and so weakens his case' (p. 219) – even though he himself argues that humans have some special responsibility towards the 'higher animals' because 'they suffer more' (p. 220). Despite what he says about my 'very loose use of biblical passages', Barclay interprets Psalm 104 as not presupposing the activity of the Spirit in relation to individual animals but only in creating 'a new generation' of life (p. 219). Is the Spirit then only the creative source of species

and not individual lives within species as well? I do not think the judgement of Karl Barth (on whom I draw heavily[9]) can be gainsaid: 'According to the Old Testament, neither soul nor Spirit can be simply denied to the beasts . . . the creative Spirit which awakens man to life is also the life-principle of the beasts . . . '.[10]

5. *Doubt and conscience.* Barclay argues that 'One of the problems with writers such as Linzey (sic) is that they manage constantly to create a situation of doubt, or possibly ill-conscience, about a responsible stewardship of the world and the use of animals' (p. 220). I am charged with this because I raise questions about the morality of pet keeping and killing wild animals. I fail to see why raising questions of doubt and conscience should be castigated in this way. Our exploitation of animals is massive: we hunt, ride, shoot, fish, wear, cage, factory farm and experiment upon millions every year. If we take seriously the biblical ideas that animals are our fellow creatures, that their lives belong to God, and that we are set in a position of God-like responsibility over them, it seems only right that our consciences should sometimes be troubled as to whether what we now do is acceptable to God.

Barclay wants under this category of 'responsible' to justify much of what we now do to animals, but he fails to see that what is *responsible* stewardship is the question which must be asked of each generation. Here, as elsewhere, Barclay ignores the long history within Christendom of profoundly negative attitudes to animals. He lists some important biblical ideas (and I have done at length elsewhere[11]), but does not allow them to illuminate his understanding. For example, if cruelty or thoughtlessness to animals is 'a serious fault' (p. 220), then we need as an urgent requirement to review all our dealings with animals – in farms, laboratories and in 'sporting' activities – which cause pain and suffering. This minimal insight alone would provide a massive agenda. As to the protest against pricking consciences, it invites the response of Albert Schweitzer that a 'good conscience is an invention of the devil'.[12]

## Notes

1. One major inaccuracy is detectable in the first line [not reproduced here – Ed.] where Singer is identified as 'one of the leading advocates of animal rights'. In fact Singer has gone out of his way to oppose the notion of animal rights and the ambiguous use of the term in his early work he now 'regrets', e.g. 'Why is it surprising that I have little to say about the nature of rights? It would only be surprising to one who assumes that my case for animal liberation is based upon rights and, in particular, upon the idea of extending rights to animals. But this is not my position at all. I have little to say about rights because rights are not important to my argument'. 'The Parable of the Fox and the Unliberated Animals', *Ethics* (1978) 88, p. 122; also discussed in Tom Regan, *The Case for Animal Rights* (London: Routledge and Kegan Paul, 1983, pp. 219–30).
2. Andrew Linzey, *Christianity and the Rights of Animals* (London: SPCK and New York:

Crossroad, 1987) p. 98. The last five pages of chapter 5 are given over to spelling out my 'theologically qualified position on rights' (pp. 94–98).

3. See, e.g., Andrew Linzey, 'The Servant Species: Humanity as Priesthood', *Between the Species: A Journal of Ethics* (1990), 6, pp. 109–117, and 'The Theological Basis of Animal Rights', *The Christian Century,* (1991), 108, p. 908.

4. *Christianity and the Rights of Animals,* op. cit., p. 29.

5. I offer a three-point definition of theos rights, *Christianity and the Rights of Animals,* op. cit., p. 69.

6. I consider six arguments at length against my rights theory (pp. 69–94) and how it differs from that of Regan (pp. 82–86) *Christianity and the Rights of Animals,* op. cit.

7. John XXIII cited in David Hollenbach, S.J., *Claims in Conflict: Retrieving and Renewing the Catholic Human Rights Tradition* (New York: Paulist Press, 1979) p. 42; discussed in Charles Villa-Vincencio, *A Theology of Reconstruction: Nation-Building and Human Rights,* Cambridge Studies in Ideology and Religion (Cambridge: CUP, 1992) pp. 131–137.

8. Dietrich Bonhoeffer, *Ethics,* ed. by Eberhard Bethge, ET N. H. Smith (London: SCM Press, 1971) pp. 127 f.; discussed in *Christianity and the Rights of Animals,* op. cit., pp. 70–72.

9. For my critique of Barth, see Andrew Linzey, *The Neglected Creature: The Doctrine of the Non-Human Creation and its Relationship with the Human in the Work of Karl Barth,* unpublished Ph.D. thesis (London University, 1986), and also *Animals and Trinitarian Doctrine: A Study in the Theology of Karl Barth* [Edwin Mellen Press, 1992].

10. Karl Barth, *Church Dogmatics,* III/2, edited by G. W. Bromiley and T. F. Torrance (Edinburgh: T. & T. Clark, 1960) p. 361n.

11. See, e.g., Andrew Linzey, *The Status of Animals in the Christian Tradition* (Birmingham: Woodbrooke College, 1985) esp. pp. 26–27.

12. Albert Schweitzer, *Civilization and Ethics* (London: Allen and Unwin, 1967) p. 221; discussed in Andrew Linzey, 'The Place of Animals in Creation – A Christian View' in Tom Regan (ed.) *Animal Sacrifices: Religious Perspectives on the Use of Animals in Science* (Philadelphia: Temple University Press, 1986) pp. 139–142.

*Dr Oliver Barclay responds*

I hope that a brief response to Andrew Linzey's 'Reply' may help to clarify a few issues. I am sorry that my original article was not more complete.

I agree that the concept of 'dominion' has been misused by some Christians. I do not, however, think that we help by reducing it to 'service' to animals. Stewardship is a more biblically-based concept for this purpose and includes elements of creative development of resources.

We may or may not agree on the nature of the distinctiveness of humankind. The statement that he quotes in his reply does not necessarily involve any ontological differences. His definition could be read as merely functional. I hope we are agreed but I am still not sure. Its relevance is that it determines the kind of dominion that God gave to humankind rather than to superior animals or even angels (see Psalm 8).

When I criticised the concept of 'Spirit filled, breathing creatures composed of flesh and blood' as those that need protection, and need to be distinguished from other animals, my point was that the biblical passages he quotes (1) do not speak of them as Spirit filled, but rather as created afresh by the Spirit and (2) they include equally all animals, however lowly. I do not at all deny the activity of the Spirit in giving and maintaining life in all creatures. To call only some animals Spirit filled is to create a weak link in the arguments for defending animals from exploitation. It also misuses the biblical concept of being Spirit filled, which is applied only to some people some of the time.

On 'theos rights' others must judge; but the confusion arises from using the concept of rights in two very different senses: God's rights and the rights of (only some) animals. A Natural Law approach to animal rights is surely something different from 'theos rights'.

On doubt and conscience I had in mind also his remarks about animal food and farming.

I am glad that we are largely agreed in the end as to the duties that humans have towards animals. I argue that we would do better to abandon the language of rights, which will be counter-productive if it is not better and more straightforwardly justifiable. The old concepts of 'welfare' and duties are more clearly biblical, and easier to grasp and define. They also apply to the whole range of animals, and indeed to the whole environment rather than to only one group of animals.

# Imaging God Through Peace with Animals: An Election for Blessing

SCOTT BADER-SAYE

'I don't trust people who don't like animals,' my mother used to say. The way to her heart was (and still is) through loving her dogs. I felt right at home, therefore, when I learned that one of the first questions my mother-in-law asked about me when I started dating her daughter was whether Demery's *dog* liked me. Finding out that I passed the dog test, she responded, 'If Maddy likes him that's good enough for me.' I guess there are worse ways to choose a son-in-law! We all know the old cliché that dogs are good judges of character, but perhaps a grain of truth lies buried in the platitude. What seems to be right is the connection of one's care for the other animals with one's character, or as the old rabbinic saying puts it, 'the way a man treats an animal is a window to his soul.'[1]

Of course, others could surely cite anecdotes in which people who are indifferent to their fellow creatures turn out to be deeply committed to serving human goods. Nonetheless, the close ties between human flourishing and proper stewardship of the other animals cannot be overlooked in the biblical witness. Twice in Genesis 1 human beings are referred to as 'imaging God,' and both times there follows a set of instructions about our relation to the other creatures. God declares, 'Let us make humankind in our image, according to our likeness; and let them have dominion over the fish of the sea, and over the birds of the air, over the cattle, and over all the wild animals of the earth, and over every creeping thing that creeps upon the earth' (Gen. 1:26; cf. 1:28). Imaging God correlates with stewarding the fish and birds and cattle. Genesis 1 pictures us standing with one hand reaching up toward God and another hand reaching out toward the animal world. This dual focus must not be reduced to a dualism of nature, in which humans are said to share a soul with God and a body with the nonhuman animals. Such a soul/body distinction is foreign to the world of Genesis. Indeed, the closest thing to the language of soul in Genesis 1 and 2 is *nephesh*, the breath of life, which in fact humans share with *all* living creatures. In short, our position between God and the other animals cannot be adequately depicted by biological or metaphysical analysis alone, but rather must be understood as the inter-

From *Studies in Christian Ethics*, vol. 14.2, pp. 1–13, (2001).

section of two mutually interpreting relations – that of image and that of dominion. These two relations are drawn together in an instructive way through the doctrine of election.

The radical calling of God's election has largely been lost in the history of Christian theology just in so far as election has been turned into a spiritualized claim about the eternal destiny of the individual soul.[2] Looking back at the witness of Israel, however, one finds that God's election is understood as the calling and forming of a people to participate in and mediate the blessings of the reign of God. In this sense we may come to understand the creation of humans in God's image as a kind of election by which humans are placed in a relationship of blessing with the nonhuman creatures.

## *Imago Dei:* **From Domination to Election**

In order to tease out the connections between *imago Dei*, divine election, and stewardship of the other animals some ground must first be cleared. Traditionally, discussions of *imago Dei* have sought to define that particular human trait or capacity that does two things – makes humans *like* God and makes us *unlike* the other creatures. It is the first of these that usually receives the attention, but I wish to focus on the second. For the practice of highlighting and elevating that particular trait which places humans above other animals in the chain of being has undermined our sense of moral responsibility toward these creatures. The logic works something like this: since other animals do not have that quality that makes humans human, that is, the quality by which we image God (and here you can fill in the blank – rationality, a soul, language, consciousness), then other animals are rightly considered instruments in the projects of those who have such a capacity. If the other animals are not like us, then they do not deserve our charity and it is justifiable to use them for whatever purpose we desire. Their stories are completely subsumed within the human story, and thus they have no story of their own by which their relation to God can be expressed . . .

It must be noted, however, that the kind of 'instrumentalism' found in premodern Christian writings differed from what was to come in modernity. For instance, it is not insignificant that Aquinas often makes reference to nonhuman animals as 'other animals,' thus expressing his awareness of the extent to which humans share an animal nature.[3] Further, it matters that Calvin envisions the animals as sharing an eschatological destiny with human beings in the reign of God. Despite the inadequacies of their formulation, these Christian writers are yoked to a narrative of creation and redemption that includes the other animals as part of God's economy. Thus, they cannot utterly lose sight of these creatures' origin and telos in God.

In modernity this narrative of origin and telos has been thrust aside or radically reinterpreted, resulting in the triumph of instrumentalism even in human relations.⁴ Such a broad acceptance of instrumentalism among humans has further deteriorated any lingering sense of moral responsibility for nonhuman creatures. Descartes, for instance, notoriously compared non-human animals to machines, and his followers justified animal experimentation by comparing these creatures' shrieks of pain to 'the noise of breaking machinery'.⁵ The pattern of denigrating nonhuman animals opens a new chapter in modernity but carries forward the basic logic that has gone before – by defining a certain quality, usually rationality of the rational soul, as that which makes us human (or, Christianly speaking, as that which constitutes the image of God in humanity), one thereby excludes from moral consideration those who lack this quality, namely the other creatures.

In the nineteenth and twentieth centuries we saw a reaction to this instru-mentalist view, and movements arose seeking 'rights' for non-human animals. While I am not averse to the goals of such groups, I am convinced that their critique of the tradition on this matter is misdirected – in short, it is not radical enough. First, the language of 'rights' does not fundamentally challenge the social structures of instrumentality. Rather it seeks to protect interests within a context where instrumentalism is presumed. Second, the animal rights advocates accept the basic presumption of their opponents – that we should have moral concern only for that part of the creation that shares certain qualities with ourselves. They simply argue the flip side of the same coin. Yes, they say, other animals *do* have rationality, or interests, or sentience, or consciousness (again you can fill in the blank). But what if, Christianly speaking, the whole basis of the argument is flawed on both sides? What if the real question is not whether other animals are sufficiently like us to warrant moral consideration, but rather what kind of people must we be to embody the claim that our lives and our dominions are images of God?

I am reminded of the way Jesus upsets the assumptions of his antagonists with the parable of the Good Samaritan.⁶ A lawyer arose to test Jesus and upon hearing Jesus enunciate the double command to love God and neighbor, he pushes for a definition of 'neighbor.' The lawyer wants to be clear who counts as an object of his moral concern; he wants to know where he can draw the line, where charity ends. But Jesus, rather than answering the question posed, tells the story of a Samaritan who, unlike the priest and Levite, cares for a wounded stranger on the road and provides for his wellbeing. Then in a climactic conclusion Jesus refuses to limit the extent of neighbor love by defining who is inside or outside the category 'neighbor.' Rather, he tells the lawyer to go and be a neighbor himself. As Richard Hays puts it, 'the point is that we are called upon to *become* neighbors to those who are helpless, going beyond conventional conceptions of duty to provide life-sustaining aid to those whom we might not have regarded as worthy of our compassion.'⁷ For too long, *imago Dei* has constituted a category that released us from concern for certain of God's creatures, put a limit on our moral vision, and placed other animals in the category of those not 'worthy of our compassion.' In this way our claims to image God have set us at odds with God's abundant and surprising charity.

I want to suggest a different way of thinking about imaging God, a way that is not driven by a search for a defining human trait, but rather attends to the narrative context of Genesis and thus makes the image of God a description that can only be understood as a specific kind of relationship between God, humans, and the rest of creation. As I have mentioned already, it is exegetically significant that both mentions of *imago Dei* in Genesis 1 are followed by the charge to have dominion over the other animals (1:26, 28). It would be inadequate to imply that this dominion constitutes the entirety of how humans image God, but as Karl Barth remarks, 'There can be little doubt that the two are brought together and that the *dominium terrae* is portrayed as a consequence of the *imago Dei*.'[8] I would suggest the connecting link here is the doctrine of election whereby human beings are chosen for a special relationship with God while being given the vocation to mediate the blessings of election to the non-elect, in this case, the nonhuman animals. Kendall Soulen makes the case that this pattern of difference and blessing is intrinsic to God's goal for creation.[9] . . .

Our reading of the *imago Dei* as a form of election situates the claim to image God and the concomitant dominion over the animals within this broader context of God's economies of blessing.

Rightly understood, election teaches us that God freely and graciously chooses to work in and with the creation through particularity. God chooses specific means by which to work out the divine plan, and the choosing of humankind to bear God's image and exercise dominion can be best understood as part of this biblical pattern of election. From among all the creation God elects humankind to represent God's rule to the other creatures. From among all humans God elects Israel to embody the ways of God before the nations. From among all the people of Israel God elects Jesus Christ to inaugurate the redemption of the world. In Jesus God elects Jews and Gentiles alike to enact the reign of God on earth. Our God is an electing God, whose choices represent God's providential commitment to bring all the creation to its good end.

We must be careful, however, with this convergence of *imago Dei* and election, for these doctrines have historically been misconstrued in similar ways: each has been distorted so as to justify hierarchy and domination. The claim of divine election has for too long underwritten the rejection and oppression of the non-elect, just as the claim that humans image God has underwritten a pattern of subjugation and destruction of the rest of creation. By bringing the two into such close relation are we not just exacerbating this danger? Here it is important to attend closely to the biblical narrative, for we find precisely this danger exposed in Genesis 3. The serpent, craftiest of all creatures, promises that if the humans eat of the tree of knowledge of good and evil they will 'be like God' (3:5). Notice that a distinction is made between 'imaging God' in Genesis 1 and 'being like God' in Genesis 3. The former is our highest calling, while the latter is our deepest rebellion. It is as if imaging God carries the intrinsic temptation to supplant God, to take God's place, to claim sovereignty where only God is sovereign. Thus, imaging God in our dominion over the other animals is a tightrope walk in which we dare not claim too much or too little for ourselves. We cannot neglect our election to give oversight to the other creatures, but surely God did not mean for us to seize possession of them. They belong to God, not to us.

## Election and Formation: Cultivating Habits of Peace

When we look at the election of Israel, the biblical paradigm of election, we see that election entails both formation and vocation. Those chosen by God are first formed and shaped into people capable of living God's ways. Like a potter molding clay, God molds the people of God into a community worthy of bearing God's name. This is why the giving of the Torah is so closely connected to Israel's identity as the elect people. Torah provides the rules and practices necessary to create a people who will be a light to the nations. So likewise, when God chooses human beings to share in the divine image, God directs us to have dominion over the animals, to name them, and with them to eat only of the vegetation of the garden. In this instruction God is seeking to produce people whose character is commensurate with the character of God, whose dominion is a truthful reflection of God's dominion. The image of God in human beings is both an indicative and an imperative, both a description and a calling. The election of humankind entails a process of formation in God's image, and thus we find that the character which images God is related to earthly dominion in a circular fashion. One needs to be shaped by the ways of God in order to enact virtuous dominion, but equally, the act of reigning virtuously creates a character that images God. The virtues and practices at work here are intertwined in such a way that each requires and produces the other.

A failure to exercise virtuous dominion over the nonhuman animals will lead to the distortion of human character and a clouding of the divine image. It should come as no surprise that violence against other animals is a strong predictor of violence against humans. Many of the young perpetrators of school shootings in recent years had a history of violence against nonhuman animals . . .

Even Immanuel Kant, who believed that 'animals are not self-conscious and are there merely as a means to an end,' was able to recognize the connection between the treatment of other animals and the formation of character. 'If he is not to stifle his human feelings,' Kant writes, 'he must practice kindness towards animals, for he who is cruel to animals becomes hard also in his dealings with men. We can judge the heart of a man by his treatment of animals.'[10] God's election of humankind to have dominion requires formation of character so that one's actions will reflect the dominion of God. In turn, a charitable dominion over the other animals will contribute to the formation of a character that faithfully images God in all relations. While peacefulness toward the other animals does not carry the same moral weight as peacefulness toward other humans, these forms of peaceful living are interconnected and together shape the virtue of peacefulness in the human heart. Charity toward nonhuman animals does not displace our concern for other humans but supports such concern by making our 'consistent ethic of life' a more comprehensive habit of living.[11]

## Election and Vocation: Blessing the Non-elect

Alongside the formation of community and character, election always carries with it a particular vocation. Those chosen by God are called to be a blessing to others, specifically to the non-elect. We find, for instance, in Abraham's calling the charge and promise that 'in you all the families of the earth shall be blessed' (Gen. 12:3). Analogously, the election of humankind is a mandate to bless the non-elect, the nonhuman animals, just as God blesses them in Genesis 1:22. Too often, election has been interpreted as a warrant for arrogance, domination and violence against the outside. But such views miss the point that election is *for the sake* of the other. It is not intended to create oppositions and hierarchies between the insiders and outsiders, the elect and the reprobate, the saved and the lost, the clean and the unclean. Election is not God's way of dividing creation into antagonistic parties; rather it is God's means of working for the consummation of all. God chooses some for a special task within the overarching goal of 'gathering up all things in Christ' (Eph. 1:10). And we have no reason to doubt that 'all things' includes the non-human animals. In so far as we see God's choice of humankind over the other animals as at least analogous to an act of election, we can see that the differences between humans and other animals, as well as the dominion given to humankind, create a relationship in which the elect are called to bless the non-elect so that they too might be drawn toward their proper eschatological fulfillment. As Stanley Hauerwas and John Berkman have noted, 'there is an analogous relation between the fact that the other animals need humans to tell them their story and the fact that we who are Gentiles need Jews to tell us our story'.[12] That is, the pattern of election gives priority to a particular portion of the creation (humans in relation to other animals, Jews in relation to Gentiles) for the sake of carrying out a calling that will bring blessing, not curse, to the other.

This vocation is bounded and directed by the central theological affirmation that 'in life and in death we belong to God' (to cite the Presbyterian Brief Statement of Faith, echoing the Heidelberg Catechism). This confession points to the heart of divine election – God's free choice to make us God's own – and it poses the following challenge: if we do not even belong to ourselves, if we are not our own, then how can we begin to claim other creatures as our own? The fact that all of creation belongs to God creates a moral boundary in our relationships with other animals. Our dominion is that of stewards. It is a vocation to care for something that belongs to another, and thus our question must always be what God desires and intends for the creature, not what we may want or find useful. Further, our limited sovereignty over the animal world must follow the paradigm of God's own dominion. Just as God rules with mercy, 'slow to anger and abounding in steadfast love and faithfulness' (Exod. 34:6), so human beings should care for other animals with mercy and faithfulness. God's sovereignty sets limits on our dominion as well as providing patterns of merciful sovereignty.

One such pattern of merciful sovereignty that emerges in the biblical story of creation is God's refusal to treat human or nonhuman creatures as mere instruments for God's pleasure. The creation stories of Israel differ significantly from those of other cultures on precisely this point. In the Mesopotamian poem *Atrahasis*, for instance, human beings are created in order to bear the burden of labor for the gods, who are wearied by their work. Humans are from their beginning instruments used to meet the needs of the gods. But in Israel's story, God does not create out of need, and humans are not made mere instruments for God's purposes.[13] God does not *require* our assistance nor seek ease at our expense. Rather God creates out of overflowing charity, desiring to covenant with the whole creation and bring it to its fulfillment. This covenant includes even the elephants, tuna, pigs, and pheasants. These animals are not created to do work for God but simply that God may delight in their flourishing. Indeed, the psalmist depicts God's relation to the nonhuman animals as one of loving provision. 'These all look to you to give them their food in due season; when you give to them, they gather it up; when you open your hand, they are filled with good things. When you hide your face, they are dismayed; when you take away their breath, they die and return to the dust. When you send forth your spirit, they are created; and you renew the face of the ground' (Ps. 104:27–30). This fellowship between God and the other animals does not require human mediation. It is a direct relationship of charity by which God oversees the lives and deaths of God's creatures. And so when Jesus affirms that not a sparrow 'will fall to the ground apart from your Father' in Matthew 10:29, he is drawing on a theme as old as the creation. God creates the world not to fill a gap or meet a need but rather to extend the fullness of blessing that is already full in the life of the Trinity. If human beings are to fulfill the vocation of our election to image God, then we will learn to approach the other animals in such a way that they are neither reduced to mere instruments in our projects nor made tools to be exploited for our good at the expense of their own.

## Naming and Misnaming the Animals

How, then, might we envision a proper dominion of service that is guided by the logic of God's electing grace and the vocation to steward the other creatures? We find a clue in Genesis 2 when God calls Adam to his first interaction with the nonhuman animals. 'Out of the ground the Lord God formed every animal of the field and every bird of the air, and brought them to the man to see what he would call them; and whatever the man called every living creature, that was its name' (Gen. 2:19). This act of naming is more than just connecting a sound to an object, for in scripture giving a name is equal to giving an identity. So, for instance, when human beings have significant encounters with God their names are often changed – Abram becomes Abraham, Sarai becomes Sarah, Jacob becomes Israel, Simon becomes Peter, and Saul becomes Paul. To name the other animals, then, is to give them an identity, and as such this act of naming provides a metaphor for proper human dominion. Here, in the act of naming the other animals, humans fulfill the calling of our election to the extent that we tell them who they are as God's creatures and thereby catch them up in the telos of glorifying and enjoying God forever.[14]

In contrast to the proper authority of naming the other animals, of shaping their identity before God and in relation to humankind, we have, especially in modern times, become complicit in a misnaming of these animals that hides our failed dominion and conceals our misuse of God's election. We regularly rename nonhuman animals today as 'commodities' for consumption or 'machines' for production; they are turned into 'experimental data'; their flesh is turned into 'meat.' As Carol Adams observes, 'In the language of "meat" and "meat eater" the issues of animal suffering and killing are neutralized. This language reveals that we have difficulty *naming the violence.* Why are we unable truthfully to name the eating of animals as such? Why do we eat animals and yet, through language, deny that this is what we are doing?'[15] . . .

## 'They Love the Sweetness of Life'

Our modern means of turning fellow creatures into meat is a process of renaming, or better, unnaming, these animals in an attempt to dislodge them from any story other than the story of their utility to human beings. But true human dominion, exemplified in the naming of the other animals in Genesis, must always refer these animals to their true source and goal, placing them within a narrative whose chief actor is not human but divine and in so doing seeking their flourishing as creatures in whom God delights. Perhaps if we came to understand *imago Dei* not primarily as the conferring of privilege or status but as an election of humans for the service and care of the other creatures, we would also begin to re-envision our practices of meat-eating, experimentation, and the harvesting of animals. We would at least have to ask ourselves the question Karl Barth puts to us on this matter, 'Who are you, man, to claim that you must venture this [killing of an animal] to maintain, support, enrich and beautify your life?'[16] Who are you, image of God, to turn the blessing of election into the curse of the other?

I close with a prayer from St Basil as a reminder that despite a flawed track record, the Christian tradition has always had those who called us to peaceful relations with the nonhuman animals: 'O God, enlarge within us the sense of fellowship with all living things, our brothers the animals to whom thou gavest the earth as their home in common with us. We remember with shame that in the past we have exercised the high dominion of man with ruthless cruelty so that the voice of the earth, which should have gone up to thee in song, has been a groan of travail. May we realize that they live not for us alone but for themselves and for thee, and that they love the sweetness of life.'[17]

## Notes

1. Andrew Linzey and Dan Cohn-Sherbok, *After Noah: Animals and the Liberation of Theology* (Herndon, VA: Mowbray, 1997), p. xviii.
2. For an extended account of this and a constructive recovery of election for ecclesiology see my book *Church and Israel After Christendom: The Politics of Election* (Boulder, CO: Westview, 1999).
3. MacIntyre, *Dependent Rational Animals*, p. 6.
4. This has resulted, to borrow Alasdair MacIntyre's phrasing, in 'the obliteration of the distinction between manipulative and nonmanipulative social relations' (Alasdair MacIntyre, *After Virtue*, 2nd edn [Notre Dame, IN: University of Notre Dame Press, 1984], p. 30).
5. René Descartes, *Discourse on Method* (Indianapolis: Bobbs-Merrill Educational Publishing, 1956), pp. 36–38; and Linzey and Cohn-Sherbok, p. 9.
6. Here I am indebted to Richard Hays' reading of this passage in *The Moral Vision of the New Testament* (San Francisco: HarperCollins, 1996), p. 451.
7. Ibid., p. 452.
8. Karl Barth, *Church Dogmatics* III/1 (Edinburgh: T&T Clark, 1958), p. 194.
9. Kendall Soulen, *The God of Israel and Christian Theology* (Minneapolis: Fortress Press, 1996), pp. 116–117.
10. Immanuel Kant, 'Duties to Animals and Spirits,' Lectures on Ethics (New York: Harper & Row, 1963), pp. 239–241, in *Animal Rights and Human Obligations*, pp. 122–123.
11. See John Berkman, 'Is the Consistent Ethic of Life Consistent Without a Concern for

Animals?' *Animals on the Agenda*, ed. Andrew Linzey and Dorothy Yamamoto (London: SCM Press, 1998), pp. 237–247.

12. Stanley Hauerwas and John Berkman, 'A Trinitarian Theology of the "Chief End" of "All Flesh",' in *Good News for Animals?* ed. Charles Pinches and Jay MacDaniel (Maryknoll, NY: Orbis Books, 1993), p. 64.

13. Of course, Christians do speak of being God's 'servants' or even God's 'instruments,' but we use these metaphors to depict the ways God is drawing us into the divine plan by which human fulfillment will be achieved. This is very different from a creation account in which the goal to be achieved has nothing to do with the good of the creatures.

14. See Hauerwas and Berkman, pp. 64, 69.

15. Carol J. Adams, 'Feeding on Grace: Institutional Violence, Christianity, and Vegetarianism,' in *Good News for Animals?*, p. 147.

16. Barth, *Church Dogmatics* III/4 (Edinburgh: T&T Clark, 1961), p. 354.

17. Cited in Richard Alan Young, *Is God a Vegetarian?* (Chicago: Open Court, 1999), p. 140. I would like to thank those who read and commented on earlier drafts of this essay: John Berkman, Charles Pinches, Stanley Hauerwas, and Emmanuel Katongole.

# CASE STUDY:
## Cc the Cloned Kitten

In 1997, Dolly the sheep was revealed to the world's media as the first mammal that was a clone – a genetically identical copy – of an already existing adult animal. Since then mice, cattle, goats and pigs have all been cloned using the same technique, known as nuclear transfer. In February 2002 a cat was added to this list. The scientists who cloned her named her 'Cc' after the project, 'Copy Cat', which led to her birth.

A variety of uses have been suggested for animal cloning. These include medical applications. For example, pigs that have been genetically modified to produce organs suitable for transplantation into humans might be cloned to increase the supply of such organs; so might genetically modified sheep that produce medically useful proteins in their milk. There may also be farming applications, for example in commercial breeding and bulk milk or meat production. Most recently, Cc's birth has led to speculation that pet owners might try to replace beloved pets that had died by cloning them. However, the success rate for all cloned mammals is currently very low, and many have had birth defects or developed health problems later in life.

## Questions
- What responsibilities, if any, do humans have towards other animals, and why?
- What uses, if any, are humans entitled to make of other animals, and why?
- Is animal cloning ever justified, and if so, for what purposes?

## Sources

Donald Bruce, 'Cloned Cat is Ethically Unacceptable', Press Release, Church of Scotland Society, Religion and Technology Project, 14 February 2002. www.srtp.org.uk.

Donald Bruce and Ann Bruce (eds.), *Engineering Genesis: The Ethics of Genetic Engineering in Non-Human Species*. 2nd ed., London: Earthscan, 2002.

*New Scientist*, 'Special Report: Cloning and Stem Cells', www.newscientist.com/hotto-pics/cloning (accessed 17 February 2002).

Taeyoung Shin et al., 'Cell Biology: A Cat Cloned by Nuclear Transplantation', *Nature* Advanced Online Publications, 14 February 2002. www.nature.com

# 9

# HUMANS AND NATURE

## Introduction

Discussions of the relation between humans and the natural world do not often have a high profile in books on bioethics: they tend to be dealt with under different headings such as 'environmental ethics'. Yet new developments in biology and biotechnology have an impact both on the traditional territory of bioethics and on environmental ethics: genetic modification, for example, has far-reaching implications for both fields. And some of the same basic theological issues lie behind ethical discussions in both. For example, to what extent are humans called simply to accept the way the world is, with all its limitations, as given by the Creator, or to what extent do we have a mandate from God to 'interfere' with nature and seek to change it for the better? This question arises both in the context of human medicine and in the context of agricultural biotechnology.

From a Christian theological perspective, what should be the proper relationship between humankind and the rest of the created world? Much Christian discussion begins from the two creation narratives in Genesis chapters 1 and 2. A key text is Genesis 1:26–28, in which God blesses the human beings he has created and gives them 'dominion' over all other living things. Critics of Christianity's record point out that the notion of 'dominion' has been used to justify the violent exploitation of nature and other living creatures, and has helped precipitate the present ecological crisis (cf. White 1967). Attempts by Christians to rehabilitate 'dominion', arguing that it should be understood as benevolent rule rather than violent domination, have not been found convincing by others (compare Osborn 1993, 87–90, with Page 1996, 122–130). Many Christians find the concept of 'stewardship' more appealing than 'dominion', though the Christian philosopher Stephen Clark dismisses it as 'fashionable cant' which may exacerbate rather than relieve the problem

(Clark 1993, 53, 106–109, 162). Some Christian thinkers argue for a radical revision of our understandings of God, ourselves and the world, drawing on neglected aspects of Christian tradition and perhaps also on other faith traditions and cultures (e.g. McFague 1993). Others argue that the Christian tradition as historically understood offers richer resources than we might think for addressing the ecological crisis of our time (e.g. Clark 1993; Northcott 1996). There is, however, widespread agreement that a response to this crisis is a task which Christian theology cannot shirk.

In the first reading in this chapter, Margaret Atkins explores a variety of understandings of nature found in classical culture and early Christianity. She argues that the traditional Christian view that the world is good but flawed, and that humans are called to use it, but use it wisely, offers more promising resources for conservation than many of the alternatives.

Aruna Gnanadason takes a more radical position in the second reading. Writing from an Indian eco-feminist perspective, she explores the connections between environmental destruction, economic injustice and the oppression of women. She argues that in an Indian context, women are among those worst affected by environmental degradation: the majority of them are poor, and are expected to bear the brunt of the work of gathering resources such as food, fuel and water to ensure the survival of their families. She is critical of the 'development' paradigm of economic growth, arguing that it does little to benefit women or other oppressed people, and in fact reinforces their subjugation. She describes women's resistance to mining, forestry and other development projects. This resistance, she argues, is animated by 'the spiritual bond between women and creation' (p. 258) recognised in traditional Indian thought, and she offers an eco-feminist vision which affirms the sacredness of all God's creation, rejects anthropocentrism and stresses the interdependence of all living beings.

## References and Further Reading

Donald Bruce and Ann Bruce (eds.), *Engineering Genesis: The Ethics of Genetic Engineering in Non-Human Species*. 2nd ed., London: Earthscan, 2002.

Donald Bruce and Don Horrocks (eds.), *Modifying Creation? GM Crops and Foods: A Christian Perspective*. Carlisle: Paternoster, 2001.

Stephen R. L. Clark, *How to Think About the Earth: Philosophical and Theological Models for Ecology*. London: Mowbray, 1993

Stephen R. L. Clark, *Biology and Christian Ethics*. Cambridge: Cambridge University Press, 2000.

Celia Deane-Drummond, *Biology and Theology Today*. London: SCM, 2001.

Sallie McFague, *The Body of God: An Ecological Theology*, London: SCM, 1993.

Michael Northcott, *The Environment and Christian Ethics*. Cambridge: Cambridge University Press, 1996.

Lawrence Osborn, *Guardians of Creation: Nature in Theology and Christian Life*. Leicester: Apollos, 1993.

Ruth Page, *God and the Web of Creation*. London: SCM, 1996.

Lynn White, Jr., 'The Historical Roots of our Ecologic Crisis', *Science*, 155 (3767), 1203–1207 (1967); reprinted in Robin Gill (ed.), *A Textbook of Christian Ethics*, 408–417. 2nd ed., Edinburgh: T & T Clark, 1995.

# Flawed Beauty and Wise Use:
# Conservation and the Christian Tradition

MARGARET ATKINS

At times it may seem as if theological debate about the environment has been hi-jacked by post-modernists, or even by post-Christians, who seek the answer to environmental problems not in the distinctive Christian story but in some spiritual consensus of the lowest 'green' common denominator of all religions. Perhaps, then, a more traditional view still might deserve a hearing. Far from being post-modern or post-Christian, I write as someone trained not in theology but in pre-Christian, Classical, philosophy. Maybe my unaccustomed viewpoint might allow me to spot something distinctive about which others may have grown blasé; at any rate, to me at least, even early Christianity can seem quite astonishingly modern and fresh!

Bearing in mind the contrast with the ancient world, I should like to discuss two things: first what it means for a Christian to say that creation is good; and secondly, what is our proper ethical response to the *fact* that creation is good. My aim will be to steer a path between the waves of rather imprecise 'green mysticism' on the one side, and the rather unfruitful rocks of indifference on the other. Or rather, I shall not argue so much for a *via media* as for a way of life that is primarily centred on God. That, however, does not mean that we can by-pass environmental issues: rather, a properly theocentric ethics should integrate within itself an effective concern for conservation.

## Marcus, Mani or Fallen Creation?

And God saw everything that he had made, and behold it was very good.'[1] The goodness of creation has become such an obvious slogan of 'green' Christianity that it is easy now to underestimate both the significance and complexity of the phrase. When I was teaching Aristotle to first-year students, they would almost all be stumped by the notion of goodness that was not *moral* goodness. A good dog, for them, was an obedient dog, not a flourishing dog. Yet the environmental crisis has initiated a quiet revolution in the philosophy of value. Suddenly, philosophers and not just theologians are

From *Studies in Christian Ethics*, vol. 7.1, pp. 1–16 (1994).

rediscovering that value is not simply created by human desires: goodness is 'out there', an independent property of other creatures. A central thesis of Genesis chapter 1 is back in fashion.[2]

'The goodness of creation' is a revolutionary idea. But it is also a complex idea. I should now like to plot, very schematically, various ways of understanding that goodness, and ask which are possible for Christians.

[Atkins then sets out various ways of understanding (I) the *scope*, and (II) the *nature* of 'the goodness of creation'. Under the heading of 'scope', she identifies three views: (Ii) 'cosmic optimism', or the claim exemplified by Marcus Aurelius that 'everything in the cosmos, just as it is, is good'; (Iii) the opposite view, exemplified by Manichaeism, that 'there is so much evil in the world that the good God cannot, after all, be in charge'; (Iiii) that 'creation is good, but flawed', as expressed in 'the Christian drama of creation, fall and redemption'. Atkins differentiates two versions of this claim: (Iiiia) that only humans are fallen, and (Iiiib) that the whole cosmos is fallen.

As to (II) the *nature* of creation's goodness, Atkins identifies two main possibilities: (IIi) that other creatures are valuable only in so far as they are of use to us, a view she calls 'anthroposolism', exemplified by the Stoic thinker Chrysippus; (IIii) that they are valuable in themselves. This second view has various versions: (IIiia) that all parts of creation are valuable because they contribute to the good of the whole; (IIiib) all the parts of the creation are to be valued in an egalitarian way, such that none is more valuable than any other; (IIiic) the 'anthropocentric' view that all creatures have their own value, but that humans have a vastly greater value than others, which entitles us to use the others as we wish – an example is Thomas Aquinas; (IIiid) a hierarchical view which claims higher value for humans but still recognises duties to creatures lower in the hierarchy, and limits to our use of them – she cites Augustine as an example.]

## The Practical Implications

Let us look now at the implications of the views I have set out, beginning with *scope*.

What of the first option: 'cosmic optimism'? The trouble with this view is that it leaves no scope or grounds for improvement. Everything is already fine, whatever it may seem like: how can one distinguish between a flourishing environment and an unhealthy one? It may be no coincidence that the pages of Marcus evoke less an atmosphere of cheery carefreeness than one of weary resignation. 'The optimist believes that this is the best of all possible worlds', as one wit put it, 'while the pessimist fears that he is right.' . . . Those Greens who ground their faith on a simple worship of nature as she is, on pure pantheism, are fooling themselves.

What then of Manichaeism? It is worth noting here that the ethical consequences of world-views are sometimes unexpected. Whereas the cosmic optimist's apparent respect for creation leads him to ignore or reinterpret genuine ills, the Manichee, far from cheerfully exterminating species, turns out to be a vegetarian ... But such considerations apart, Manichee dualism hardly provides a solid grounding for an ethic of respect for material creation.[3]

What of the third view of the scope of goodness in creation, that of orthodox Christianity? Both of the variations on this view offer a contrast between what creation is and what it ought to be, and therefore both offer a possibility for making real judgements about when to improve and when to let well alone. The view that only humanity is fallen focuses its critique on human sin and its consequences, and will aim to check, say, human greed and violence. It will not be tempted to intervene, say, to adjust the balance between competing populations of wild animals.

On the other hand, the view that all creation is fallen may lead to a more interventionist view: humanity is likely to see itself as having a more wide-ranging responsibility for the redemption of fallen creation. At any rate, both views will have serious practical consequences for our treatment of non-human creation.

So much for different views of the scope of goodness. What about its *nature*? Chrysippus' anthroposolism will have some effect on conservation, but only in so far as human welfare is directly affected ... hard-headed practical conservationists will naturally employ this type of argument when they think it will work; but it is not, in the end, enough for them. It is difficult to defend very rare creatures from extinction on the grounds that, small as their numbers and local as their distribution might be, they contribute significantly to human welfare.

Next, then, what are the environmental consequences of the various versions of the view that other creatures are valuable in themselves? Obviously all of them ought to have some practical effect on our behaviour. The choices generated by the holistic approach will be unpredictable; at any one time any particular species may be more or less vital in sustaining the 'biotic community'. At the very least, all our ordinary intuitions about the value of individual creatures, human and others, will be questioned ...

The egalitarian view would seem to generate more plausible ethical consequences. One of its valuable elements is the recognition that decisions do not always involve deciding conflicts: if one can act cooperatively rather than competitively, then it may be possible to respect the needs of all relevant creatures.

Important as that insight is, however, it remains the case that we are constantly having to choose between several courses, all of which will harm the interests of some creatures. Whether or not we like it, we have inherited Adam's dominion, and to an extent undreamed of by the writers of Genesis.

There are real dangers in setting ourselves up simply as 'responsible' for conservation;[4] yet, realistically, we no longer have the choice (if we ever did) simply to 'live and let live'. In practice, much of our collective behaviours will harm parts of our environment; we need some principles, some guidance in choosing less damaging or more justifiable courses of action. Otherwise how can we ever weed a garden or manage a forest? How can we know if we are justified in offering special assistance to one endangered species to the disadvantage of another? How do we weigh priorities for minimising our damaging impact on the environment, and for integrating human flourishing with that of other creatures? Some kind of hierarchy of value seems necessary if we are to be stewards rather than simply another group of equal citizens; and the latter, I fear, is not a genuine option: in practice if we are not gentle stewards we will be oppressive landlords.

In so far as we will in practice need to exercise stewardship, what are the consequences of believing in an anthropocentric hierarchy of goodness? Again, as in the case of anthroposolism, we should recognise that this view does not lead simply to environmental destruction: human needs and those of other creatures are so interdependent that even here conservation is important. Moreover, a Thomist might further contribute to the myriad revelation of God in creation. Where there is no conflict with human wants, the conservation of creatures for their intrinsic goodness and beauty ought to have a high priority.

I suggested earlier however, that this position may lead to an ambiguous attitude to conservation: if the value of other creatures is seen to lie *primarily* in their contribution to human welfare, the motivation for serious changes in human behaviour for the sake of non-human creatures will be relatively slight. However, if combined with other elements of Christian ethics such as simplicity of life-style, such a theory might prove to have some healthy teeth.

If the value of the anthropocentric view lies in its recognition of the distinctive role of humanity, and that of the egalitarian view in its forceful advocacy of our common creatureliness, is it possible for a hierarchical, but not simply anthropocentric, position to combine the strengths of each? Such a view might recognise that all creatures have value and that some are more valuable than others; it will accept that creatures are permitted to use each other, without ignoring the real costs of that use.

Of course, the hierarchy will need to be more complex than Augustine's simple *scala naturae*. It might, for example, integrate both the concerns of theorists of animal rights for creatures with greater intelligence, autonomy or sensitivity, and the conservationists' twin concerns for rarity and for environmental importance. Different creatures may have different values in different contexts: there are few simple rules.[5] However, it should be possible to devise some clear principles of priority within this schema, and there is room to be realistic about the value of human as against other needs.

Importantly, it would be possible to give priority to genuine human needs without thereby neglecting the real value elsewhere: we have to choose between humans and oysters in one particular situation; but that is no reason for simply ignoring oysters' welfare in all situations.

The brighter, or more suspicious, of my readers may have noticed that the views for which I have claimed most have been those that correspond most closely to traditional orthodox Christianity. That is not, I hope, as a result of slippery argument; in sharp contrast to the well known thesis of Lyn White, my own considered view is that such a standpoint offers our best hope for wise environmental attitudes and practices. I leave it to others to develop and assess the schemata I offer as they see fit.

## Wise Use and the Virtues of Restraint

Let me now turn to human beings themselves. How in our way of life as Christians are we to respond to the view of creation that our faith entails?

What I want to talk about particularly now is *use*. In the world of practical conservation, the latest buzz-phrase is 'wise use'.[6] That does not seem surprising. But it is striking how little the word is used in theological theorising about environmental issues. It is as if we are rather coy about the fact we actually *use* created things. We will touch on the subject occasionally, with reference to, say, sustainability, or, more negatively, consumption. But in the end, we are talking about *using* other creatures in order to sustain a way of life; we might as well say so straightforwardly.

There are two elements involved in choosing ways of using things. We need to consider the impact of courses of action on the environment; and we need to consider the real value of making use of the object in the proposed way. Information about the likely environmental effect of a course of action can only come from scientific experts. But it is the ethicist who can give guidance about the real importance of certain goals, about whether such a course of action is really needed, or really valuable.

The word 'need' keeps creeping into my discussion. In short, I am suggesting that we ought to revive the distinction (so beloved of ancient moralists) between need and luxury; or at least discover a way of grading needs and wants as to their seriousness. To destroy a forest to build a golf course is less clearly justifiable than to destroy a forest to feed starving families. The point is obvious, but we can only theorise it by being prepared to say unambiguously that some desires are trivial, others vital.

But how do we decide which are which? The passionate golfer will take a rather different view of the value of the forest from the ornithologist. Do we simply, in the end, count votes? (The idea may seem absurd theoretically speaking; but in practice political decisions are usually made in favour of those who shout the loudest.) What is needed to determine more and less serious issues, I suggest, is a rich model of what it is for a human being to flourish, a model within which the values of food and shelter, health and education, and indeed prayer, culture, leisure, play and celebration can be integrated. One specific community may, in a real sense of the word, *need* a football ground; the opportunity for children to play is not simply an optional extra. But that need will not override all the other possible considerations. The needs of a starving village which requires the ground for cultivation will take priority. Such decisions, however, must be grounded upon a rounded understanding of flourishing that incorporates the realisation that many human desires are too trivial to be described as needs. Wise use, then, depends on an understanding of real human flourishing. Such an understanding can generate serious purposes, for which things may freely be used.

It is worth noting here that the concept of use (as opposed to consumption) is valuable for the conservationist precisely because it entails limit. One uses x for purpose y. One needs to use only as much of x as will achieve purpose y. It is no wonder that in a society characterised largely by a loss of sense of purpose we have lost also a sense of the proper limits to consumption.

At this point I should like to turn for assistance to the perhaps unlikely figure of St Augustine.[7] Augustine makes an important distinction between two verbs: *utor* and *fruor*. These can be translated roughly as 'use' and 'enjoy' – but it is important to remember that this is a rough translation. Thus, when he asks in one of his treatises[8] 'whether everything has been created for the use (*utilitas*) of human beings' he is not asking whether the point of creating animals was so that human beings could eat them. His question is quite different: ought created things to be enjoyed by us in and for themselves? Or ought they rather to be used as a means to some greater, indeed, all-encompassing good? When we make use of other creatures, he tells us, we should refer that use to the enjoyment of God. *Utor* is the proper verb for those goals that are intermediate only; the society of other human beings quite as much as relation with animals falls into the category of *utenda* rather than *fruenda*. Everything has been created for human 'use', Augustine tells us, just in this sense, that with regard to everything except God we must use our rational judgement to assess its value and our proper use of it by referring it to God.

Does such a view make Augustine exploitative? Does it mean that Augustine thinks we can do anything we like with created things, justifying our actions by the claim that our true end is service of God, not of creatures? Of course not, just as Augustine does not think we can treat human beings however we like. Rather, his theocentricity gives him a model of good living that sets strict limits to an individual's use of other creatures. One might recall the traveller who tramps the pages of *The City of God* with his gaze fastened firmly on his ultimate goal, 'making use of earthly and temporal things like a pilgrim in a foreign land who does not let himself be taken in by them or distracted from his course towards God, but rather treats them as supports . . . they must on no account be allowed to increase the load.'[9] The other-worldly goal of a pilgrim is precisely what limits his material wants. The selfish or exploitative amassing of wealth would simply be a distraction.[10] (It is interesting to note here that the way of the pilgrim who travels lightly sits comfortably with the egalitarian's concern to *allow* other creatures space to live their own lives, even more so perhaps than with the more interventionalist approach of stewardship.)

But there is, of course, more than this. The way that the Christian pilgrim progresses on the route is precisely by living the Christian life, the life of charity. This adds both a more urgent and a broader dimension to the question of the use of wealth and resources. As Augustine put it in one of his letters: 'If we personally own sufficient for ourselves then such things [sc. extra possessions] belong not to us, but to the poor; we have the responsibility for administering them, so to speak, but we do not seize them, claiming ownership for ourselves (which would be unforgivable).'[11]

In sum, (a) it is precisely because the Christian's motivational centre of gravity is outside the material, created world that he or she can treat it with the detachment that avoids exploitativeness: theocentricity frees one for concern for creation; (b) the form of the Christian life, that is charity, positively demands that our personal use of created things is limited so that we can share goods with the needy.[12]

In Augustine's day, of course, the environmental dimension of concern for the needy simply did not exist. Yet the basic ethical scheme shared by the Fathers is easily adaptable in the light of contemporary experience and insight; we simply need to understand both that environmental catastrophe will damage poor human beings above all others, and also that charity in the sense of love of God's creatures can be extended to non-human creatures in their own right. But the structure of the theocentric ethics of use remains the same.[13]

My implicit contrast has been with an ethics that is based simply upon undisciplined human desires. If the goal of public policy is human happiness, and if that happiness is assessed only by considering what people say they want, then there is no limit to the consumerism that attempts to quench its own boredom by yet more consumption. Without individual and public goals and purposes beyond those of acquisition (which in our society means beyond those of status, wealth and pleasure) there can be no distinction between serious and trivial desires, between needs and superfluous luxuries.

Even more important practically, perhaps, is this: without clear goals and purposes there is not motivation to live a life of discipline, self-restraint, charity, the sort of life, that is, that we will, collectively, have to learn to lead if we are to reduce the damaging impact of our treatment of the rest of creation.

In arguing the value of a distinctively Christian ethics for wise environmental practice I am not advocating an instrumental attitude to religion. Christianity might save the earth; but that provides no grounds for believing or disbelieving it.[14] The claims of Christian revelation must stand or fall on their own terms. However, if one accepts them it is entirely reasonable to point out that their observance rather than their neglect tends to lead to the flourishing of humanity and of the rest of creation.

## Asceticism, Gratitude and Joy

I have suggested so far that the hallmarks of Christian ethics are theocentricity and charity, which in combination can restrain unnecessary desires for wealth, pleasure, and so on, both limiting and redirecting the use of goods by the Christian. Traditionally, Christian practice has gone even further: asceticism and poverty have been valued as Christian virtues in their own right. Green critics of Christianity have sometimes characterised Christian asceticism as Manichee, world-rejecting, inimical to creation. What is it, we ought therefore to ask, that prevents a healthy Christian asceticism from succumbing to hostility to the material that it denies to itself?

A Christian ascetic, let me suggest, ought to give up goods – marriage, luxurious food, rich clothing, personal freedom and so on – not because he or she thinks them bad, but precisely because he or she recognises that they are indeed good. It is because wine is a glorious gift of God that it is worth our giving it up, occasionally at least, out of love for Him . . .

St Francis, the patron saint of ecologists, provides us here with an ideal model. Many have noted his enthusiastic embrace of his fellow creatures as brothers and sisters. But Francis' love of birds and animals and the rest of the natural world cannot be separated from his devotion to a life of abject poverty, focused utterly on God, and characterised, despite its darker moments, by a spirit of ebullient joy and gratitude . . .

If poverty and asceticism are unfashionable, so are their corresponding virtues. Indeed, it is hard to translate into English the terms that a classical or mediaeval writer might have used for these virtues. Their literal equivalents are unfortunate: temperance conjures up images of earnest tee-totallers, while continence is used almost exclusively in its privative form, and then with an extremely narrow reference! What about self-denial, self-control, restraint, self-discipline? They are the nearest we get; and all of them conjure up a picture of a desperate struggle to repress those desires and emotions that our liberal, post-Freudian society thinks of as healthy and natural.

There are perhaps two points to make here; the first that while there is indeed a healthy way to fulfil most emotions and desires, not every way is healthy. Discipline, training, education, involve learning, individually and communally, to feel and be moved in a truly healthy way. Secondly, *temperantia* does not, as 'self-control' does, suggest a divided personality struggling against itself. Indeed (as Aristotle well recognised) the persons (and, we might add, the society) whose desires and emotions are well trained, is precisely the one not so divided; they want the things they ought to want, they feel emotions as they ought and as much as they ought.[15]

It is because Christians, who are less sanguine than Aristotle about natural perfectibility, realise quite how difficult it is for fallen human nature to learn such a lesson, that they have seen the disciplinary, that is the *educational*, value of asceticism, thought of it in this context as penance, as learning to 're-pent', to think and to feel in a new way.

Asceticism was also thought valuable as a way of removing distractions, of avoiding entanglements in the kind of unnecessary practical concerns that interrupted single-minded concentration upon God. Such a view may seem unworldly; but again, it is worth remembering those who are less occupied with satisfying their own inflated material wants have more time and energy for the practical as well as the contemplative life.

Asceticism, then, was thought valuable for training someone in Christian virtues, and for allowing someone to concentrate on God. But the saints never lost sight of the link between asceticism and charity, as the quotation from Augustine suggests. 'Otherworldliness' – if that is the right word for it – and 'thisworldliness' are not in practice in conflict. The pilgrim who travels light has more to give away, or simply needs to use less.

Am I suggesting a revival of hair-shirts and bread-and-water fasts? We might perhaps be able to be more imaginative about our modern, environmentally sensitive, asceticisms. Fasting on occasion may provide a salutary reminder of the stark fact that we live in an age and a society strikingly unusual for the fact that we take our daily bread for granted. (How much more does the Lord's Prayer mean to someone in Ethiopia?) But we also take for granted so much else: the variety and quality of food and every other good we can buy; the speed of communications and transport that enables us to live lives with a busyness inconceivable to our fathers; continual comfort with respect to temperature, space, household utilities.

Perhaps the very real efforts of those individuals who try their best to live in a 'green' way in an ungreen society, the banal routine of the bike trip to the bottle bank; the extra costs of organic food; the boring attention to fuel consumption – perhaps these can be dignified as sacrifices for the love of God, as much as was the grinding daily asceticism of the desert fathers. But perhaps we should also be thinking communally; as a society are we prepared to accept limitations on not only consumption but also speed, noise, convenience? Are we prepared to use the language of temperance, restraint, even sacrifice, in the areas of transport and use of power and land? Surely a Christian ethics rooted in respect for asceticism and poverty can assist us here.[16]

My model throughout has been not creation-centred but theocentric. Creation, for the Christian, I argued, is good, but not simply god. Creation is not to be enjoyed as an ultimate goal (Augustine's *fruor*) but rather 'used' in Augustine's sense of the word, i.e. referred to the service of God. But this should be done in such a way that (a) respects the independent value of creation; and (b) makes a real difference to practice by setting limits to use and priorities for use.

Why not, someone might object at this balanced point, have a *simply* creation-centred ethic? After all, are we not more likely to solve the problems of this world if we concentrate on them alone? . . . Why not substitute simply 'green living' for 'Christian living' as one's ideal? I have no time for a full-scale critique of this alternative. But perhaps it is worth suggesting one or two weaknesses: in the first place, such a practice is inevitably, at least in this society, confined to the few zealots; most of us have a complex range of responsibilities to family, work etc. which means that concern for the environment can be at most one element integrated into an ethical whole. Secondly, we need to face the difficult questions about the relative priorities of concern for ourselves as against other humans, and for human beings as against other creatures. Do we refuse to use a car ever, even to help a person in need? Do we always eat only what we need to live, and never, say, indulge ourselves for the human and religious purposes of communal celebration? Of course, in practice, all but a few fanatics integrate Green and other concerns; the theocentric Christian ethical model can provide a wider framework within which to do so. Thirdly, if efficiency is our only aim in our response to environmental problems, we are likely to end up missing the point. The hard-headed practitioner is likely to forget just what he does not know, what he cannot predict and control. As Robin Grove-White argued . . . recently, the element of mystery, of the unknown, will be ignored.[17] But there is little that non-believers can do about the unknown; therefore, it is ignored in their calculations. The believer, on the other hand, accepting the existence of the unknown and uncontrollable, can still act for the best, within his or her limited knowledge, while relying ultimately not on humanity but on the Lord. Anxiety can thus be replaced by trust, though not concern by complacency.

Finally, then, and perhaps most importantly, is the question of attitude. The believer has resources for dealing with guilt that might otherwise overwhelm, and grounds for hope and trust in the face of a task that often seems insurmountable. Faith in a personal creator allows one to exercise restraint not out of mechanical duty, or scrupulous fearfulness, but with gratitude and with joy. The other face of asceticism is thankfulness; our fasting should be punctuated by the rhythm of feasts. Otherwise the Christian will forget that he or she is in fact a pilgrim whose goal is foreshadowed in celebration. I shall give the last word, therefore, to Jean Vanier, who reflects on a life-time of living and working in a community with the handicapped:

'Celebration is the sign that beyond all the sufferings, purifications and deaths, there is the eternal wedding-feast, the great celebration of life with God. It is the sign that there is a personal meeting which will fulfil us, that our thirst for the infinite will be slaked, and that the wound of our loneliness will be healed.'[18]

## Notes

1. Genesis 2:31.
2. See e.g. T. Regan, 'The nature and possibility of an environmental ethic', in Regan, *All that Dwell Therein* (London 1982); Holmes Rolston III, 'Are values in nature subjective or objective?', in R. Elliot and A. Gare (ed.), *Environmental Philosophy* (St Lucia 1983); K. Goodpaster, 'On being morally considerable', *Journal of Psychology*, June 1978.
3. For details, see S. Lieu, *Manichaeism in the Later Roman Empire and Medieval China* (Manchester 1985). For a brilliant, if tendentious, modern critique of Manichaeism from a Catholic Christian perspective, see Christopher Derrick, *The Delicate Creation* (London 1972).
4. See especially S. R. L. Clark in 'Amando il mondo vivente', *Cenobio* 40, 1991; a shorter version in *Argument* 1, 1990.
5. One of the reasons that environmental questions pose problems for ethicists is that they can rarely be answered using simple rules; there are few, if any, absolute prohibitions. What is required in any specific situation is to assimilate and assess an indefinite amount of information of both a scientific and a social nature, and to balance an indefinite number of needs and wishes. The most promising type of ethics for dealing with such questions is one based on virtue, emphasising in particular the virtues of understanding, attentiveness, fairness and *prudentia*, wise practical judgement.
6. I owe this point to conversations with Mark Spalding of the World Conservation Monitoring Centre, Cambridge.
7. Augustine has been criticised as hostile to creation, most notoriously by Matthew Fox. See in response Margaret Atkins, 'The Hippo and the Fox: a cautionary tale', *New Blackfriars*, October 1992, and Angela West, *Matthew Fox: Blessing for Whom?* (Blackfriars publications 1993).
8. On Diverse Questions 83 no. 30. On the distinction between *utor* and *fruor* see J. Burnaby, *Amor Dei* (London 1938), pp. 104–110.
9. *The City of God* XIX. 17.
10. It is frequently said that Augustine's Neoplatonic metaphysics leads him to devalue the material creation. Even non-Christian Neoplatonism is not, however, unambiguously hostile to matter: while the non-spiritual is relatively inferior to the spiritual, it also *reflects* the goodness of its source. Plotinus himself was ambiguous about the goodness of matter; it is arguable, however, that Neoplatonic thought placed a high value upon the cosmos as revelatory of God (see e.g. A. H. Armstrong, *Plotinian and Christian Studies* (London 1979), chapter XXII). Augustine may have been influenced to some degree by the negative as well as the positive aspects of Neoplatonic metaphysics, but he was also well aware that Neoplatonism needed to be modified in the light of incarnational and creational theology. It may also be true that his interest in interiority shifted the focus of the tradition away from creation; but it is important not to neglect his consistent interest in the created order, in particular in his commentaries on Genesis (see further Atkins, *art. cit.*, n. 21).

11. *Letter* 185.35.
12. On the Fathers in general, see J. L. Gonzalez, *Faith and Wealth* (San Francisco 1990).
13. See Derrick, *op. cit.*, pp. 79ff.
14. Cf. Derrick, *op. cit.*, p. 91: 'We shall be acting unwisely therefore, if we embark upon some kind of anti-Manichaean crusade, seeing this primarily as a means towards survival and the good life, as an instrument by which we can master our present difficulties. That old itch for mastery is responsible for half the trouble: it is one of the first things we shall need to sacrifice.'
15. For Aristotle's distinction between *sophrosyne* and *encrateia* see *Nicomachean Ethics* VII. IX. 6, 11151a, 32ff.
16. Cf. Derrick, *op. cit.*, especially pp. 113ff.
17. 'The Christian "person" and environmental concern', *Studies in Christian Ethics*, vol. 5, no. 2, 1992.
18. *Community and Growth* (London 1979), p. 248. I should like to take this opportunity to thank members of the Society for the Study of Christian Ethics for inviting me to speak to them and for their constructive discussion of this paper and others throughout the conference in 1993.

# Women, Economy and Ecology

ARUNA GNANADASON

For too long, those of us involved in issues of justice have tended to treat concern for creation as secondary to what we presume to be priority issues. In India in the last few years, however, the environmental movement and the women's movement have revitalized this concern, which has engaged people throughout our history. The urgency with which we need to act cannot be overemphasized. Forests in India are disappearing (we lose 1.3 million hectares per year); soil conditions are deteriorating; water and wind produce erosion (56.6 percent of India's land has suffered); floods and drought cause serious damage each year; indiscriminate use of water resources is causing a fall in the level of ground water. Pollutants and chemical wastes as well as fertilizers and pesticides are eating into the core of our environment.

Bina Agarwal helpfully describes some of the key factors which have brought about this situation.[1]

*'Scientific' forest-management.* Since colonial times, the state has taken over the forests and land curtailing the community's traditional customary rights. These forestry programmes, unfortunately, concentrate on growing commercially profitable species. There has been indiscriminate felling of trees for profit and for building a service infrastructure of trains, bridges and ships, benefiting a few. Women had in many communities been the protectors of forests as they had derived livelihood from them.

*Privatization.* In earlier times, members of a community nurtured the piece of land to which they communally had a right. What the government termed 'land for the landless' programmes have in fact encouraged exploitation by individuals, most of whom of course are men.

*Erosion of community resource management.* Traditional institutional arrangements for resource use have been undermined. When the community worked the land, responsibility for resource management was linked to resource use, which was controlled by the community, and women had access to the resources.

*Population growth.* While this is one cause, it is not the primary reason.

From David G. Hallman (ed.), *Ecotheology: Voices from South and North*, pp. 179–185. Geneva: World Council of Churches, 1994.

Poverty associated with environmental degradation induces a range of fertility-increasing responses. The direct link between the low status accorded to women and increasing population and environmental degradation cannot be overlooked. But women would assert that an anthropocentric view of creation is what damages creation the most.

*Agricultural technology and production systems.* The choice of these systems cannot be separated from the dominant 'scientific agriculture', which is part of the development paradigm that has ignored the integrity of creation and is based on the abuse of the land. Over the years there has also been a systematic devaluation and marginalization of indigenous knowledge about species varieties, processes of nature and sustainable forms of interaction between people and nature. Women's knowledge and creativity have been completely ignored.

I have intentionally included the word 'economy' in the title of this paper as reminder that for women in India, as in most of the Third World, ecology and the protection of the environment and its resources are issues of livelihood and survival. The majority of women in India are poor. They are the backbone of the subsistence economy which sustains rural India. As feminist ecologist Vandana Shiva puts it, poor women in many parts of India are those who 'work daily in the production of survival'.[2] Although victims of the degeneration of the environment, they are also active in movements to protect it from the onslaughts imposed by 'development' on the earth and its resources.

Women and girl children are most affected by environmental degradation because sex role divisions of labour ensure that women do the most strenuous kinds of work related to the resources of the earth: food-gathering, water-collecting and fetching of water from distant places. They are expected to cater for the needs of their families, often single-handedly, in contexts where men live wasteful lives. When resources are depleted, women need to go even further in search of food, water and livelihood. Bina Agarwal also speaks of

> Systematic gender differences in the distribution of subsistence resources (including food and health care) within rural households, as revealed by a range of indicators: ... mortality rates, hospital admissions data and the sex ratio (which is 93 females per 100 males for all India).[3]

Added to this is the fact that women in India do not have access to resources, land or production technology. Women have been unable to compete in the labour market, being seen as a cheap reserve army of unorganized, unskilled labour. The development pattern adopted by India ensures that women are pushed to the periphery where they must engage in a daily struggle for survival.

This has engaged the women's movement in a critique of the entire 'development' paradigm, from which neither women nor any of the other subjugated identities, Dalits or tribals, have benefited. A model that views 'development' largely from the perspective of economic growth operates to the detriment of large sections of marginalized people, including women, and all of creation. Thus it is clear why women articulate their fears in this way. To quote Vandana Shiva again:

> We perceive development as a patriarchal project because it has emerged from centres of Western capitalist patriarchy and it reproduces those patriarchal structures within the family, in community and throughout the fabric of Third World societies. Patriarchal prejudice colours the structures of knowledge, as well as structures of production and work, that shape and are in turn shaped by 'development' activity. Women's knowledge and work as integrally linked to nature is marginalized or displaced, and in its place are introduced patterns of thought and patterns of work that devalue the worth of women's knowledge and women's activities and fragment both nature and society.[4]

Yet often we hear governments and development agencies attempting to integrate women into this dominant development process, using phrases like the 'women's component' or 'women in development' – even though this dominant model does not in fact 'develop' them in any way. Because of their frustration and disillusionment with these processes, many rural women in India have formed their own cooperatives, trusting in their organized power to opt out of mainline development processes and setting up their own small-scale informal structures to afford some small respite.

## New Economic Policy: The Environment and Women

The discussion of the effects of the economy on both women and creation take on special significance in India in the context of recent economic policy shifts along the lines of recommendations from the World Bank and the International Monetary Fund. The resulting trend towards privatization and monetarization is posing a tremendous burden on the people and the resources of the earth. Gabriele Dietrich warns that:

> Ecological concerns get usurped in the process and the regulations on intellectual property rights outlined by the General Agreement on Tariffs and Trade (GATT) violently curtail and appropriate people's alternative knowledge systems.[5]

A market-oriented, industrial economy requires increased energy production, which implies more dams and nuclear energy projects. Recent history has shown how these affect the environment and people's lives in deleterious ways. Women will no doubt be most affected, as they are the ones who must deal with the shortages of water and food that result.

The Chipko movement, in the Utharkhand region of the Himalayas, is a largely tribal women-centred struggle, in which local people clung to trees in order to protect them from the saws of the contractor's men. They had also struggled against mining operations in the mountain region. This long struggle, which is a symbolic call to heed the knowledge of women, is beautifully described by Vandana Shiva:

> The Chipko movement started mobilizing for a ban on commercial exploitation throughout the hill districts of Uttar-Pradesh because the over-felling of trees was leading to mountain instability everywhere. In 1975, more than 300 villages in these districts faced the threat of landslides and severe erosion.
>
> The movement for a total ban was spurred by women like the 50–year-old Hima Devi, who had earlier mobilized public opinion against alcoholism, in 1965, and was now moving from village to village to spread the message to save the trees. She spoke for the women at demonstrations and protests against auctions throughout the hill districts: 'My sisters are busy harvesting the kharif crop. They are busy in winnowing. I have come to you with their message. Stop cutting trees. There are no trees even for birds to perch on. Birds flock to our crops and eat them. What will we eat? The firewood is disappearing: how will we cook?'
>
> Bachni Devi of Adwani led a resistance against her own husband who had obtained a local contract to fell the forest. The forest officials arrived to browbeat and intimidate the women and Chipko activists, but found the women holding up lighted lanterns in broad daylight. Puzzled, the forester asked them their intention. The women replied, 'We have come to teach you forestry.' He retorted, 'You foolish women, how can you who prevent felling know the value of the forest? Do you know what forests bear? They produce profit and resin and timber.' And the women immediately sang back in chorus:
>
> > What do the forests bear?
> > Soil, water and pure air
> > Soil, water and pure air
> > Sustain the earth and all she bears.

The Adwani satyagraha created new directions for Chipko. The movement's philosophy and politics now evolved to reflect the needs and knowledge of the women. Peasant women came out openly, challenging the reductionist commercial forestry system on the one hand and the local men who had been colonized by that system, cognitively, economically and politically, on the other.[6]

I have quoted extensively here to illustrate how any act against creation breaks the spiritual bond between women and creation. In pre-Aryan thought in India, nature was symbolized as the embodiment of the feminine principle. The dynamic feminine principle *shakti* (energy, power) is the source and substance of everything. *Prakriti* (nature) manifests this primordial energy. Throughout the centuries women have drawn their *shakti* from *prakriti*. Common concepts such as *bhudevi* (goddess earth) and *bhumatha* (mother earth) emphasize this.

Itwari Devi, a woman leader in the struggle against mining operations, describes how women have drawn energy from nature to sustain their struggles:

> Our power is nature's power, our *shakti* comes from *prakriti*. Our power against the contractor comes from these inner sources, and is strengthened by his trying to oppress and bully us with his false power of money and muscle. We have offered ourselves, even at the cost of our lives, for a peaceful protest to close this mine, to challenge and oppose the power that the government represents. Each attempt to violate us had strengthened our integrity. They stoned our children and hit them with iron rods, but they could not destroy our *shakti*.[7]

## The Shattered Bond

But this intrinsic bond has been broken and abused. Indian culture, which is in essence very patriarchal, has reduced women to subordinate roles through the traditional mothering and nurturing. This has contributed substantially to the abuse of both women and creation. It is assumed in the Indian Patriarchal mindset that since women are able to give birth and suckle new life, and since they have traditionally been the ones most affected by the depletion of natural resources, their responsibility is to care for children and to find the water and fuel the family needs. This has imposed restrictions on women, domesticating them and holding them in hostage to the precarious survival of their families. It has also been the basis for associating women and nature with the base, the inferior, the degraded – to be appropriated, used, abused and discarded. Indian religions have given quasi-divine legitimation to this abuse.

## A Holistic Vision of Interdependence

One important characteristic of the feminist paradigm is that although women are the special victims of environmental degradation, they do not speak merely as victims when they participate in environmental movements. They speak here of a whole new creative way of understanding life and doing theology and resolving conflicts, schisms and dualisms that have been generated. The new insight provided by the participation of rural and tribal women in struggles to save the earth makes clear that women contribute not in passive resignation to the hard life they bear, but in creative actions for sustaining life.

The eco-feminist vision emphasizes the life that is in everything, the value of all God's bounty. It challenges limited views of development that measure the value of the gifts of creation only in terms of their use in the marketplace. Many of the environmental resources we should value (the clean air we breathe, the poetry of a tree or of a mountain) are excluded from economic measurement. Yet their exploitation (as in the tourist industry) or destruction and the costs of cleaning up after the destruction are labelled 'growth' and 'production'.

An eco-feminist theological vision therefore affirms the sacredness of all God's gifts in creation – the animate and the inanimate. It rejects anthropo-centric worldviews, which legitimate and even seek biblical sanction for the extraction of more and more from the life-giving mother earth.

In Jesus we see an affirmation of the 'small things' of life. He drew in-spiration from them in his teachings and his ministry – a lily in the field, a stone, a child, a mustard seed, grains of wheat, fish and loaves of bread, pigs, spit and mud, the birds in the air. Women in the dailiness of their lives have also been in close contact with life's little things, tending and caring for an environment which will enhance the growth and health of their families or communities.

An eco-feminist theological vision also emphasizes the connectedness between women and nature, as between humanity and nature. This poses radical challenges to the Aristotelian dualisms of mind-body, spirit-flesh, culture-nature, man-woman which have informed much of Western patri-archal theology and to the hierarchical theories of 'chain of being' and 'chain of command'. Such a philosophy has legitimated the domination of humanity over the rest of nature and other forms of domination based on gender, race, class and caste. The colonial expansion, the white man's urge to 'civilize' the world, the growth of market-based industrial development, the exploitation of the labour of the marginalized in our societies, the gross forms of violence and injustice against women – all these are consequences of this.

Five thousand years ago India was an agricultural country in which the bonds between humanity and the soil were nurtured and the earth therefore gave her plenty. India continues to be an agricultural country. This must be protected from attempts to destroy the basis of life by senseless acts of aggression in the name of progress and development. The earth our mother cries out for protection. The church and all concerned people will have to heed the voice of women and the environmental movement before it is too late.

## Notes

1. Bina Agarwal, *The Gender and Environment Debate: Lessons from India*, Vacha Study Circle Readings no. 16, SETV Centre for Social Knowledge and Action, 1992, pp. 131–35.
2. Vandana Shiva, *Staying Alive: Women, Ecology and Survival in India*, Delhi, Kali for Women, 1998, p. 210.
3. Agarwal, *op. cit.*, p. 137.
4. Shiva, *Let Us Survive: Women, Ecology and Development*, Sangarsh, 1985, p. 5.
5. Gabriele Dietrich, 'Emerging Feminist and Ecological Concerns in Asia', *In God's Image*, XII, no. 1, Spring 1993.
6. Vandana Shiva, *op. cit.*, pp. 74f., 27.
7. Cited by Shiva, *ibid.*, pp. 208f.

# CASE STUDY:
## Direct Action Against GM Crops

In July 1999, Lord Melchett, Executive Director of Greenpeace UK, and 27 other activists attempted to uproot a crop of genetically modified maize being grown in a field trial for the agrochemical company AgrEvo. The other activists included a Baptist minister. All 28 were arrested and charged with theft and criminal damage, but at trials in April and September 2000, they were all acquitted of both charges. The defence case was that the protestors had lawful excuse under the Criminal Damage Act (1971), because leaving the GM crop to flower and pollinate would have led to a greater crime, the contamination of other crops nearby.

Lord Melchett was reported as saying after the trial, 'We have known for a long time that people don't want to eat GM food; supermarkets won't sell GM food and now the time has come for people to stop planting GM food.' A spokesman for the Department of the Environment said that GM field trials would continue: 'If we halted our strictly controlled research there would be widespread GM crop planting without us getting the evidence we need . . . Our top priority is to protect the environment and human health.'

## Questions
- What responsibilities do humans have concerning the 'environment', and why?
- Can genetic modification of crops be consistent with these responsibilities, and if so, under what conditions?
- Are field trials of GM crops morally justified at the present time?

**Source**
Paul Kelso, 'Greenpeace Wins Key GM Case', *The Guardian*, 21 September 2000.

# 10

# CHRISTIANS AND PUBLIC DEBATE ON BIOETHICS

## Introduction

In previous chapters, we have seen a great variety of Christian theological engagement with the basic issues behind bioethical controversies and debates: what importance human life has and why, what we understand by health and disease, how we should regard non-human animals, what our attitude should be towards the natural world, and so on. The readings addressing these issues reflect in many different ways the conviction that there is *distinctively* Christian thinking to be done in these areas – that is, that Christians are called to think about these things in ways that are faithful to their basic theological convictions. They reflect varying views about the *specificity* of Christian ethics – that is, the extent to which Christian theology says anything *different* about moral obligations from what might be known by a morally aware non-Christian (on distinctiveness and specificity, see MacNamara 1998). The case studies in preceding chapters have offered opportunities to work out the significance of these basic convictions for some particular questions and controversies.

But there is a further question to be asked. As I pointed out in the Introduction, many bioethical debates are not only questions of individual moral choice but also of 'public' ethics – policy-making and legislation. Assuming it is possible to articulate a distinctively Christian response to these questions, what part should that Christian response play in public policy in a society such as the UK in which only a minority are active Christians? Is it the business of Christians and churches to engage in these debates? What should they hope to achieve if they do, and what strategies and methods should they adopt?

In this chapter I give brief sketches of various possible Christian approaches to public ethical debates. There is something of the 'ideal type' about some of these positions – at times I sketch them with sharper outlines than they have in the work of any real theologian, for the sake of setting out the options as clearly as possible. Although I quote real authors as examples, it is important to remember that these authors' writings may not be limited to any one of the 'ideal types', but may contain elements of more than one. For example, I cite Duncan Forrester as an example of the 'theological fragments' approach, but he also makes some use of liberationist perspectives (Forrester 2000, 21–31). Not all of the 'ideal types' are incompatible with each other, though some certainly are. The chapter concludes with a case study which the reader is invited to use to consider the strengths and weaknesses of each approach in relation to a specific example.

## I. Seeking the Moral Common Ground

According to the first approach, if Christians articulate a position explicitly based on Christian convictions, they are unlikely to persuade anyone who does not share those convictions. Therefore they should instead seek the moral common ground: instead of appealing to specifically Christian sources or assumptions, they should base their moral arguments in the public sphere on premises shared by everyone, Christian or not. Some would argue that Beauchamp and Childress' four principles, outlined in the introduction to chapter 1, are a good example of common moral ground in bioethics. There may be a place for specifically Christian arguments within the Christian community, but not outside it.

Something like this position is held by the so-called 'autonomy' school of Roman Catholic ethics. This school of thought holds that distinctively Christian sources (the Scriptures and Christian tradition) teach nothing specific about the *content* of Christian morality: the moral obligations that Christians acknowledge could also be recognised by a morally aware person of any faith or none. Christian sources, however, may supply a specifically Christian *context* for these moral teachings and a specifically Christian *motivation* for doing what any person of good will could discover that they ought to do (MacNamara 1998). Those who argue for an 'autonomy' view may do so on the basis of a concept of 'natural law': that human beings can acquire some understanding of the good or of God's laws by the use of their reason and their experience of the created world (see chapter 1 introduction).

## 2. Seeking Wisdom

A second approach that has something in common with the first is based on the theological notion of *wisdom* (e.g. Deane-Drummond 2001a). God is the source of all wisdom, and the created order reflects the wisdom of God. Human wisdom, originating in the wisdom of God, may be found in many places and people: it is not the sole preserve of any one community or tradition. However, human wisdom can never encompass the totality of divine wisdom, and for the Christian, human understanding is radically challenged by the surprising wisdom of Christ's cross.

In contrast to the fragmented, atomistic nature of much modern knowledge, and particularly modern science, wisdom has the capacity to integrate different areas of knowledge and kinds of understanding, for example the empirical and the intuitive. Wisdom also has a moral quality: in some of the biblical sources of the concept (such as the book of Proverbs), folly is not merely stupidity but a kind of moral deficiency, and may be seen as a choice to ignore 'God's whisper' to the world (cf. Deane-Drummond 2001a, 148–149). Because of its moral quality, wisdom can offer a way of re-integrating not only different kinds of knowledge, but also knowledge and goodness, which have become split off from one another in our modern scientific age (Hardy 1998).

Such a view should encourage Christians to listen for expressions of wisdom from all the participants in public debates, but to be ready to challenge those debates when wisdom is forgotten or ignored. A striking example of such an approach can be found in the interpretation, by Deane-Drummond and her colleagues, of public reactions to the GM food controversy (Deane-Drummond et al. 2001b).

## 3. A Dogmatic Christian Ethics

The third approach stands in sharp contrast to the first two: it is what Michael Banner, in his essay 'Turning the World Upside Down', refers to as a 'dogmatic Christian ethics' (Banner 1999, 1–46). 'Dogmatic' in this context does not mean doctrinaire or authoritarian, but rather refers to an account of ethics that is firmly rooted in the self-revelation of God in Jesus Christ. For Banner, one of the most important exponents of this approach to ethics was the great Protestant theologian Karl Barth, whose account of health and disease can be found in chapter 4.

Banner follows Barth in advocating this approach. He is highly critical of what he calls 'apologetic Christian ethics'. By this he means any account of Christian ethics which seeks to justify itself and its conclusions in terms of any other system, for example what I have called the 'common moral ground' approach. For Banner, the only accountability that Christian ethics should acknowledge is to 'the kingdom of Jesus Christ' (Barth, *Church Dogmatics* II.2, 527; cited by Banner 1999, 9).

This does not mean, however, that Christian ethics is incapable of engaging with other systems and positions in the public arena. It can do so in a variety of ways: for example, by '[asserting] what it knows to be good and right' (Banner 1999, 36–37), by denouncing what it knows to be wrong, and by exposing the weaknesses and inconsistencies of other systems and approaches. But whenever dogmatic Christian ethics enters the public arena, 'it does so on the basis of its own distinctive premise . . . of faith in the life, death and resurrection of Jesus Christ' (ibid., 39).

## 4. A City Set on a Hill

The fourth approach is similar in many ways to the third, though Banner is careful to differentiate his account from it. It is particularly associated with Stanley Hauerwas, who is represented in this book by one of the readings in chapter 5. Hauerwas draws on many diverse influences, including George Lindbeck's 'postliberal' view of theology as the distinctive language of a faith community and Alasdair MacIntyre's recovery of virtue theory in moral philosophy (Lindbeck 1984, MacIntyre 1985).

For Hauerwas, Christian ethics is not so much concerned with rules or principles as with character and virtue – put simply, it is not first and foremost about what we should do, but about the sort of people and communities we should be. We do not develop virtue and character by rational deliberation, but by belonging to a 'community of character' (Hauerwas 1981) – a community that shares a narrative or story which gives it a distinctive moral identity. The Church is called to be a 'community of character' whose identity is formed by the Christian story: 'Christian ethics is not first of all an ethics of principles, rules or values, but an ethics that demands we attend to the life of a particular individual – Jesus of Nazareth' (Hauerwas 1984, 76).

Hauerwas, therefore, has little time for Christian strategies of public debate that seek common moral ground. The contribution Christians are called to make is of a very different kind: 'the first social ethical task of the church is to be the church' (Hauerwas 1984, 99). In other words, it is called to be an alternative *polis* or political community, displaying a different way of living together in faithfulness to its distinctive story. And this acted-out witness to the possibility of a different way of life is the most important and helpful thing that the church can offer to the world.

## 5. Theological Fragments

The next approach is in a sense a middle way between some of the positions I have already outlined. The role of Christians in public debates is to contribute 'theological fragments', a term that comes from Duncan Forrester (1997; see also Forrester 2000, 143–157). Forrester is highly sympathetic to thinkers like Hauerwas, but is hesitant to draw such sharp lines between church and public arena. In his book *Christian Justice and Public Policy* he examines the problem of justice in a pluralist society – the difficulty both of saying what justice *is* and of *practising* it. He finds secular theories wanting, but is also aware that Christianity has a mixed record where justice is concerned, and does not think that the Church of today either can or should try to produce a comprehensive theological theory of justice. What it *can* do is to offer 'theological fragments'. By 'fragments' he means ideas and insights and practices which come from a 'quarry' of coherent Christian thought, which when introduced into the public arena can act as irritants, challenges and insights that move debate and practice in new directions. Forrester's examples are wide-ranging, including statements of faith like the Barmen Declaration produced in 1934 by Christians opposed to Nazi ideology, insights such as the need for a concept of forgiveness in a criminal justice system and examples of practice like the South African Truth and Reconciliation Commission. Fragments in isolation from their quarry can be misunderstood or abused, so Christians have a twofold task of contributing fragments to the public arena, while at the same time continuing to do the basic theological work to maintain and develop the theological 'quarry' (Forrester 2000, 155–156).

## 6. Middle Axioms

A very different middle way from Forrester's makes use of what are rather misleadingly known as 'middle axioms' (Preston 1986; 1991, 107–109). This approach was very influential in Anglican social thought in the second half of the twentieth century, though Malcolm Brown (1997) suggests that it is in need of radical reworking, at the very least. It takes very seriously the gap between general theological affirmations and detailed policy prescriptions. Theology of itself is not able to bridge this gap, and attempts to read policy decisions directly off theological principles are apt to be naïve, ridiculous or even dangerously misleading. To steer a course through the middle ground between theological generalities and detailed policies, it is necessary to bring together those with various kinds of relevant expertise, including theologians but also (for example) economists, scientists and so on. It is also necessary to attend to the experience of those affected by the issues being discussed, and particularly to 'those marginalized in society, who frequently fail to get a hearing' (Preston 1991, 108).

## 7. The View from Below

Finally, a very different way of setting up the relationship between Christian reflection and public debate is suggested by the many and varied 'theologies of liberation'. As I remarked in chapter 1, it is dangerous to generalise about liberation theologies, since they are by nature contextual and particular.

However, a liberationist approach would most likely be sceptical of discussion that was dominated by elites, experts and the powerful. A better starting point for reflection is the experience of the poor and oppressed – for example, the economically poor, those denied political power, ethnic minorities that experience racism, and women who experience sexism. A theology of liberation is a theology done 'from below', by the poor and oppressed and those who stand with them, not by the privileged on their behalf. It also emphasises the priority of 'praxis' – that is, doing God's will by acting in solidarity with the oppressed – over theory. The role of theology is to reflect on praxis, and so to inform and direct one's future action, but this theological reflection cannot be done abstractly in advance of action and involvement with the oppressed (see Gutiérrez 2002 for a brief summary). Laurie Green (1990) has outlined a theological method that has much in common with some liberationist approaches, which moves from *experience*, through *analysis* using whatever tools or disciplines are relevant (e.g. psychology, sociology, economics and other human sciences) to clarify the experience and define it better, to theological *reflection* on the experience using the resources of the Christian tradition, which gives rise to proposals for *action* in response to the experience and reflection; this action gives rise to new experience, which begins a new cycle of reflection and response. The action or praxis which is essential to such approaches could be anything that is in line with the 'kingdom of God', where that is understood at least partly in terms of freedom, justice and human flourishing in this present world – for example, grass-roots community action or the formation of a self-help group, campaigning for political or institutional change, or protest and direct action. In this book, readings by Boff (chapter 1), Hull (chapter 4), Lebacqz (chapter 6), Fabri dos Anjos (chapter 7) and Gnanadason (chapter 9) reflect some of these emphases.

The theological approaches outlined in this chapter suggest that Christian theological traditions, as well as having rich resources for bioethical reflection, suggest a wide range of possible strategies for engagement with wider public debate and action. As I have already observed, some of these strategies are mutually exclusive, but others can be combined. Whatever the approaches and strategies chosen, Christians and the churches have every reason to think clearly about bioethical questions and to engage vigorously with public debate and practice.

## References and Further Reading

Michael Banner, *Christian Ethics and Contemporary Moral Problems*. Cambridge: Cambridge University Press, 1999.
Malcolm Brown, 'Some Thoughts on Theological Method', in Council of Churches for

Britain and Ireland, *Unemployment and the Future of Work: An Enquiry for the Churches*, 293–298. London: Council of Churches for Britain and Ireland, 1997.

Celia Deane-Drummond, *Creation Through Wisdom: Theology and the New Biology*. Edinburgh: T & T Clark, 2001 (a).

Celia Deane-Drummond, Robin Grove-White and Bronislaw Szerszynski, 'Genetically Modified Theology: The Religious Dimensions of Public Concerns about Agricultural Biotechnology', *Studies in Christian Ethics*, 14.2, 23–41, 2001 (b).

Ian C. M. Fairweather and James I. H. McDonald, *The Quest for Christian Ethics: An Inquiry into Ethics and Christian Ethics*. Edinburgh: Handsel Press, 1984.

Duncan Forrester, *Christian Justice and Public Policy*. Cambridge: Cambridge University Press, 1997.

Duncan Forrester, *Truthful Action: Explorations in Practical Theology*. Edinburgh: T & T Clark, 2000.

Robin Gill, *Moral Leadership in a Postmodern Age*. Edinburgh: T & T Clark, 1997.

Laurie Green, *Let's Do Theology: A Pastoral Cycle Resource Book*. London: Mowbray, 1990.

Gustavo Gutiérrez, 'The Task and Content of Liberation Theology', in Andrew Bradstock and Christopher Rowland (eds.), *Radical Christian Writings: A Reader*, 335–342. Oxford: Blackwell, 2002.

Daniel Hardy, 'The God Who Is With the World', in Fraser Watts (ed.), *Science Meets Faith: Theology and Science in Conversation*. London: SPCK, 1998.

Stanley Hauerwas, *A Community of Character: Toward a Constructive Christian Social Ethic*. Notre Dame: University of Notre Dame Press, 1981.

Stanley Hauerwas, *The Peaceable Kingdom: A Primer in Christian Ethics*. London: SCM, 1984.

George Lindbeck, *The Nature of Doctrine: Religion and Theology in a Postliberal Age*. Philadelphia: Westminster Press, 1984.

Alasdair MacIntyre, *After Virtue: A Study in Moral Theory*. 2nd ed., London: Duckworth, 1985.

Vincent MacNamara, 'The Distinctiveness of Christian Morality', in Bernard Hoose (ed.), *Christian Ethics: An Introduction*, 149–160. London: Cassell, 1998.

Ronald Preston, 'Middle Axioms', in John Macquarrie and James Childress (eds.), *New Dictionary of Christian Ethics*, 382. London: SCM, 1986.

Ronald Preston, *Religion and the Ambiguities of Capitalism*. London: SCM, 1991.

# CASE STUDY:
## Vote for the Common Good

In March 2001, in advance of that year's General Election, the Catholic Bishops of England and Wales produced a booklet entitled *Vote for the Common Good*, a shortened and updated version of a document produced before the 1997 election. The document drew attention to a wide range of issues including abortion, euthanasia, family life, criminal justice, the treatment of asylum seekers, and world poverty. It invited voters to bear these issues in mind when deciding how to vote and to question candidates about some of them.

Much of the secular newspaper coverage focused on the document's comments about abortion, euthanasia, embryo experimentation and human cloning: the sections on criminal justice, asylum seekers and poverty received much less attention. Accusations of 'playing party politics' were reported, the bishops' comments on abortion were said to have provoked 'fury', and hostile reactions to the sections on other bioethical issues were also quoted.

## Questions
- What priority should the churches give to influencing public policy on bioethical issues, and why?
- What should the churches aim to achieve when they enter public and political debates on these issues?
- What strategies should they employ to achieve their aims?

## Sources
Anon, 'Anger over Catholic Anti-abortion Poll Call', *Yorkshire Post*, 23 March 2001, p. 6.
Anon, 'Cardinal Virtue' (editorial), *The Mirror*, 24 March 2001, p. 6.
Catholic Bishops' Conference of England and Wales, *Vote for the Common Good*. London: Catholic Media Office, 2001.
Ruth Gledhill and Sam Coates, 'Bishops Accused of Party Politics in "Life" Crusade', *The Times*, 23 March 2001, p. 4.
Andrew Sparrow, 'Put Morality First, Bishops Tell Voters', *Daily Telegraph*, 23 March 2001, p. 2.
Nicholas Watt, 'Fury over Cardinal's Voting Advice', *The Guardian*, 23 March 2001, p. 10.

# Glossary

In this glossary, I have tried to define as many as possible of the terms which may be unfamiliar to many readers. Some of the terms listed have a range of related meanings, depending on the context, and I have attempted to give definitions that are related to the contexts in which the terms appear in this book.

Agape: (Greek) Self-giving love, divine or human.

Anthropology: Study, theory or doctrine of humanity.

Asceticism: Spiritual discipline, particularly discipline of the physical appetites.

Autonomy: The right or ability to make significant decisions for oneself.

Beneficence: Doing good.

Brain stem: The lowest part of the brain, including centres which regulate vital functions such as heartbeat and breathing.

Carcinogen: Cancer-causing chemical or other agent.

Charity: Love of neighbour; see also *Agape*.

Chrismation: Anointing with oil.

Christology: The doctrine or theological study of the person of Christ.

Chromosome: Self-replicating structure found in almost all living cells, made up of DNA in association with proteins. Most of an organism's genetic information is carried in its chromosomal DNA.

Clone: Genetically identical copy of a living organism.

Competence: The ability to make important decisions affecting one's life and health, e.g. about consent to medical treatment.

Consistory: Gathering of church leaders or church court.

Contingent: Description of an event or circumstance that could have been other than it is; the opposite of 'necessary'.

Covenant: Solemn agreement or pledge, between God and humans or between humans.

Dalit: (Bengali) Literally 'crushed'; member of an oppressed group in India.

Dalkon shield: A form of intra-uterine contraceptive device marketed in the USA until 1975, when it was withdrawn because it was associated with a high rate of complications.

Dialysis (haemodialysis): Treatment for kidney failure in which waste products normally removed by the kidneys are artificially removed from the blood.

Demythologisation: Attempt to re-express biblical or theological ideas without using mythical language or imagery.

Deontology: A theory of ethics based on duty.

Deoxyribonucleic acid (DNA): Large biological molecule which acts as the medium of genetic information in most living organisms.

*Dominium terrae*: (Latin) Dominion over the earth.

Ecclesiology: Study, theology or doctrine of the church.

Ectopic pregnancy: Pregnancy in which the embryo becomes implanted somewhere other than the mother's womb. It cannot develop very far, and will endanger the mother's life if not terminated.

Election: Theological term for choice, particularly God's choice of God's people.

Electroencephalogram (EEG): Reading of the electrical activity of the brain.

Embryo: Individual formed by cell division of a fertilised egg; it is known as an embryo between about two and eight weeks after fertilisation.

Encyclical: Papal teaching document.

Enlightenment: Intellectual and cultural transition in eighteenth-century Europe and America, characterised by an emphasis on reason, science and human autonomy.

Eschatology: Theology or doctrine of the 'last things', the end of time and the fulfilment of God's purposes.

Essentialism: Claim that objects and beings have certain essential properties without which they would not be what they are.

Eucharist: Literally 'thanksgiving'; specifically, Christian rite in which believers eat bread and drink wine in remembrance of Christ's death.

Eugenics: Project of 'improving' the human species genetically.

Evangelical: To do with the gospel (good news) of Christ; also, Protestant theological tradition which emphasises (among other things) biblical authority and the believer's personal commitment to Christ.

Extraordinary means: In medicine, means of treatment which go beyond the 'ordinary' means that any reasonable doctor could be expected to employ.

Fall: The story told in Genesis 3 of human disobedience to, and alienation from, God.

Fiduciary relationship: Relationship of trust.

Foetus: Individual growing in the womb, after two months' gestation.

Gene: Unit of genetic inheritance; a sequence of DNA which codes for a particular protein.

Genetics: The science of biological inheritance.

Genetic engineering, genetic modification: Artificially altering the instructions encoded in an organism's DNA so that the biological characteristics of that organism are changed.

Genome: The totality of an individual's genetic information.

Globalisation: The phenomenon that economic, political and social forces operate increasingly at an international level and their effects are not limited to a particular community or nation state.

Gospel: The good news of Jesus Christ; also one of the first four books of the New Testament.

Grace: God's free, undeserved love for human beings, made known particularly through Christ, which transforms the conditions and possibilities of human life.

Hagiography: Story of a saint's life.

Hermeneutics: Theory of interpretation, particularly of biblical or other texts.

Holy Unction: Rite of anointing a dying person with oil.

Hubris: Self-deceiving and destructive pride.

Hypostasis: Greek word often translated 'person', especially with reference to the persons of the Trinity.

Hysterectomy: Surgical removal of the womb.

Immanent: Present and active in the world; used particularly of God.

*Imago Dei*: (Latin) The image of God.

In vitro fertilisation (IVF): Artificial fertilisation of an egg by sperm in the laboratory.

Incarnation: Christian doctrine that in Jesus Christ, the eternal Son of God has assumed human nature.

Incompetence: Opposite of *Competence*.

Infarction: Damage to an area of tissue caused by lack of oxygen in that area; e.g. myocardial infarction, or 'heart attack', caused by interruption of the blood supply which carries oxygen to an area of the heart muscle, resulting in death of that part of the heart muscle.

Intersubjectivity: Relationship or communication between persons (or 'subjects').

Jubilee: in ancient Israel, year of celebration in which debts were to be cancelled, slaves set free and land restored to its original owners (Leviticus 25); Christian churches called for 2000 to be a 'year of jubilee' marked by the cancellation of Third World debt.

Libertarianism: Opposition to any social or political constraints on human freedom.

Manichees: In the ancient world, followers of Mani (216–276 CE), who taught a radical cosmic dualism of light and darkness, good and evil, and spirit and matter.

Mammography: X-ray screening of the breast, particularly to detect signs of cancer.

Messianism: False pretension of an individual, group or system to the role of a 'messiah' or saviour.

Metaphysics: Study or theory of the character of reality and existence as a whole.

Modernism, modernity: Cultural and intellectual era which began with the Enlightenment, characterised by reason, science and technology.

Naturalism: Theory of ethics based on nature or the way the world is.

Neo-cortex: Outer part of the brain, associated with consciousness, thought, etc.

Neurotransmitter: Chemical, produced by nerve cells, which plays a part in transmitting signals within the nervous system.

Non-maleficence: Not doing harm.

Ontic: To do with being.

Ontology: Study of being or existence.

Ordinary means: In medicine, those means of treatment which any reasonable doctor would be expected to employ.

Pantheism: Doctrine or theory that all that exists is divine.

Paradigm: An overarching conceptual framework which guides the study of a subject.

Patriarchy: Male dominance and oppression of women.

Patristic: To do with the 'Fathers', i.e. the leaders and theologians of the early Church.

Placenta: Structure which develops from some of the cells of the embryo, through which the growing embryo and foetus receives oxygen and nourishment from the mother's blood.

Post-modernism, post-modernity: The present intellectual and cultural era, according to some observers; in some ways a development of modernity, but in some ways a reaction against its emphasis on objective reason, science and technology.

Pre-embryo: Fertilised egg before cell division begins.

Proteins: Large biological molecules which perform many thousands of structural and biochemical functions in living organisms.

Proxy: Person empowered to make decisions or act on behalf of another.

Prudence: The virtue also known as 'practical wisdom', which enables a person to choose the right means to an end.

Psychic: To do with the soul, mind or spirit.

Repentance: Change of heart, mind and life; in particular, turning away from sin.

Ribonucleic acid (RNA): Biochemical compound similar to DNA which acts as the medium of genetic information in a few viruses, and performs many molecular genetic functions in all organisms.

Sacrament: A visible sign of God's grace, particularly in the context of worship; almost all Christian traditions recognise baptism and eucharist as sacraments; some also include others such as confirmation, penance and holy unction.

Sanctity: Holiness, sacredness.

Sanctification: Growth in holiness.

Semantic: To do with the meaning of words or signs.

Shalom: (Hebrew) Sometimes translated 'peace', but conveys a much more wide-ranging sense of well-being.

Somatic: To do with the body.

Stem cells: Cells, e.g. from early embryos, that have the potential to differentiate into many or all of the different kinds of cell found in the body; they could in theory be used to repair or replace damaged tissues or organs.

Stoicism: School of ancient Greek philosophy which held that the good consists in living in accordance with reason and nature.

Telos: (Greek) End, purpose or goal.

Teleology: Theory of ends or goals; a teleological theory of ethics judges right and wrong in terms of the ends, purposes or consequences of actions.

Temporal: To do with time; existing in the present time or present world.

Theocentric: Centred on God.

Theodicy: Theological attempt to show that God is just, and particularly to address the problem of the existence of evil and suffering.

Total depravity: The doctrine that no aspect of human nature is unaffected by sin.

Transcendent: 'Outside' the world, not limited by space, time or physical existence; particularly used of God.

Trinity: Christian understanding of God as one God in three persons, traditionally called Father, Son and Holy Spirit.

Utilitarian: To do with usefulness or utility.

Utilitarianism: Ethical theory which judges actions according to the 'principle of utility': that the happiness or preferences of those affected should be maximised.

Vice: Opposite of virtue.

Virtues: Habits, dispositions or skills that contribute to a good life.

Vitalism: Belief that life has an absolute, unlimited value.

Zygote: Cell formed by the fertilisation of an egg by a sperm.

## Sources

In compiling the glossary, I have been particularly helped by the following works:

Mukti Barton, *Scripture as Empowerment for Liberation and Justice*. Bristol: Centre for Comparative Studies in Religion and Gender, 1999.

Sinclair B. Ferguson and David F. Wright (eds.), *New Dictionary of Theology*. Leicester: IVP, 1988.

Antony Flew (ed.), *A Dictionary of Philosophy*. 2nd ed., London: Macmillan 1983/Pan 1984.

Gerhard Kittel and Gerhard Friedrich (eds.), *Theological Dictionary of the New Testament*. ET, Grand Rapids: Eerdmans, 1964–1976.

Colin E. Gunton (ed.), *The Cambridge Companion to Christian Doctrine*. Cambridge: Cambridge University Press, 1997.

Alister E. McGrath, *Christian Theology: An Introduction*. 2nd ed., Oxford: Blackwell, 1997.

John MacQuarrie and James Childress (eds.), *A New Dictionary of Christian Ethics*. London: SCM, 1986.

*MedTerms Medical Dictionary*, www.medterms.com (accessed 14 March 2002).

*CancerWeb On-line Medical Dictionary*, www.graylab.ac.uk/omd (accessed 14 March 2002).

# Acknowledgements

## Chapter 1

Gilbert Meilaender, from *Bioethics: a Primer for Christians*, pp. 1–10. Grand Rapids: Eerdmans, 1996/Carlisle: Paternoster, 1997.

John Breck, *The Sacred Gift of Life*, Introduction, pp. 11–18. Crestwood, NY: St Vladimir's Seminary Press, 1998.

John Paul II, *Evangelium Vitae*, pp. 3–9. ET, London: CTS, 1995.

Leonardo Boff, 'Science, Technology, Power and Liberation Theology', from *Ecology and Liberation: A New Paradigm*, pp. 123–130. Maryknoll: Orbis, 1995.

## Chapter 2

Richard McCormick, 'The Quality of Life, the Sanctity of Life', from *How Brave a New World? Dilemmas in Bioethics*, pp. 395–401. London: SCM/NY: Doubleday, 1981.

John Breck, *The Sacred Gift of Life*, Introduction, pp. 5–11. Crestwood, NY: St Vladimir's Seminary Press, 1998.

Karen Lebacqz, 'Alien Dignity: The Legacy of Helmut Thielicke for Bioethics', in Allen Verhey (ed.), *Religion & Medical Ethics: Looking Back, Looking Forward*, pp. 44–60. Grand Rapids: Eerdmans, 1996.

## Chapter 3

Maureen Junker-Kenny, 'The Moral Status of the Embryo', from Maureen Junker-Kenny and Lisa Sowle Cahill (eds), *The Ethics of Genetic Engineering: Concilium 1998/2* pp. 43–53 London: SCM/Maryknoll, NY: Orbis.

Ian A. McFarland, 'Who Is My Neighbor? The Good Samaritan as a Source for Christian Anthropology', *Modern Theology* vol. 17.1, pp. 57–66 (2001).

Lisa Sowle Cahill, '"Embodiment" and Moral Critique', in Lisa Sowle Cahill and Margaret A. Farley (eds.), *Embodiment, Morality and Medicine*, pp. 199–215. Dordrecht: Kluwer Academic Publishers, 1995.

**Chapter 4**

Karl Barth, from *Church Dogmatics*, vol. III/4, §55.1, pp. 356–374. Edinburgh: T & T Clark, 1961.

John M. Hull, from *In the Beginning There Was Darkness: A Blind Person's Conversations with the Bible*, pp. 107–113, London: SCM 2001.


**Chapter 5**

Stanley Hauerwas, 'Religious Concepts of Brain Death and Associated Problems', from *Suffering Presence: Theological Reflections on Medicine, the Mentally Handicapped and the Church*, pp. 87–99. Edinburgh: T & T Clark, 1988.

Vigen Guroian, 'The Vision of Death', from *Life's Living Towards Dying*, pp. 41–61. Grand Rapids: Eerdmans, 1996.


**Chapter 6**

William F. May, 'The Medical Covenant: An Ethics of Obligation or Virtue?', in Gerald P. McKenny and Jonathan Sande, (eds.), *Theological Analyses of the Clinical Encounter*, pp. 29–44. Dordrecht: Kluwer Academic Publishers, 1994.

Karen Lebacqz, 'Empowerment in the Clinical Setting', in Gerald P. McKenny and Jonathan Sande, (eds.), *Theological Analyses of the Clinical Encounter*, pp. 133–147. Dordrecht: Kluwer Academic Publishers, 1994.


**Chapter 7**

Paul Ramsey, 'A Human Lottery?' from *The Patient as Person: Explorations in Medical Ethics*, pp. 252–259. New Haven: Yale UP, 1970.

Márcio Fabri dos Anjos, 'Power, Ethics and the Poor in Human Genetics Research', from Maureen Junker-Kenny and Lisa Sowle Cahill (eds), *The Ethics of Genetic Engineering: Concilium* 1998/2, pp. 73–82. London: SCM/Maryknoll, NY: Orbis.


**Chapter 8**

Oliver R. Barclay, from 'Animal Rights: A Critique', *Science and Christian Belief*, vol. 4.1, pp. 57–61, 1992.

Andrew Linzey, 'Animal Rights: A Reply to Barclay', and response by Oliver Barclay, *Science and Christian Belief*, vol. 5.1, pp. 47–51, 1993.

Scott Bader-Saye, 'Imaging God through Peace with Animals', *Studies in Christian Ethics*, vol. 14.2, pp. 1–13, T & T Clark 2001.

## Chapter 9

Margaret Atkins, 'Flawed Beauty and Wise Use: Conservation and the Christian Tradition', *Studies in Christian Ethics* 7.1, pp 1–16. Edinburgh. T & T Clark, 1994.

Aruna Gnanadason, 'Women, Economy and Ecology', in David G. Hallman (ed.), *Ecotheology: Voices from South and North*, pp. 179–185. Geneva: WCC, 1994. Available from WCC Publications, World Council of Churches, P.O. Box 2100, CH–1211 Geneva 2.

The editor and publishers would like to thank all those who have granted permission for the use of material in this book. Every effort has been made to trace and identify copyright holders and to secure necessary permission for reprinting. If we have erred in any respect, we apologise and would be glad to make any necessary amendments in subsequent editions of this book.

# Index

abortion 4, 19, 20, 23, 25, 28, 37, 49, 60,
  65, 66, 75, 78, 82, 102, 131, 138, 158,
  185, 186, 270
agape 51, 55, 56, 57, 58, 59, 271
age 17, 92, 93
AIDS 183, 205, 212–213
Alder Hey 153, 155, 188–9
alien dignity 38, 50–62, 277
Andersen, Edward B. 24, 25
angels 129
animals 3, 4, 6, 33, 38, 69, 107, 137, 141,
  202, 215–38, 249, 263, 278
anthropocentrism 243, 245, 255, 259
anthropology 48, 72, 76–84, 85, 139, 271,
  277
Aquinas, Thomas 83, 84, 100, 161, 229,
  243
Aristotle 154, 159, 242, 250
asceticism 10, 19, 22, 25, 47, 48, 86, 87,
  221, 249–52, 271
Athanasius 141
Atkins, Margaret 240, 242–53, 279
Augustine of Hippo 88, 98, 137, 245,
  247–9, 251, 252
autonomy 9, 13, 14, 59, 60, 61, 62, 71,
  85, 86, 93, 158, 180, 187, 204, 264, 271

Bader-Saye, Scott 216, 228–37, 278
Banner, Michael 192, 194, 265, 268
baptism 13, 14, 16, 46, 80, 84, 96, 143,
  147, 150, 158, 274
Barclay, Oliver R. 215, 216, 217–22, 223,
  224, 225
Barth, Karl 104, 105, 106, 107–16, 225,
  226, 231, 236, 265, 278
Basil 143, 236

Beauchamp, Tom L. 7, 9, 12, 155, 191,
  192, 194, 264
beneficence 9, 13, 158, 271
Bevans, Steven B. 12
Bible 10, 66, 76–7, 105, 117–22, 219
biotechnology 6, 33, 239, 269
birth 73, 98, 139, 144, 177, 182
Bland, Tony 126
blindness 105, 117–22
body 5, 13, 14–16, 20, 23, 24, 28, 46,
  65–102, 107–10, 112, 113, 131, 132,
  142, 144, 150, 165, 174, 185, 186, 188,
  228, 259
Boethius 76, 83
Boff, Leonardo 11, 12, 31–6, 193, 268,
  277
Bonhoeffer, Dietrich 224, 226
brain death 125, 127, 128–38, 278
Breck, John 10, 19–25, 38, 45–9, 277
British Deaf Association 123
Brown, Peter 86, 91, 94, 96, 97, 99
Bruce, Ann 216, 240
Bruce, Donald 216, 240
Bynum, Caroline Walker 94, 100

Cahill, Lisa Sowle 67, 68, 85–101, 202,
  277
Callahan, Daniel 104, 105, 136–7, 138
Campbell, Alastair V. 12
cancer 136, 183–5, 187
catholicism see Roman Catholicism
celibacy 96
chaos 111
character 5, 26, 28, 42, 51, 57, 68, 74, 75,
  157, 158, 168, 228, 232, 233, 266, 269

Childress, James 1, 3, 4, 7, 9, 12, 155, 158, 191, 192, 264
christology 81, 82, 224, 271
church 3, 6, 7, 10, 11, 14, 21, 22, 24–31, 33, 45–7, 80, 81, 83, 84, 96, 98, 105, 107, 118, 128, 141, 142, 147, 150, 151, 226, 236, 237, 260, 263, 265–74, 278
Clark, Stephen R. L. 216, 217, 221, 239, 240, 252
cloning 2–4, 74, 238, 270, 271
cochlear implants 123
coma 20, 43, 65, 76, 82, 204
Commandments *see* Ten Commandments
communication 33, 34, 175–7
communion 14, 15, 23, 26, 29, 30, 33, 45–7, 67, 80–3, 99, 141, 144, 148, 151
community 13, 14, 23, 29, 70, 96–8, 105, 117, 121, 179, 180, 206, 218, 232, 233, 254, 266, 268
conception 19, 22, 47, 48, 72, 88
conscience 25, 28, 30, 55, 98, 148, 159, 220, 221, 225
consciousness 65, 69, 72, 92, 95, 126, 130–2, 134, 229, 230, 273
consent 3, 23, 24, 70, 78, 85, 86, 88, 89, 92, 154, 172, 180–1, 188, 209, 211, 271
conservation 240, 242–53
consumption 246, 247
contraception 25
contracts 20, 154, 168, 169
covenant 59, 60, 68–71, 75, 105, 117, 118, 147, 154, 156–71, 222, 234, 271, 278
creation 15, 22, 53, 100, 111, 117, 129, 140, 144, 150, 218–20, 224, 226, 229–31, 233, 234, 237, 239–44, 246, 248, 249, 251, 252, 254–6, 258, 259, 269
Creator 15, 28, 104, 112, 113, 115, 140, 216, 218, 224, 239, 251
cross 94, 132, 145, 265
Crossan, John Dominic 91, 95, 100
crucifixion 16, 139, 143

Dalits 256, 271
damnation 80

deafness 118, 120, 123
Deane-Drummond, Celia 240, 264, 265, 269
death 2, 5, 13, 17, 22, 23, 37, 39, 46, 55, 84, 86, 87, 92, 94, 98, 99, 110, 111, 115, 116, 125–52, 144, 145, 149, 158, 179, 187, 198, 200, 234, 252, 266, 278
deification 21, 45
dementia 16
demons 111, 112, 117
deontology 15, 271
Descartes, René 86, 132, 230, 236
devil 111, 112, 225
Diaz, Maria 180, 181
Dieter, Theodor 11, 12
dignity 38, 50–62, 133, 277
disability 11, 37, 102, 105, 117, 173, 174, 183, 278
discipline 67, 94, 248, 249
discrimination 40, 41, 54, 56, 59
disease 5, 17, 18, 27, 92, 95, 99, 104, 121, 160, 203, 205
disempowerment 154, 172, 173
distinctiveness of Christian ethics 12, 263
diversity 56, 61, 105, 123
divorce 97, 181
domination 86, 93, 229, 231, 239
dominion 218–20, 223, 226, 229, 231–6, 239, 244, 272
Donaldson, Liam 2, 7
Douglas, Mary 86, 91, 92–5, 100
Down's syndrome 41, 63
drug companies 163, 203–6, 212, 213
dualism 14, 67, 85–9, 91, 228, 244, 259

ecclesiology 236, 272
ecology 4, 12, 33–5, 222, 239–41, 249, 254–60, 277, 279
economics 5, 31–3, 34–6, 191–213, 229, 240, 254–60, 268, 279
Eddy, Mary Baker 110
egg 68, 70, 72, 73, 75
election 31, 228, 229, 272
Eliot, T. S. 144, 145

embryo 3, 19, 65, 66, 67, 68–75, 187, 270, 272, 274, 277

empowerment 172, 278

Engelhardt, H. Tristram 24, 70, 75

environment 102, 227, 239, 240, 242, 244–6, 248, 249, 251–61

equality 35, 86, 197, 216

eschatology 142, 233, 272

Eucharist 94, 97, 272

eugenics 20, 56, 62, 104, 272

euthanasia 2–4, 19, 23, 25, 28, 37, 65, 77, 88, 125, 126, 133, 152, 270

exorcism 95

experience 10

experimentation 20, 65, 74, 77, 82, 187, 235, 270


Fabri dos Anjos, Márcio 193, 202–11, 268, 278

Fairweather, Ian C. M. 11, 12, 269N

faith 87, 111–16, 136, 147, 240, 251, 263, 266

family 42, 96, 97, 179, 188, 250, 270

Farley, Margaret A. 85, 100

Farrer, Austin 139, 150

feminism 52, 59, 61, 66, 69, 71, 100, 184, 240, 255, 259, 260

fidelity 154, 162–4, 168, 169

Fitzmyer, Joseph 83, 84

Fletcher, Joseph 66, 67

Flexner, Abraham 159, 164

Florovsky, Georges 139, 141, 150

foetus 19, 65, 66, 68, 70, 72, 75, 82, 271

food 33, 92, 94, 98, 122, 221, 222, 234, 247, 249, 250

forgiveness 147, 267

Forrester, Duncan 264, 266, 267, 269

Foucault, Michel 86, 92, 93, 95, 100

Francis 249


gamete 74

gender 89, 90, 97, 99, 156, 259, 260

genetic modification 239, 272

genetics 56, 88, 158, 193, 202–11, 238, 272, 278

Gentiles 97, 233

Gill, Robin 7, 127, 269

Glover, Jonathan 38

GM crops 2, 261, 265

Gnanadason, Aruna 12, 240, 254–60, 268, 279

goodness 11, 27, 39, 49, 86, 116, 161, 169, 242, 243

Gospel 24, 26, 27, 29, 30, 31, 33, 46, 87, 98, 272

grace 27, 112, 114, 235, 272

Greenpeace 261

Grove-White, Robin 251

Gunton, Colin E. 66, 67

Guroian, Vigen 126, 127, 139–51, 278

Gutiérrez, Gustavo 12, 268, 269

gynaecology 182, 184, 185


Habgood, John 66, 67, 126, 127

Hardy, Daniel 265, 269

Hare, Richard 104, 105

Harris, John 65–70, 73, 75

Hauerwas, Stanley 2–4, 7, 9, 12, 84, 105, 125, 126, 128–38, 154, 155, 233, 237, 266, 269, 278

Hays, Richard B. 10, 12, 230, 236

healing 17, 18, 86, 87, 94, 104, 121, 147–9, 174, 183

health 5, 17, 18, 23, 32, 33, 92, 103–24, 174, 202, 247, 261

health professionals 2, 3, 5, 6, 17, 18, 20, 24, 28, 42, 99, 103, 104, 153–89, 196

hierarchy 86, 97, 101, 231, 233, 243, 245, 259

holiness 46

Holy Spirit 14, 23, 26, 46, 47, 76, 77, 79, 80, 82, 83, 87, 96, 143, 147

homoeroticism 89

homosexuality 29

hope 170

hospital 42, 92, 165–7, 169, 177, 179, 182, 188, 195, 208

Hull, John M. 12, 105, 117–22, 268, 278

Human Genome Initiative 20, 56, 60

hysterectomy 182, 183, 187, 273

illness 86, 87, 94, 95, 103, 106, 148, 160, 173

image of God [*imago Dei*] 47–9, 50–2, 60, 61, 141, 216, 219, 228–37

immortality 141–3

in vitro fertilization 19, 60, 73, 158, 273

incarnation 27, 252, 273

incompetence 42, 273

information 21, 154

instrumentalism 54, 61, 74, 229, 230

intersubjectivity 71

intimacy 89, 92

Irenaeus 45, 46

Isasi-Diaz, Ada Maria 50, 60, 61

Israel 17, 156, 229, 231, 232

James 98

Jesus Christ 13, 14, 16, 17, 23, 24, 26, 27, 45–8, 51, 66, 77, 78, 80–2, 84, 94–6, 98, 112, 115, 126, 129, 136, 139, 143, 144, 220, 223, 224, 230, 231, 234, 265, 266

Jews 78, 97, 156, 157, 158, 223, 233

John of Damascus 141, 142

John Paul II, Pope 11, 26–30, 32, 38, 277

John the Evangelist 46

John XXIII, Pope 224, 226

Jonas, Hans 172, 187

Jonsen, Albert R. 1, 7

joy 26, 118, 142, 146, 147, 179, 249–52

judgment 43, 46,104, 110–13, 115, 116, 145, 146, 168, 196, 200

Jungel, Eberhard 136–8

Junker-Kenny, Maureen 66, 68–75, 202, 277

just war 85

justice 9, 13, 30, 32, 58, 85, 117, 158, 166, 167, 172, 187, 195, 254, 267–70

Kant, Immanuel 179, 232, 233, 236

Kapp, M. B. 172, 176, 180–2, 187

Kevorkian, Jack 60

kidney dialysis 1, 20, 55, 62, 191, 195, 196, 198, 271

kingdom of God 23, 46, 95, 96, 98, 100, 101, 111, 268

Kübler-Ross, Elisabeth 135, 138

Kuhse, Helga 37, 38

Lammers, Stephen E. 4, 7

Lebacqz, Karen 12, 38, 50–62, 100, 154, 172–87, 268, 277, 278

legislation 2, 28, 188, 196, 197, 206, 207, 209, 263

liberation theology 11, 12, 31, 36, 52, 57, 58, 267, 268, 269, 277

life 2–4, 7, 9, 12, 26–30, 35, 36, 39–41, 46, 49, 70, 98, 99, 107, 115, 116, 126, 129, 131, 132, 133, 136, 139, 142, 143, 149, 150, 152, 197, 198, 200, 202, 203, 225, 234, 259, 263, 265, 270, 277, 278

Lindbeck, George 266, 269

Linzey, Andrew 216–20, 222, 223–6, 236

Locke, John 83

Lonergan, Bernard 83

lottery 192, 195–201, 278

love 14, 24, 27, 30, 46, 49, 51, 53, 54, 55, 57, 59, 60, 62, 66, 70, 71, 77, 91, 95, 98, 104, 129, 135, 137, 143, 146, 156, 157, 164, 234, 248

McCormick, Richard 37, 38, 39–44, 277

McDonald, James I. H. 11, 12

McFadyen, Alistair I. 66, 67

McFague, Sallie 240

McFarland, Ian A. 66, 76–84, 277

MacIntyre, Alasdair 236, 266, 269

McKenny, Gerald P. 154, 155, 156, 172

MacNamara, Vincent 12, 263, 264, 269

magisterium 11, 32

Maguire, Marjorie Reiley 66, 68, 70, 71

manichaeism 243, 244, 249, 252, 253, 273

marriage 19, 20, 82, 88, 96, 97, 157, 221, 249

martyrdom 94, 98

Marxism 58

May, William F. 39, 43, 154, 156–71, 278

Meilaender, Gilbert 10, 13–18, 277

Melchett, Lord 261

Menninger, Karl 21
mercy 49, 97, 113–15, 117, 146, 147
Merleau-Ponty, Maurice 90, 100
Messiah 26
middle axioms 267, 269
Midgley, Mary 216, 222
Mieth, Dietmar 72, 75
mind 28, 67, 85, 86, 87, 89, 259
miracles 95, 117, 121, 122, 148
Moltmann, Jürgen 104, 105

narrative 3, 229, 236
natural law 11, 27, 227, 264
nature 4, 15, 89, 239–61, 263
Nazis 1, 20, 267
New Testament 10, 94, 95, 98, 103, 104,
    110, 145, 219
newborn infants 37, 65
non-maleficence 9, 158, 273
Northcott, Michael 240
Nuremberg 1, 88

obstetrics 90, 182, 184
Old Testament 10, 110, 225
omnipotence 52
ontology 59
ordinary/extraordinary means 41, 133,
    272, 273
Origen 87
Orthodoxy, Eastern 10, 19, 139–42, 145,
    148, 150, 246
Osborn, Lawrence 240

Page, Ruth 239, 241
pain 17, 49, 86, 87, 92, 94, 99, 125, 136,
    217
pantheism 243, 273
Parsons, Susan 66, 67
patents 206, 209
paternalism 24, 188
patience 116
patients 5, 23, 84, 90, 99, 169, 173, 188,
    191, 192
patriarchy 61, 90, 100, 256, 258, 259, 274
Pattison, Stephen 103, 105, 106

Paul 46, 47, 48, 80, 87, 96, 98, 101, 105,
    129, 131, 135, 140, 141, 144
peace 117, 216, 232, 278
penance 144, 145, 147–9, 250
Persaud, Rajendra 192, 194
Persistent Vegetative State (PVS) 20, 42,
    126
person 3–5, 11, 14–16, 23, 28, 38, 40,
    47–9, 65–102, 108–10, 119, 141, 142,
    215, 216, 224, 250, 278
physician-assisted suicide 49
Pieper, Josef 169, 170
placenta 68, 74, 274
Plato 86, 87
policy 1, 2, 192, 248, 263, 267, 269, 270
Potter, Van Rensselaer 1
poverty 5, 27, 29, 31–4, 58, 97, 180, 184,
    193, 203, 205–7, 209, 210, 248–50, 268,
    270
praxis 268
prayer 23, 111, 112–16, 147, 247, 250
pregnancy 70, 88, 102, 121, 184, 272
Preston, Ronald 267, 269
Pretty, Diane 152
principles 9, 10, 13, 225
procreation 19, 89, 97
prostitution 28, 54, 87, 101
Protestantism 2, 10, 20, 224
prudence 154, 159–62, 168, 252, 274
psychology 21, 109, 135, 142, 218, 268
public-spiritedness 154, 164–70

Quality Adjusted Life Year (QALY) 192
quality of life 37, 38, 39–44, 48, 49,
    192, 202, 277
Quinlan, Karen Ann 42, 126, 130

race 50, 56, 60, 89, 90, 99, 156, 180, 259,
    268
Ramsey, Paul 1, 2, 7, 20, 38, 129, 132–4,
    138, 153–5, 158, 191–4, 195–201, 278
rape 70, 101
rationality 32, 51, 57, 65, 66, 86, 87, 88,
    90, 132, 180, 181, 186, 229, 230
reason 10, 11, 76, 83, 186

reasonable/unreasonable treatment 41–3

redemption 27, 36, 229, 243

Regan, Tom 215, 216, 218, 219, 223, 224, 225, 252

relationship 3, 5, 14, 24, 28, 33, 51, 56, 59–62, 66, 70, 75–7, 82, 91, 92, 97, 109, 126, 180, 185, 187, 202, 230, 231, 234

repentance 127, 144, 145–7, 250, 274

reproduction 92, 100

reproductive technology 25, 88, 187

research 1, 5, 54, 169, 172, 193, 202–11, 215, 217, 261

resource allocation 5, 191–4, 213

resurrection 87, 94, 98, 99, 139, 142–4, 149, 150, 220, 266

rights 13, 23, 24, 29, 31, 32, 38, 57, 58, 70, 75, 99, 130, 137, 197, 215, 216, 217–27, 230, 245, 278

ritualism 93

Roman Catholicism 11, 37, 75, 101, 224, 226, 252, 264, 270

rules 10, 192, 193, 195, 232, 245

Sacks, Oliver 154, 173–183, 187

sacrament 46, 148, 150, 274

saints 143

salvation 139, 143, 145, 146

sanctification 21

sanctity of life 29–30, 37, 38, 39–44, 45–9, 131–3, 274, 277

saviour 17, 26, 32, 144

scarcity 191

Schiedermayer, David 53, 54, 60, 61, 62

Schmemann, Alexander 139, 142, 150, 151

Schweitzer, Albert 225, 227

science 12, 35, 75

Scripture 10–11, 19, 21, 25, 76, 110, 122, 139, 164, 264

self 65, 85, 87, 88, 89, 90, 99, 100

Sermon on the Mount 10, 95

sex 19, 25, 50, 53, 54, 56, 85, 89–94, 96, 97, 100, 140, 180, 185, 187, 255, 268

Shiva, Vandana 255, 256, 257, 260

sin 14, 21, 87, 97, 106, 110, 111, 112, 129, 127, 131, 140–2, 143, 144, 146, 147, 221

Singer, Peter 37, 38, 66, 69, 215, 216, 223, 224, 225

single-parenting 20

slavery 28, 97

solidarity 30, 33, 35, 93, 95, 97, 98, 118, 180, 208

soul 107, 108, 112, 113, 131, 132, 142, 150, 161, 165, 228, 229

specificity of Christian ethics 12, 263

sperm 68, 72, 73, 75

spirit (human) 14–16, 67, 87–9, 111, 132, 146, 147

stem-cell 2, 274

Stephen 98

sterilisation 180, 181

stewardship 46, 47, 220, 225, 226, 228, 235, 239, 245

Stoics 243

suffering 16, 17, 49, 87, 98, 99, 126, 147, 235, 252, 278

suicide 19, 21, 49, 60, 88, 125, 152

sustainability 246

Taylor, Charles 88, 91, 100

teleology 23, 59, 274

telos 45, 147, 229, 274

Ten Commandments 20

theocentricity 242, 247, 251, 274

theosis 10, 45

Thielicke, Helmut 38, 50–62

Tolstoy, Leo N. 148, 151

tradition 3, 10, 19, 21, 24, 43, 94, 179, 224, 236, 264

transcendence 52, 159, 169, 275

transgression 114, 146

transplant 1, 20, 25, 55, 62, 158, 191, 201, 238

triage 199, 200

Trinity 23, 24, 45, 47, 66, 67, 76, 77, 79, 80, 83, 234, 237, 274

truth 11, 22, 23, 30, 86, 92, 146, 161, 164, 169, 175

uterus 71, 90
utilitarianism 54, 55, 69, 157, 192, 274

Vanier, Jean 252
Vaux, Kenneth 61
Veatch, Robert 2, 7, 41, 44, 129, 130, 133,
    134, 137, 138
vegetarianism 237, 244
Verhey, Allen 4, 7, 50
virtue 150, 154, 200, 232, 249, 252, 266,
    269, 275, 278

vitalism 37, 40, 49
vocation 47, 231, 232–5

Warnock, Baroness Mary 73
welfare 57, 181, 184, 221, 227, 246
White, Lynn Jr. 222, 239, 241, 246
wisdom 75, 146, 264, 265, 269
womb 70, 73, 87

Zizioulas, John D. 66, 67, 83
zygote 68, 71–3, 75